KU-261-565

Contents

all being briefly discussed in intro & importance of nutrition @ very stage of the life cycle

14932

Preface

This is a nutrition textbook for people who are not nutrition experts. In recent years the importance of nutrition in relation to health and disease has been stressed, and dietary change is considered essential if *Health of the Nation* targets are to be met. At the same time, the trend towards shorter periods of hospitalisation and increased community care means that many acute and chronic disorders with nutritional implications are now managed within the primary care setting. As a result, GPs, practice nurses and other health care professionals increasingly find themselves required to give dietary advice. Many find it quite difficult. Some have received little formal training in the subject of nutrition, and much of what they have had may be out-of-date. Others have some theoretical nutritional knowledge but find it difficult to interpret this in terms of what people should or should not eat. Many are confused by the seemingly conflicting theories or recommendations emanating from both government sources and the media. Few have the time to seek out and read the mass of scientific literature which might clarify the situation.

This book attempts to provide a balanced overview of the relationships between diet, health and disease and to bridge the gap between the classic textbook of nutrition and resource material available at local level. Where possible, dietary needs and strategies have been explained in terms of foods rather than as quantified amounts of nutrients. While it may be interesting to know that, for example, an average adult woman requires 14.8 mg iron/day, for the non-dietetic expert this

information is not particularly helpful. Most primary care workers are unlikely to have the time, resources or expertise to make an accurate assessment of individual iron intake in quantitative terms and even if they did, the figure of 14.8 may not necessarily be the dietary iron requirement of that particular individual. What the health professional needs to be able to assess is whether an individual's need for iron is likely to be particularly high or low, whether that person is eating the types of foods which are likely to meet this need, and if not, what should be eaten instead. All this can be done much more easily and effectively in terms of food intake rather than by detailed nutritional calculations. Throughout this book much use has been made of the recently developed National Food Guide *The Balance of Good Health* (© Health Education Authority) which forms an ideal practical model for both dietary assessment and modification in the primary care setting.

The book is divided into three parts:

- Part 1 *Diet and Health* looks at the fundamental links between nutrients, foods, diet and health. It explains what nutrients do, what the dietary balance between them should be, and how this can be assessed and, if necessary, modified in practice.
- Part 2 *Diet and People* considers the particular needs and problems of various sectors of the population from infancy to old age and includes different ethnic groups and people with specific needs.

■ Part 3 *Diet and Disease* focuses on the dietary aspects of the prevention and management of diseases which are commonly encountered in the primary care setting.

For reasons of simplicity and space, references have been kept to a minimum and mainly confined to those which are either particularly important or contentious. For those who wish to pursue a subject further, suggested further reading will usually contain details of readily available reviews or briefing papers which will point the way to the relevant literature.

This book is not intended to be a substitute for the expertise of dietitians. On the contrary, it stresses the circumstances in which dietetic referral is either advisable or essential, and perhaps may also reveal the complexity of some dietetic problems. Instead its aim is to highlight the types of problems which can be managed by the non-dietetic expert and the nature of the guidance which should be given. It also explains the dietary management of some disorders which normally are under qualified dietetic supervision so that appropriate supporting guidance can be given by the primary care team if necessary. Above all, this book tries to ensure that all health professionals give the same dietary messages to an increasingly confused general public.

Briony Thomas

PART 1

Diet and Health

1

Nutrients

In order to survive, the human body requires oxygen, water and nutrients, and in that order of priority. Without oxygen, survival is limited to a few minutes, without water, to a few days and without nutrients, to a matter of weeks.

In practice, people do not eat 'nutrients'; they eat 'foods' containing a mixture of nutrients. Most people have heard of terms such as protein, fibre and saturated fatty acids but relatively few know what these do, where they are found or how much they should consume. Nor is it necessary to know in order to eat a healthy diet. People require dietary guidance in terms of food intake, not nutrition or biochemistry. However, those who give the dietary advice do require a sound understanding of the effects of nutrients on health and disease. Without this knowledge, it is impossible to translate theory into practice and the information given is more likely to be inaccurate, inappropriate, or ineffective.

In order to grow and maintain health, humans require a diet which provides sufficient:

Energy which can be derived from:
   protein
   fat
   carbohydrate
   alcohol.
Nitrogen from protein for construction of tissues.
Micronutrients (vitamins and minerals) to maintain the structure and function of the human machine.
Dietary fibre (non-starch polysaccharide) for

functional efficiency and protection of gastrointestinal tract.

ENERGY

The most fundamental nutritional need is for a supply of energy. The human body is a machine and like all machines it requires a source of energy in order to function. Energy is needed for:

- The basic processes of life (e.g. breathing, heart beat, peristalsis, metabolism, organ function, thermoregulation).
- Muscular movement (e.g. walking, physical exercise).
- The creation of new tissues (growth and cell replacement).

This energy is derived from food. Protein, fat, carbohydrate and alcohol all contain chemical energy which can be released and harnessed for the body's needs when these compounds are metabolised following digestion and absorption.

Without a dietary supply of energy, the body will in effect cannibalise itself in order to meet its energy needs. Initially energy will be derived from body fat stores but as these decline, muscle, including muscle from vital organs such as the heart, will also be used as an energy source. Ultimately, prolonged starvation will result in organ dysfunction and death.

Because a supply of energy is so important for survival, the body will attempt to conserve any surplus energy consumed by storing it as fat. In the days when man was a hunter-gatherer and food availability ranged from the plentiful to the non-existent, this was an important protective measure. Nowadays, in affluent Western societies where it is easy to eat more than is required on a daily basis, it is much more of a disadvantage and surplus energy tends to be stored to such an extent that it results in overweight and obesity.

The amount of energy provided by a diet is measured either in kilojoules (kJ) or kilocalories (kcal). Expression in kilojoules is scientifically more correct but the term kilocalories (usually known as 'calories') is more familiar to most people, and certainly the general public.

The four energy-bearing nutrients do not all provide the same amount of energy:

1 g of protein provides	4 kcal (17 kJ)
1 g of carbohydrate provides	4 kcal (17 kJ)
1 g of fat provides	9 kcal (37 kJ)
1 g of alcohol provides	7 kcal (29 kJ)

Fat is thus the most energy dense nutrient providing over twice as much energy on a weight for weight basis as protein or carbohydrate. Alcohol can also be a significant source of energy. These may be relevant considerations for those who need to lose weight.

Although all these nutrients are energy providers, the amount of energy derived from each source has important metabolic and health implications (see Chapter 2, *Dietary Targets*). The body has a specific requirement for protein, and in normal circumstances needs both fat and carbohydrate in order to operate effectively. Alcohol is different; it can be utilised as a source of energy but there is no physiological requirement for it.

Dietary energy intake is a primary determinant of dietary adequacy. The amount of energy consumed is closely associated with the intake of many other nutrients; a low energy intake is often a marker of low micronutrient intake.

Energy requirements

On average, an adult man requires 2550 kcal/day and an adult woman 1940 kcal/day[1] but there is enormous variation in the energy requirements of individuals as a result of differences in age, body weight and activity level and variation in metabolic efficiency. Energy needs can be more accurately quantified by multiplying estimated Basal Metabolic Rate (BMR – derived from prediction equations) by the estimated Physical Activity Level (PAL)[1]. In the primary care setting it is usually neither necessary nor helpful to do this. Whether or not an individual's diet is appropriate in terms of energy content and composition can be more easily assessed by considering body weight and adiposity, and the balance of food groups within the diet (see Chapter 6, *Assessing Nutritional Adequacy*). If dietary energy content needs to be adjusted, advice needs to be given in terms of food intake not number of calories. Complex calculations of energy needs and intakes may seem more scientific but in the hands of the inexperienced are fraught with inaccuracies and tend to divert attention from the real problem which is dietary food imbalance.

PROTEIN

Protein is an essential energy-bearing nutrient because it provides nitrogen, vital for the formation of cells and new tissue. Since these structures are constantly being broken down and replaced, an equally constant supply of protein is necessary. In addition infants, children, and pregnant and lactating women have an additional need for protein for the creation of new tissue.

Sources of protein

In the average diet, about two-thirds of the protein intake is obtained from animal foods. Most of the remaining third comes from cereal foods with about 10% being derived from vegetable sources.

Principal sources of protein are:

Meat
Fish
Eggs
Milk
Cheese
Cereals
Nuts
Pulses (beans, peas and lentils).

Protein quality

Proteins are large complex molecules comprised of individual units called amino acids linked together in long chains. Dietary protein is broken down into its constituent amino acids which are then used by the body as building blocks to create the proteins it needs such as enzymes and structural tissues.

The human body requires 20 different amino acids for its structure and function (see Table 1.1). Eight of these are nutritionally essential (or 'indispensable'), i.e. they cannot be made by the body so must be obtained from the diet. Another amino acid, histidine, is essential during infancy. The remainder are classified as non-essential (or 'dispensable') because they can be synthesised from other amino acids.

Protein quality depends on its content of amino acids. Dietary proteins from animal foods (such as meat, fish, eggs, milk and cheese) contain significant amounts of *all* the essential amino acids and are sometimes referred to as High Biological Value (HBV) proteins. Proteins derived from plants (such as cereals, peas, beans and pulses) usually lack one or more of the essential amino acids and, on an individual basis, have lower biological value. However, plant proteins of different botanical origin tend to lack different amino acids (e.g. cereals lack lysine while pulses lack methionine) so combinations of plant proteins can balance out deficiencies and create complete amino acid mixtures. This is an important aspect of vegan diets (see Chapter 21).

For practical purposes, amino acid content is not a concern other than in those on vegan or synthetic (e.g. intravenous) diets or in severely protein restricted diets sometimes necessary in the management of renal or liver disease. Protein quality is unlikely to be inadequate in anyone who consumes a normal mixed diet or a vegetarian diet containing milk products or eggs.

Protein requirements

Because of its structural function, protein requirement depends on body weight. The average adult requires 0.6g protein/kg body weight/day and a daily intake of 55g protein (in men) or 45g (in women) will meet the protein needs of most adults[1]. Pregnant and lactating women will require more. Infants and children have a higher requirement for protein per kg body weight than an adult, although their smaller size means that the actual amount needed will be less.

Protein can only be used for growth or tissue replacement if there is a sufficient supply of energy. The body's need for energy will always take priority over that for growth and repair and if both energy intake and energy reserves are low (for

Table 1.1 Amino acids.

Essential ('indispensable') amino acids	Non-essential ('dispensable') amino acids
Isoleucine	Alanine
Leucine	Arginine
Lysine	Asparagine
Methionine	Aspartic acid
Phenylalanine	Cysteine/cystine
Threonine	Glutamic acid
Tryptophan	Glutamine
Valine	Glycine
	Proline
Histidine (in infants)	Serine
	Tyrosine

example in those who are chronically ill or under-fed) dietary protein will tend be used as an energy source instead. The undernourished child who is failing to grow or a chronically ill person with muscle wasting usually needs an increased energy intake rather than an increased protein intake.

Conversely, the body can only use a certain amount of protein per day and is unable to store any surplus. If more protein is consumed than required, the excess will be broken down and converted into energy. There are thus no health benefits from consuming excessive amounts of protein (surplus protein will ultimately boost body fat stores not the size of the muscles) and there may be some long-term health disadvantages, particularly in terms of renal function. In this country, most people consume far more protein than they need. The recommended maximum protein intake for adults is 1.5 g/kg body weight/day but many exceed this level.

FAT

Fat is the most concentrated source of energy and most people in the UK consume too much of it. However, dietary fat is not a uniformly undesirable compound but a complex mixture of substances, some of which are harmful if consumed to excess but others being either beneficial or even essential to health.

Most dietary fat is present in food in the form of triglyceride, a storage form of fat. A triglyceride is comprised of a molecule of glycerol to which three fatty acids are attached. It is the nature of these fatty acids which is of key relevance to health and disease.

Main types of fatty acids

A fatty acid is a chain of carbon and hydrogen atoms. The length of the carbon chain and the way in which the carbon and hydrogen atoms are linked together determines the way in which fatty acids are metabolised and hence their physiological significance. Fatty acids are classified by their degree of 'saturation' (in chemical terms, the number of hydrogen atoms attached to the carbon chain):

- *Saturated fatty acids* (also known as saturates) are so called because they are molecules which are fully saturated with hydrogen atoms; chemically, there are single bonds between all the carbon and hydrogen atoms.
- *Unsaturated fatty acids* are not fully saturated in terms of hydrogen content because there is one or more double bond at some point in the carbon chain:
  - □ *Monounsaturated* fatty acids have one double bond
  - □ *Polyunsaturated* fatty acids have two or more double bonds in their structure.

There are two main types of polyunsaturated fatty acids, omega-6 (or n-6) and omega-3 (or n-3) (see below). Most dietary polyunsaturates (e.g. vegetable oils and polyunsaturated spreads) are in the n-6 form.

All food fats are a mixture of saturated, monounsaturated and polyunsaturated fatty acids. No food contains only one type alone; polyunsaturated margarine contains some saturated fatty acids and butter contains some polyunsaturated ones. For simplicity though, food fats can be broadly classified as follows:

- *Foods with the highest proportion of saturated fatty acids*
  Hard margarine, milk fat and derivatives (butter, cheese, cream), meat fat and derivatives (lard, suet) and products which contain these such as pies, pastry, meat products, cakes and biscuits.
- *Foods with the highest proportion of monounsaturated fatty acids*
  Olive oil, rapeseed oil, groundnut oil and margarines/spreads made from them.
- *Foods with the highest proportion of polyunsaturated fatty acids*
  - □ n-6 polyunsaturates: sunflower oil, soya oil,

safflower oils, corn oil and margarines/ spreads made from them.

□ n–3 polyunsaturates: fatty fish and fish oils. Soya oil and rapeseed oil have a higher content of n–3 polyunsaturates than other vegetable oils.

In general, fats derived from animals contain more saturated fatty acids than vegetable fats and oils but this is not always the case (e.g. coconut oil is highly saturated). The consistency of a fat or oil at room temperature also provides some guidance on fatty acid content; harder fats tend to be more saturated although the manipulations of modern food technology mean that this is not an infallible guide.

Terminology of fatty acids

The different terminology used to describe fatty acids can be confusing although it is not as complicated as it may appear. In medical literature, fatty acids may be described either by a common name (e.g. linoleic acid) or by a form of chemical shorthand (e.g. 18:2n-6). In any such abbreviation, the first number denotes the length of the carbon chain and the second the number of double bonds it contains. Thus 18:0 is an 18 carbon atom with no double bonds (i.e. a saturated fatty acid), 18:1 is an 18 carbon monounsaturated fatty acid while 18:2 is a polyunsaturated fatty acid.

The n-suffix (an abbreviation for 'omega') will only apply to mono- or polyunsaturated fatty acids because it denotes where the first double bond occurs on the carbon chain (e.g. n-6 means the first double bond is 6 carbon atoms from the methyl end of the molecule). The position of this double bond is relevant because it determines the way in which the fatty acid is metabolised and its physiological effect.

Unsaturated fatty acids may also be described as either *cis* or *trans*. This refers to their geometrical configuration and these differences in shape can affect the way the molecule is metabolised. Most fatty acids are in the *cis* configuration. The implica-

tions of *trans* fatty acids are discussed further on in this chapter.

Essential fatty acids

Two polyunsaturated fatty acids, linoleic and alpha-linolenic acids, have a vital role in cell membrane synthesis, particularly in nerve tissue, but unlike other fatty acids cannot be synthesised by the body and so must be supplied by the diet. They are therefore known as essential fatty acids. The requirement is small but vital; about 1% of dietary energy should come from linoleic acid and 0.2% from alpha-linolenic acid. Both of these fatty acids originate from vegetable oils; the primary sources of linoleic acid are sunflower, corn and safflower oils; alpha-linolenic acid is more predominant in rapeseed and soya oils.

Omega-6 and omega-3 (or n-6 and n-3) fatty acids

These terms denote the fact that the essential fatty acids (linoleic and alpha-linolenic) are metabolised by different pathways with different end products and different effects.

The omega-6 pathway
Linoleic acid is an omega-6 fatty acid (often written as n-6) and the fatty acids derived from it are called omega-6 fatty acids. Important derivatives of the omega-6 pathway are gamma-linolenic acid (GLA) and arachidonic acid (see Fig. 1.1).

The omega-6 pathway influences the production of prostaglandins and other biological regulators affecting inflammatory processes, immune function and hormone balance. A deficiency of linoleic acid, or impairment of its metabolic pathway, may affect these functions. Diets rich in saturated fats or low in certain vitamins and minerals (particu-

Linoleic acid $\rightarrow$ Gamma-linolenic acid $\rightarrow$ Dihomogammalinolenic acid $\rightarrow$ Arachidonic acid

18:2 n-6   (GLA) 18:3 n-6   20:3 n-6   20:4 n-6

Fig. 1.1 The omega-6 pathway.

Alpha-linolenic acid $\rightarrow$ 18:4 n-3 $\rightarrow$ 20:4 n-3 $\rightarrow$ Eicosapentaenoic acid $\rightarrow$ 22:5 n-3 $\rightarrow$ Docosahexaenoic acid

18:3 n-3   (EPA) 20:5 n-3   (DHA) 22:6 n-3

Fig. 1.2 The omega-3 pathway.

larly B_6, zinc and magnesium) have been reported to reduce enzyme activity at various points in these pathways, as may other external factors such as smoking, alcohol and viral infections. Supplements of evening primrose oil or borage oil (starflower oil) which supply a ready-made source of one of the intermediate fatty acids, GLA, may overcome any impairment in production and any effects of deficiency. Evening primrose oil is prescribable for the treatment of atopic ezcema and cyclical mastalgia. It may also have benefits in the treatment of premenstrual syndrome and some inflammatory disorders although these effects are currently poorly documented.

The omega-3 pathway

The metabolism of alpha-linolenic acid (an omega-3 fatty acid) results in the production of eicosapentaenoic acid (EPA) and docosahexaenoic acid (DHA) (see Fig. 1.2) which have beneficial effects on blood clotting mechanisms and may have an important role in helping to prevent thrombosis (see Chapter 22, *Coronary Heart Disease*).

The omega-3 pathway is extremely active in marine animals so fish oils are rich sources of these long chain derivatives.

EPA may reduce the inflammatory response, possibly by inhibiting the production of certain interleukins. For this reason, increased consumption of fish oil (either from oily fish or supplements) may help people suffering from inflammatory disorders such as rheumatoid arthritis (see Chapter 38).

Trans fatty acids

Trans fatty acids are unsaturated fatty acids with an unusual shape. As a result they are metabolised in a way which makes them more like saturated fatty acids in metabolic effect.

Small amounts of *trans* fatty acids are produced by cows and sheep as a result of a hydrogenation process which occurs in the rumen. Therefore foods such as milk, dairy products, lamb and beef contain small amounts of *trans* fatty acids. However, most dietary *trans* fatty acids originate from the manufacturing process of hydrogenation when vegetable oils are artificially hardened to form margarine. This hydrogenated fat has been used extensively in recent years in manufactured food products such as cakes, biscuits, pastry, etc., resulting in a considerable increase in *trans* fatty acid intake (in the USA this has been reported to be as much as 8% of energy intake).

Concern about *trans* fatty acids was heightened when an American prospective study reported that *trans* fatty acid intake was significantly related to coronary heart disease risk, independently of other known risk factors[2]. The significance of this, particularly in the UK where *trans* intake is much lower than in the USA, remains a matter of debate[3]. A diet high in *trans* fatty acids may simply be a marker of a diet containing a high proportion of ready meals and highly processed convenience foods and hence relatively few protective foods such as fruit and vegetables. Current guidelines are that *trans* fatty acid intake should not increase above the current estimated average of 4–6g/day or 2% of dietary energy. People whose diet contains a high proportion of manufactured foods probably exceed this level.

Dietary cholesterol

A very small proportion of dietary fat intake (about 0.5–1%) is comprised of dietary cholesterol, mainly derived from meat, dairy products and eggs.

Contrary to popular belief, dietary cholesterol usually has little effect on serum cholesterol. The body synthesises its own cholesterol (for cell membrane structure and hormone synthesis) and normally produces 2–4 times as much as is consumed in the diet. The level of cholesterol circulating in the blood (relevant to the development of atheroma and coronary heart disease) is primarily influenced by total fat intake, in particular the consumption of saturated fat. Dietary cholesterol has to be reduced to extremely low levels before it has any significant impact on the blood cholesterol level. Since cholesterol in an integral part of animal cell membranes, it is impossible to achieve such a low intake other than on a strict vegan diet. Within the range of normal intake (200–450mg/day), the effect of dietary cholesterol on blood cholesterol is small.

Most people do not need to worry about dietary cholesterol and should be encouraged to modify their dietary fat intake instead. The only people who may be advised to lower their cholesterol intake are:

- Those with the rare genetic disorder Familial Type 2 Hyperlipidaemia (characterised by extremely high levels of blood cholesterol).
- Those who have unusually high intakes of foods rich in cholesterol (eggs – several per day, fish roes, offal, shellfish).

Fat requirements

It is generally agreed that the typical UK diet contains both too much fat in total and an inappropriate balance of fatty acids. A high intake of total and saturated fat elevates serum cholesterol which is one of the major risk factors for coronary heart disease. It is therefore recommended that total fat intake should be reduced from its current average level of about 40% of dietary energy to 35%, and saturated fatty acids from 16% of dietary energy to 11% (see Chapter 2, *Dietary Targets*).

Unsaturated fatty acids tend to lower serum cholesterol levels although it is not now recommended that n-6 polyunsaturated fatty acid intake should exceed current levels (7% of dietary energy) as this may be detrimental in terms of lipid membrane peroxidation (see Chapter 22, *Coronary Heart Disease*). However, current average intake of n-3 polyunsaturates (from fish oils) should be doubled (from 0.1g/day to 0.2g/day) because of their anti-thrombotic benefits.

Mono-unsaturated fatty acids appear to have some of the cholesterol-lowering advantages of polyunsaturates without some of the disadvantages. Mono-unsaturate-based oils and spreads are a useful substitute for cooking/spreading fats rich in saturated fatty acids.

Guidance on dietary fat alteration is given in Chapter 3, *Healthy Eating*.

CARBOHYDRATE

Carbohydrate provides a readily available source of fuel for the human body. For practical purposes carbohydrates are usually divided into sugars and starches although chemically all carbohydrates are comprised of units of single sugars (monosaccharides) and, following digestion, are absorbed in this form. Sugars are either monosaccharides or disaccharides (i.e. two monosaccharides joined together). Starches are polysaccharides and comprised of hundreds or thousands of monosaccharide units.

- *Monosaccharides*
  Glucose
  Fructose
  Galactose
- *Disaccharides*

Sucrose ('sugar')	comprised of glucose + fructose
Lactose (milk sugar)	comprised of glucose + galactose
Maltose	comprised of glucose + glucose

- *Polysaccharides*

  | Starch | comprised of hundreds of glucose units |

Many types of polysaccharides exist in nature but starch is the only one which is digestible by man. Those which are indigestible are called 'non-starch polysaccharides' and have an important role as 'dietary fibre' (discussed later in this chapter).

Virtually all dietary carbohydrate originates from plant foods. Starch (a storage form of energy in plants) is principally found in:

Cereal grains and flours and the wide range of products made from them (e.g. flour, pastry, bread, breakfast cereals, pasta, rice)
Tubers and root vegetables (e.g. potato, carrot, swede).

Sugars are primarily found in:

Fruit
Green vegetables
Milk (as lactose).

However, in nature, there is considerable interaction between starch and sugar content. In general, seeds lose sugars and store starch as they mature (so young peas contain more sugars and less starch than fully ripened peas). In contrast, the flesh of fruit loses starch and increases in sugar content as it ripens. Most root vegetables (e.g. potato) contain nearly all their carbohydrate in the form of starch but this is not always the case; pars-

nips contain up to 50% in the form of sugars. Runner beans, bulbs (leeks, onions) and leafy vegetables contain more sugars than starch.

The significance of this is that nature intends us to eat a mixture of sugars and starches because this is an ideal form of readily utilisable energy. There is nothing inherently wrong with sugar. Any problem associated with sugar consumption arises from the fact that man has distorted the natural balance between sugars and starches by extracting sucrose (i.e. 'sugar') from its sources and adding it to foods.

Non-Milk Extrinsic Sugars (NMES)

This term was introduced in the Department of Health report on dietary sugars – *Dietary Sugars and Human Disease*[4] – as a way of distinguishing between sugars naturally present in the structure of foods and those added to it. Dietary sugars can be classified as:

- *Intrinsic sugars* i.e. those naturally incorporated into the cellular structure of foods such as those present in fruit and vegetables.
- *Extrinsic sugars* i.e. those present in a free form within a food. This group was subdivided into:
  - □ *Milk sugars* i.e. lactose
  - □ *Non-milk extrinsic sugars* (NMES) i.e. sugars which have been released or extracted from cellular structures such as:
    Table sugar present in sweetened foods and drinks
    Fruit juice
    Honey
    Jam
    Confectionery
    Glucose and invert sugar syrups.

It is important to realise that this is an arbitrary distinction, not a physiological one. Ultimately the body cannot distinguish between a molecule of glucose derived from an apple or from a bar of chocolate. Nor is the distinction entirely practical; the intracellular sugars present in fruit soon become extrinsic sugars when chewed or cooked. The significance of the NMES classification is that it is a marker for dietary quality – a diet where a high proportion of its energy content comes from NMES (e.g. sugary drinks, snacks, confectionery) tends to be low in other important dietary components such as vitamins, minerals and dietary fibre. Foods containing intrinsic sugars (fruit and vegetables) have other nutritious or protective properties, such as antioxidant nutrients or dietary fibre, but the sugars themselves are the same as those in extrinsic sources.

A high consumption of NMES often reflects the fact that sugars are consumed at frequent intervals and this will increase the risk of dental caries (see Chapter 28). There is no evidence that sugars have a causal role in the development of coronary heart disease, obesity or diabetes although diets high in NMES may indirectly exacerbate these disorders if they result in a dietary energy surplus or nutrient imbalance.

Carbohydrate requirements

There is no specific metabolic requirement for carbohydrate although a diet containing very little carbohydrate will result in unpleasant ketotic side effects as the body attempts to meet its fuel needs from fat metabolism. In contrast, there may be considerable benefits from a diet obtaining a relatively high proportion of its energy from carbohydrate, partly as a result of the accompanying intake of other important dietary components associated with carbohydrate foods (such as antioxidant vitamins and fibre) but principally because it will displace high-fat foods from the diet.

Current recommendations are that 50% of dietary energy should be obtained from carbohydrate, most of which should come from starches and sugars naturally present in cereals, fruit, vegetables and milk. Only 11% should come from non-milk extrinsic sugars. At present few people achieve either of these targets.

ALCOHOL

Alcohol is used by the body as a source of energy but there is no physiological requirement for it.

Moderate amounts of alcohol do not appear to be harmful and in some respects are beneficial, but the health risks in terms of liver and pancreatic disease accelerate sharply once intake exceeds a certain level. These aspects and guidance on the sensible use of alcohol are discussed in Chapter 4.

DIETARY FIBRE/NON-STARCH POLYSACCHARIDE (NSP)

Dietary fibre is not a 'nutrient' as such because its benefits derive from the fact it is not absorbed by the body, but it is an important component of the diet. Dietary fibre can be regarded as the undigested remains of plant materials. It is not a single substance but a complex mixture of different types of unavailable polysaccharides and plant cell wall constituents with differing effects, some of which have not yet been fully evaluated in chemical or physiological terms.

Terminology is also a matter of some confusion. Older generations will think of this dietary component as 'roughage'; food labels and most healthy eating literature refer to it as 'dietary fibre' while nutritionists prefer the term 'non-starch polysaccharide' (NSP) which is chemically more accurate. At the moment, 'fibre' is the term best understood by the general public and non-dietetic health professionals and is the one generally used in this book.

Whatever the definition, the functionally important constituents of dietary fibre are the non-starch polysaccharides. These are structural components of plant cell walls, mainly cellulose (present in the cell walls as microscopic fibres) or the non-cellulosic polysaccharides (which form a matrix surrounding the cellulose fibres).

Older methods of 'fibre' analysis also include other components which are less relevant in physi-ological terms. These are:

- *Lignin* A woody plant cell wall material thought to be of little physiological significance.
- *Resistant starch* This is ordinary starch but present in a form which makes it resistant to normal digestion. This may be because it is enclosed in enzyme-resistant granules (e.g. in raw potato or unripe banana) or because the starch retrogrades after being heated and cooled into a digestive-resistant form (e.g. in some breakfast cereals or cold cooked potatoes). Resistant starch is usually fer-mented by colonic bacteria into short-chain fatty acids (acetic, butyric and propionic acids).

Sources of fibre

Fibre is only found in foods derived from plants, i.e. cereals (and bread and flour derived from them), grains, seeds, pulses, fruit and vegetables. There is no fibre in animal foods such as meat, fish, cheese and eggs (unless mixed with plant-derived ingredients such as flour used to make pastry).

The amount of fibre present in a food depends on the extent to which it is still intact; cereal foods which still contain the outer layers of the grain (wholemeal or wholegrain cereals) and fruit and vegetables consumed with their skins will provide the most. However, it is a mistake to assume that fibre is only found in foods containing 'bran'; all plant foods provide some fibre.

In terms of physiological effect, dietary fibre can be divided into two types: soluble and insoluble fibre.

Soluble fibre

Soluble fibre comprises water-soluble non-cellulosic polysaccharides (e.g. pectin) and gums and mucilages (e.g. guar gum). These dissolve in the fluid contents of the gut forming a viscous gel which slows down the rate of absorption of some nutrients, particularly glucose. The type of soluble fibre found in oats, peas, beans and lentils also has a hypocholesterolaemic effect (probably because it binds bile acids and so increases cholesterol excre-tion) although large amounts have to be consumed before any noticeable reduction in blood choles-terol occurs.

Soluble fibre can be fermented by colonic bacteria to short-chain fatty acids (acetic, propionic and butyric acids), CO_2, hydrogen and methane. These fatty acids are absorbed and provide a small amount of energy to the body. This fermentation process may also be protective in terms of carcinogenesis in the colonic mucosa (see Chapter 41, *Cancer*).

Soluble fibre is present in:

Fruits, including dried fruit
Vegetables
Pulses (e.g. red kidney beans, baked beans and lentils)
Foods containing oats, barley or rye.

Insoluble fibre

Insoluble fibre (e.g. cellulose, arabino-xylans, xylo-glucans) has a sponge-like effect within the intestine, soaking up water and swelling in size. This produces a sensation of satiety and adds bulk to the intestinal contents, stimulating peristalsis and increasing faecal mass, thus reducing the risk of constipation. Insoluble fibre is not significantly fermented by colonic bacteria and hence is a better stool bulking agent than soluble fibre and the most effective at treating constipation. Insolu-ble fibre may be protective against colo-rectal cancers because of its effects in shortening intes-tinal transit time and hence reducing the exposure to carcinogens.

Insoluble fibre is primarily that found in cereals and grains, especially wholemeal varieties:

Bread
Flour

Breakfast cereals
Rice
Pasta
Fibrous vegetables (e.g. carrots, celery).

Fibre supplements

Bran
Bran is a concentrated source of insoluble fibre but merely adding it to foods is not a good way of increasing fibre consumption because it will not provide any of the vitamins or minerals present in fibre-containing foods. Unprocessed bran is also rich in phytic acid which impairs the absorption of minerals such as calcium, iron and zinc. In addition, if consumed without sufficient liquid, bran can cause obstructive problems and is unsuitable for those with intestinal disease, children or elderly people because of the risk of faecal impaction.

Fibre-containing drinks and supplements
The value of isolated sources of fibre marketed in the form of drinks and other products (often containing soluble fibre such as beta-glucan from oats or pectins) is uncertain. Although these appear to be an easy way for people to increase their fibre intake, the effects of isolated forms of fibre may not be the same as when they are consumed as an integral part of food. It also seems likely that some of benefits associated with fibre consumption, particularly that from fruit and vegetables, may in part be due to the associated consumption of other nutrients such as carotenoids and other antioxidants. Isolated fibre supplements will not provide these.

Fibre requirements

Recommendations for fibre intake are given in terms of non-starch polysaccharide (NSP) because this is acknowledged to be the important component of dietary fibre.

Average adult intake of NSP in the UK is about 12 g/day, but this varies widely between individuals. Women usually consume less than men as they tend to eat less food in total. It is recommended that average NSP intake should increase to about 18 g/day (i.e. a 50% increase), the NSP being obtained from a variety of sources. However, this level of intake may not be appropriate for those with small appetites or those whose diet is marginal in terms of micronutrients. In practice this means children and some ill or elderly people.

It should be noted that 'dietary fibre' figures given on nutrition labels often include other fibre components (such as resistant starch) as well as NSP and so can be considerably higher than true NSP content. This is particularly likely to be the case with processed cereal foods (e.g. breakfast cereals) which can contain significant amounts of resistant starch.

General dietary guidance on increasing fibre consumption is given on p. 40.

MICRONUTRIENTS

Vitamins and minerals have many roles within the body. Many are essential for normal metabolic function because they act as co-factors or constituents of enzyme and hormonal systems. Some also have a structural function (e.g. as a constituent of bone), others act in a functional capacity (e.g. helping to maintain fluid balance regulation). Many act together to fulfil a common purpose, (e.g. create blood or to provide antioxidant protection).

Although each essential micronutrient has unique effects, it is important to realise that each one rarely operates in isolation and that a surplus or deficiency of one may have implications for another.

VITAMINS

Vitamins are a diverse array of chemicals required in only minute amounts but nevertheless are essential for survival. Vitamins operate at the cellular level affecting enzyme activity and chemical reactions. Most cannot be made by the body so must be provided by diet. The only exceptions are vitamin D (synthesised by the action of sunlight on skin), vitamin K (synthesised by gut bacteria) and niacin which can to some extent be made from the amino acid tryptophan.

In the past, interest in vitamins has tended to focus on the deficiency diseases which can result from severe deficiency (such as scurvy, beri-beri and pellagra). Because these problems are rarely seen in the UK, there has been a general assumption that dietary vitamin content is of little concern in people who are well fed. Recent evidence suggests this is not necessarily the case; sub-optimal intake of many vitamins may have a more subtle but highly significant influence on health and disease.

Vitamins have traditionally been classified according to whether they are soluble in fat or water. This distinction has some value because it provides some guide to the type of foods which contain them, some of their properties and their potential toxicity.

- *Fat-soluble vitamins*   A   D   E   K
- *Water-soluble vitamins*   B group   C

Fat-soluble vitamins are, as their name suggests, usually found in foods which contain fats or oils. There is therefore a risk of deficiency on very low fat diets. They tend to be robust vitamins, stable to heat and light and not easily destroyed by cooking. Excess intakes tend to be stored rather than excreted so overdosage is more likely to have toxic effects.

Water-soluble vitamins are much more fragile and can often be destroyed by poor storage or prolonged cooking. They are less likely to be stored in the body so tend to be required on a daily basis.

At normal ranges of intake, surplus amounts are rapidly excreted in the urine so the risk of overdosage is low. However, toxic effects can occur with megadoses of some of them.

Fat-soluble vitamins

Vitamin A (retinol)

Necessary for

- Healthy skin and mucous membranes (e.g. lining of mouth, airways and digestive system).
- Vision, especially in dim light.

Principal sources of vitamin A

Liver
Full-fat milk, cheese, butter
Margarine and most fat spreads (these are fortified with vitamin A in the UK)
Egg yolk
Fatty fish (e.g. herrings, sardines, mackerel)
Fish liver oils

Vitamin A can also be synthesised in the body from beta-carotene, the yellow pigment present in some fruit and vegetables. By this route 6 mg of beta-carotene produce 1 mg of vitamin A. Sources of beta-carotene can thus be regarded as a source of vitamin A although, unlike the vitamin itself, excessive quantities of beta-carotene are not toxic because the body only converts it to vitamin A when it is required.

Principal sources of beta-carotene

Orange/yellow/red vegetables (e.g. carrots, swedes, red peppers)
Orange/yellow/red fruits (e.g. apricots, mangoes, tomatoes)
Dark green leafy vegetables

Beta-carotene is thought to have an important role in its own right as an antioxidant (see p. 29).

Requirements

Average vitamin A requirements for adults are in the region of 400–500 μg retinol equivalents per day. The RNI (Reference Nutrient Intake, the level which covers the needs of virtually the whole population – see Chapter 5) has been set at 700 μg/day for adult men and 600 μg/day for adult women. Most people consume considerably more than this, on average about twice as much[1].

Deficiency

- Risk: Low.
- Most likely to occur in:
  - Young children not given vitamin A drops.
  - People on very low fat diets.
- Symptoms of deficiency:
  - Reduced night vision.
  - Loss of vision due to gradual damage to cornea.
  - Reduced resistance to infection due to loss of integrity of skin and mucous membranes.

Potential toxicity

- Risk: High.
- Recommended maximum intake:
  - Men   9000 μg/day
  - Women   7500 μg/day

Excess amounts of vitamin A are stored in the body and can cause damage to the liver and to bone. Excessive vitamin A may be also teratogenic and pregnant women are advised to avoid foods such as liver due to its high content of vitamin A (see Chapter 12, *Pregnancy*).

Vitamin D (cholecalciferol)

Necessary for

- Absorption of calcium.
- Mineralisation of bones and teeth.

In many ways vitamin D acts more like a hormone than a vitamin. Vitamin D itself (cholecalciferol) is an inactive substance which circulates in the blood as 25-hydroxyvitamin D and is converted in the kidney to the active form of the vitamin 1,25-dihydroxyvitamin D (calcitriol). It is this compound which regulates the amount of calcium absorbed from the intestine and its deposition in bone.

Principal sources of vitamin D

Most vitamin D is obtained by the action of ultra-violet light on the skin. There are very few natural dietary sources of vitamin D, the most significant sources are foods fortified with the vitamin:

Fortified margarines and fat spreads
Fortified breakfast cereals
Oily fish (e.g. herrings, kippers, mackerel)
Egg yolk
Full cream milk and dairy products

Requirements

People in the age range 4–64 years are assumed not to require a dietary source of the vitamin as long as they are exposed to sunlight during the summer months. The RNI for elderly people and for pregnant and lactating women is 10 μg/day.

Deficiency

- Risk: Low in most of the population but high in particular groups.
- Most likely to occur in:
  - Institutionalised or housebound elderly people.
  - Asian women and children.
- Symptoms of deficiency:
  - Inadequate calcification of bone.
  - Skeletal deformity (rickets and osteomalacia, see Chapter 37).

Potential toxicity

Risk: High, particularly in infants. 50 μg/day can cause hypercalcaemia in children.

Vitamin E (tocopherols)

Vitamin E is in fact a group of compounds called tocopherols. Alpha-tocopherol is the most biologically active form. Gamma-tocopherol is the most abundant form of vitamin E in the diet and accounts for about 50% of vitamin E intake.

Necessary for

■ Protecting cell membranes from oxidative damage.

Vitamin E is an important antioxidant. Being fat soluble, it is able to position itself within the lipid layers of membranes and is able to break the chain of events in which a free radical is passed from one molecule to another causing progressive oxidative damage. Such damage is thought to be part of the degenerative processes leading to the development of cardiovascular disease, cancer and other degenerative disorders associated with ageing. The antioxidant effects of vitamin E are enhanced by other antioxidants such as vitamin C and selenium.

Principal sources of vitamin E

> Vegetable oils (especially sunflower and safflower oils)
> Nuts
> Vegetables such as spinach and broccoli
> Wholegrain cereals and wholemeal bread
> Wheatgerm

Although natural and synthetic vitamins are normally considered to be equivalent because their chemical structures are identical, this may not be the case with vitamin E. The types of vitamin E compounds present in natural sources of vitamin E (e.g. sunflower and corn oils) may have higher biological potency than those from synthetic sources.

Some polyunsaturated margarines and spreads contain added vitamin E although this is mainly to protect the polyunsaturated fatty acids present from oxidation and the type of vitamin E added may have lower biological activity than alpha-tocopherol.

Requirements
Because of its function as an antioxidant, requirements are largely determined by the level of polyunsaturated fatty acids in the diet and hence

present in biological lipids. Because this level of intake varies, no Dietary Reference Values (see Chapter 5) for vitamin E have been set. Each gram of polyunsaturated fatty acid is thought to require an intake of about 0.4 mg vitamin E. If polyunsaturated fatty acid comprises 7% of total energy intake (as recommended), someone consuming 2000 kcal/ day would require a vitamin E intake of about 6 mg/day.

Levels which are thought to be adequate to prevent deficiency are:

Men	in excess of 4 mg/day
Women	in excess of 3 mg/day

Deficiency

■ Risk: Inadequate intakes of vitamin E may be more common and more significant than has been previously appreciated.
■ Most likely to occur in:
   ☐ People consuming a high intake of polyunsaturated fatty acids.
   ☐ Premature infants.
   ☐ People with malabsorption.
■ Symptoms of deficiency:
   ☐ May increase the risk of coronary heart disease and some types of cancer.
   ☐ May accelerate the development of some degenerative diseases, e.g. cataract, rheumatoid arthritis and ageing.

Potential toxicity
Unknown but believed to be low.

Vitamin K

Necessary for

■ Formation of blood clotting proteins especially prothrombin.

Principal sources of vitamin K

> Synthesis by bacteria in the gut
> Dietary sources:
>   Dark green leafy vegetables
>   Margarines and vegetables oils (especially those containing soya oil)

Milk
Liver

Requirements

There is insufficient information to enable dietary requirements to be estimated. Intakes of $1\,\mu g/kg$ body weight/day are believed to be safe and adequate for adults.

Deficiency

- Most likely to occur in:
  - □ Newborn infants. The gut is sterile at birth so it takes time for vitamin K to be manufactured. Additionally, infants are born with low vitamin K stores as it is poorly transferred across the placenta.
  - □ Deficiency is rare in adults. It is most likely to occur in those with bowel disorders or malabsorption.
- Symptoms of deficiency:
  - □ Deficiency in infants causes haemorrhagic disease which can be fatal. To minimise the risk, newborn infants are usually given a prophylactic dose of vitamin K.
  - □ Vitamin K deficiency in adults may increase blood clotting time.

Potential toxicity

Naturally-occurring forms of vitamin K are believed to be safe even at 100 times the safe intake. However, some synthetic forms of vitamin K may not have this margin of safety.

Water-soluble vitamins

Vitamin C (ascorbic acid)

Necessary for

- Prevention of oxidative damage in tissues.
- Immune function and resistance to infection.
- Wound healing.
- Integrity of skin, gums, blood vessels and other tissues.

- Synthesis of collagen (a constituent of connective tissue), hormones, neurotransmitters and other biologically important substances.
- Detoxification of harmful substances.
- Assisting absorption of non-haem iron.

Vitamin C has a vital role in the repair of damaged tissues and in wound healing.

It is also an important antioxidant because it can scavenge for, and intercept, free radicals present in the aqueous component of tissues before they can attack unsaturated lipids in cell membranes. In addition vitamin C regenerates vitamin E after it has reacted with a free radical.

Vitamin C also helps to maintain immune function. In particular it may reduce inflammation associated with infection by helping to neutralise oxidising compounds released by phagocytic leucocytes. Vitamin C is no longer believed to have a direct effect in preventing the common cold but it may well modify the severity or duration of such infections.

Principal sources

Fruit and vegetables especially:
Citrus fruit (oranges, lemons)
Soft fruits (blackcurrants, blackberries, raspberries)
Fruit juice
Potatoes
Green vegetables
Salad vegetables

Requirements

In adults, 10 mg/day prevents signs of scurvy but average requirements are about 25 mg/day. The RNI for the adult population has been set at 40 mg/day. Individual requirements are increased by illness, surgery, pregnancy, lactation and cigarette smoking.

Deficiency

- Risk: High in some groups.
- Most likely to occur in:
  - □ Those with a low of intake of fruit and vegetables.

□ Cigarette smokers.
□ Chronic illness.
□ Post-operative patients.
□ Elderly people.
Sudden cessation of megadoses of vitamin C
may cause a rebound scurvy.
■ Symptoms of deficiency:
□ Poor wound healing.
□ Lowered resistance to infection.
□ Bleeding gums, fragile capillary blood
   vessels.
□ Damage to bone and connective tissue.

Toxicity
Risk: Low.
   Surplus vitamin C is rapidly excreted in urine.
However, continual megadoses of vitamin C (in
excess of 1g/day) can cause oxalate stones in the
kidney.

B group vitamins

B vitamins are a group of substances which usually
act as co-factors for different enzyme systems in
the body, particularly those concerned with the
release of energy from food. Each of the B vitamins
has its own role but their functions tend to interact.
It is therefore important to consume a balanced
intake of the whole group.

   Deficiency tends to result in symptoms which
are diffuse such as tiredness, muscle weakness, and
loss of appetite. B vitamin adequacy should always
be considered in cases of anaemia or poor growth in
children.

   Thiamin, riboflavin and niacin are closely involved with energy metabolism, in particular the
metabolic pathways by which carbohydrate and fat
are turned into energy at the cellular level. Deficiency in children can result in poor growth.

   Vitamin B_{12} and folic acid are particularly
important in rapidly dividing cells such as blood-
producing cells in bone marrow so can affect blood
formation and, in the case of folic acid, embryo
development. B_6, closely associated with amino
acid metabolism, is also linked with blood formation via its effects on haemoglobin synthesis.

   Because B group vitamins are water soluble,
excess intakes of most of them are excreted in the
urine. The two exceptions are B_{12} and folic acid
which can be stored in the liver.

Thiamin (vitamin B_1)

Necessary for

■ Release of energy from carbohydrates, alcohol
   and fats.
■ Central nervous system function.

Principal sources

Wholegrain cereals (e.g. brown rice and whole-
   meal bread)
Fortified breakfast cereals
Meat (especially pork)
Pulses (peas, beans and other pulses)
Yeast extract (e.g. Marmite)
Nuts
UK produced white flour and bread (fortified
   with thiamin)

Requirements
This is dependent on the energy content of the diet
and the RNI is 0.4mg/1000kcal. In practice this
means that an intake of about 1.0mg/day will be
sufficient for adult men and 0.8mg/day for adult
women.

Deficiency
Common in alcoholics causing neurological dysfunction and Wernicke-Korsakoff syndrome. Mild
deficiency may result in tiredness, muscle weakness
and gastrointestinal disturbances and poor growth
in children.

Toxicity
Low.

Riboflavin (vitamin B_2)

Necessary for

■ Release of energy from protein, fats and
   carbohydrates.
■ Healthy skin and mucous membranes, particularly the cornea.

Principal sources

Milk and dairy products
Fortified breakfast cereals

Eggs
Yeast extract (e.g. Marmite)
Liver
Green leafy vegetables

Requirements
Average adult requirements are between 0.9 mg/day (women) and 1.0 mg/day (men). Signs of deficiency can appear on intakes below 0.8 mg/day. The RNI is 1.3 mg/day for adult men and 1.1 mg/day for adult women.

Heavy drinkers, smokers and women taking the contraceptive pill may have increased requirements.

Deficiency
Characterised by cracks and sores in the skin around the mouth and nose. Severe deficiency is unlikely in the UK.

Toxicity
Low.

Niacin (nicotinic acid and nicotinamide)

Necessary for

■ Energy metabolism.

Principal sources

Meat
Fortified breakfast cereals
UK produced white flour and bread (fortified with niacin)
Yeast extract (e.g. Marmite)

Niacin can also be synthesised in the body from the amino acid tryptophan (60 mg tryptophan are required to produce 1 mg niacin).

Requirements
The RNI for all ages is 6.6 mg niacin equivalents per 1000 kcal (i.e. either niacin itself or niacin derived from tryptophan). This means that about 13–16 mg niacin equivalents will meet the needs of most adults.

People who consume enough protein to maintain nitrogen balance will be able to generate sufficient niacin for their needs from tryptophan alone and an additional dietary supply will not be necessary.

Deficiency
Rare.

Toxicity
Doses of 20 mg/day can cause pharmacological effects such as tingling sensations and dilation of blood vessels. Intakes of 3–6 g/day can cause liver damage.

Pyridoxine (vitamin B_6)

Necessary for

■ Protein metabolism.
■ Central nervous system function.
■ Haemoglobin production.
■ Antibody formation.

Principal sources

Meat (especially beef and poultry)
Fish
Wholemeal bread
Fortified breakfast cereals

Requirements
These are related to protein intake and the RNI for both children and adults is 15 μg/g protein per day. In an average adult diet containing 15% of dietary energy from protein, this would require an intake of 1.2 mg/day (in women) and 1.4 mg/day (in men).

Requirements may be increased in women premenstrually and in those taking the contraceptive pill.

Deficiency
Can exacerbate anaemia.

Toxicity
Relatively high.

Pharmacological doses of pyridoxine can help alleviate some of the side effects induced by the contraceptive pill and possibly some of the symptoms associated with premenstrual syndrome. However, sensory nerve function can be impaired at intakes of 50mg/day (a level which is easily attainable with some of the pyridoxine supplements available).

Vitamin B₁₂ (cyanocobalamin)

Necessary for

- Red blood cell formation.
- Nerve sheath formation and central nervous system function.

Principal sources
Vitamin B_{12} is found in small amounts in virtually all foods of animal origin. It does not occur in plant foods unless added artificially.

Requirements
The RNI for adults is $1.5\,\mu g$/day. Unlike most water soluble vitamins, B_{12} can be stored in the liver so larger amounts can be consumed (or, if necessary, injected) at infrequent intervals.

Deficiency
This results in pernicious anaemia characterised by large immature blood cells and nerve dysfunction. This rarely results from dietary deficiency alone, it usually occurs only in vegans who avoid all animal foods and do not consume food fortified with B_{12}.

Pernicious anaemia is more likely to be caused by lack of intrinsic factor, a glycoprotein secreted by the stomach and essential for B_{12} absorption. Intrinsic factor may be absent either congenitally or following total gastrectomy. Either requires treatment with B_{12} by injection.

Toxicity
Low.

Folic acid (folates)

Folates are a group of compounds of which folic acid is the basic structure. Different compounds have varying degrees of biological activity; tetrahydrofolates are the most easily absorbed and the most active. Folic acid itself is rarely found in nature but is added to foods and supplements in this form because of its comparative stability.

Necessary for

- Nucleotide synthesis and cell division.
- Formation of red blood cells.
- Embryonic development of the nervous system.

Principal sources

Green leafy vegetables (especially broccoli, spinach and Brussels sprouts)
Fortified breakfast cereals
Wholemeal bread and fortified white bread
Yeast extract (e.g. Marmite)
Fruit (especially oranges, grapefruit and bananas)
Pulses (e.g. baked beans, peas)
Nuts

The folate content of foods can vary considerably. Folate is readily oxidised to an inactive form during harvesting and storage and can also be destroyed by overheating. Much of the folate content of green vegetables can be lost by prolonged boiling.

Requirements
Average adult folate requirements are $150\,\mu g$/day and the RNI has been set at $200\,\mu g$/day. However, women who may or intend to become pregnant are advised to take an additional $400\,\mu g$ (0.4mg) of folic acid per day (i.e. $600\,\mu g$ or 0.6mg/day in total) to minimise the risk the neural tube defects (NTD). Women with a history of NTD are advised to take a daily supplement of 4mg folic acid.

Deficiency
Because folate is needed for DNA synthesis, deficiency manifests itself where there is active cell division (e.g. in the developing fetus) or where there is rapid cell turnover (e.g. red blood cell production). In children, deficiency may result in poor growth; in adults, a megaloblastic anaemia is the most likely manifestation. An adequate supply of folate may be especially critical in the embryo at the

time of neural tube closure (about 28 days after conception), see Chapter 12, *Pregnancy*.

Toxicity
Low.

Biotin and pantothenic acid

These are also B vitamins which are involved in energy metabolism. Both are ubiquitous in the diet and deficiency is unlikely.

Other vitamin compounds

Choline, inositol, bioflavonoids and carnitine may be necessary in the diet although overt deficiency is unknown.

Pangamic acid (so-called vitamin B_{15}) is not a vitamin and some forms of it may be harmful.

Vitamin supplements

There is little risk of overdosage from vitamins consumed as part of a normal mixed diet. There is a considerable risk of overdosage from vitamins consumed in the form of supplements and these can cause effects ranging from the undesirable to the hazardous.

There are circumstances in which supplements of some vitamins are a sensible precaution, e.g. A, D, C drops in children, folate in women who may become pregnant, vitamin D in housebound people or vitamin C in immunocompromised people. However, vitamin supplements should never be regarded as an optional alternative to healthy eating; a vitamin C tablet is not, for example, an adequate substitute for fruit and vegetables because it will not provide the other beneficial dietary components such as antioxidant carotenoids or soluble fibre. There is also plenty of evidence to suggest that people who buy multi-vitamin supplements

are usually those who least need them, i.e. those who are relatively affluent and well nourished. In such circumstances, supplements are a waste of money.

MINERALS AND TRACE ELEMENTS

These are essential substances required for a variety of functions:

- Tissue structure (e.g. for the formation of bones and blood).
- Components of enzyme systems.
- Regulation of body fluids.
- Nerve function.

Those which are required in relatively large quantities are usually referred to as 'minerals'. Others which are required in much smaller quantities tend to be known as 'trace elements'. Those of most importance to the body are given in Table 1.2.

Other elements such as boron, nickel, and vanadium have been shown to have a role in metabolic processes but it is unclear whether a dietary requirement exists or deficiency ever occurs.

Table 1.2 Minerals and trace elements.

Minerals	Calcium
	Phosphorus
	Magnesium
	Sodium (and chloride)
	Potassium
Trace elements	Iron
	Zinc
	Fluoride
	Selenium
	Iodine
	Copper
	Manganese
	Chromium
	Molybdenum

Minerals

Calcium

Necessary for

- The structure of bones and teeth (these contain 99% of the calcium present in the body).
- Muscle contraction and cell function.
- Nerve conduction.
- Blood clotting.

Principal sources

Milk (full-fat, semi-skimmed and skimmed)
Cheese
Yogurt (both full-fat and low-fat varieties)
Canned fish (e.g. pilchards, sardines)
Green leafy vegetables
UK produced white flour and bread (fortified with calcium)
Pulses (including baked beans)
Tap water in hard water areas

Only about 30% of the calcium consumed is absorbed although this varies according to its bioavailability (calcium in milk is more easily absorbed than that in cereals and vegetables) and other factors such as dietary protein and phosphate content, the total amount of calcium consumed and the level of requirement. Calcium absorption and excretion are controlled by several hormones and vitamin D.

Requirements
As with many minerals, requirements are difficult to quantify because of variability in the bioavailability of calcium and its rate of absorption. Taking these factors into account, 700 mg/day has been deemed to be sufficient to meet the needs of most adults. The RNI for adolescent boys (11–18 years) is 1000 mg/day and for girls 800 mg/day, reflecting the high demand for calcium during these years. There is also a marked increase in requirement during lactation.

Deficiency
Low calcium intakes in childhood and adolescence may result in failure to achieve peak bone mass and increase the risk of osteoporosis in later life (see Chapter 36).

People at risk of low calcium intakes are:

- Vegans.
- Pregnant teenagers.
- Slimmers.
- Infants or children on parentally imposed milk-free diets (i.e. without dietetic advice).
- Anyone who consumes little milk or few dairy products (either full- or low-fat types).

Toxicity
Low since the body adapts to high calcium intakes by reducing the amount absorbed. Calcium supplements of 1–2 g/day may increase the risk of calcium stones in some people.

Phosphorus

Necessary for

- Formation of bone.
- Many metabolic reactions.

Principal sources
Phosphorus is present in all plant and animal cells and so is present in most foods except fats and sugars. Dietary deficiency is therefore unlikely. Most dietary phosphate is found in foods with a high content of calcium (e.g. milk and dairy products) or animal protein (e.g. meat and fish).

Requirements
About 60% of phosphorus consumed is absorbed and this necessitates an intake of about 400 mg/day in order to maintain normal plasma phosphate levels. In practice, dietary phosphate intake usually greatly exceeds this level.

Deficiency
Unknown.

Toxicity
Not known in adults. However, infants cannot handle excessive loads of phosphorus and unmodified

cows' milk can cause problems in young infants for this reason. The ratio of calcium to phosphorus is an important consideration in the formulation of infant milks.

Magnesium

Necessary for

- Bone structure.
- Neuromuscular transmission.
- Energy metabolism.

Principal sources
Magnesium is present in most foods. Dark green leafy vegetables contain large amounts but much of it is not available for absorption. Other vegetables and cereals are the most significant sources.

Requirements
The metabolic requirement for magnesium in adults is thought to be about 50 mg/day but because of variability in absorption, an average dietary intake of about 200–250 mg/day is required to meet this. The RNI has been set at 300 mg/day in adult men and 270 mg/day in adult women.

Deficiency
This is rare and usually caused by severe diarrhoea or excessive urinary losses resulting from diuretic drugs or renal disease. Severe magnesium depletion can cause muscle dysfunction including that of the heart.

Toxicity
Oral magnesium is not toxic since amounts in excess of 2 g/day are not absorbed from the intestine.

Sodium (and chlorine)

Necessary for

- Regulation of body water content.
- Maintenance of acid–base balance.
- Maintenance of blood volume and blood pressure.
- Neuromuscular transmission.

Principal sources
Many foods in their natural unprocessed state contain small amounts of sodium but none contain large amounts. The sodium content usually increases considerably once these foods are preserved or processed in some way. Mostly this results from the use of salt (sodium chloride) but other additives comprised of sodium salts, such as sodium bicarbonate, sodium nitrite or monosodium glutamate, supply additional amounts. The sodium content of foods will also be increased by the addition of salt during cooking or at the table.

On average, sodium intake is derived from:

Sodium naturally present in food	15–20%
Salt used in cooking or directly added to food	15–20%
Salt added during food processing or manufacture	60–70%

Some manufactured foods with a high sodium content are obvious because of their salt taste, for example:

Ham
Bacon
Smoked fish (kippers, mackerel)
Products canned in brine (e.g. frankfurters, fish)
Cheese
Butter (unless unsalted)
Salted foods (e.g. nuts, salted biscuits)
Yeast extract (e.g. Marmite)

Less obvious but significant sources of dietary sodium are:

Bread
Breakfast cereals
Ready meals or meat products (e.g. pies, beefburgers, sausages)
Canned meats (e.g. corned beef, spam)
Savoury snacks and crisps
Packet soups and sauces
Canned soups, spaghetti, baked beans, vegetables
Bottled sauces (e.g. tomato ketchup, soy sauce, brown sauce)
Stock cubes

Requirements

Sodium intake normally greatly exceeds sodium requirement. Most people actually need about 20 mmol sodium/day (460 mg sodium), equivalent to about 1 g of salt. In the UK, average salt consumption ranges between 3–18 g/day with an average of about 9 g/day, i.e. 9 times more than is necessary. Current recommendations are that this should be reduced by about one-third to 6 g salt/day.

It should be noted that this target intake figure relates to *salt* intake, but that nutrition information provided on food labels is (by law) expressed as *sodium* content. These figures are not interchangeable. Sodium only comprises 40% of the salt molecule so the figure on a nutrition label has to be related to a target *sodium* intake of 2.4 g/day, rather than 6 g salt/day.

Deficiency

Dietary deficiency is unlikely in normal circumstances.

Sodium depletion can result from excessive losses due to sweating during strenuous sporting activities or in a hot climate or by severe vomiting and diarrhoea (especially in infants and young children). The symptoms of this include fatigue, nausea and muscle cramps.

Toxicity

Habitually high salt intakes may be linked with the development of hypertension (see Chapter 24).

Sea-salt

Sea-salt contains as much sodium as refined table salt.

Salt substitutes

Some products are being marketed as alternatives to table salt. These contain either potassium or ammonium salts as a partial or total substitution for sodium. In general, it is probably preferable that people become accustomed to food tasting less salty but for inveterate salt-eaters they may be helpful. A more significant reduction in salt intake may be achieved by a lower consumption of processed convenience foods.

Salt substitutes have a high potassium content

and are contraindicated in people with hypertension secondary to renal disease.

General dietary guidance for salt reduction is given on p. 41.

Potassium

Necessary for

- Regulation of fluid balance in conjunction with sodium. Potassium maintains water within body cells whereas sodium maintains extracellular fluid volume.
- Essential for proper functioning of cells including nerves.
- Neuromuscular transmission.

Principal sources

Present in all foods except fats, oils and sugar. Particularly good sources are:

Fruits, especially bananas, oranges
Vegetables
Potatoes
Coffee/Tea/Cocoa

Requirements

Adults require between 2–3.5 g/day (50–90 mmol/day) and average intakes are in this region. Because potassium counteracts the effects of sodium, it has been suggested that increasing potassium intake (from fruit and vegetables) may be a protective measure in terms of hypertension, stroke and coronary heart disease[5].

Deficiency

Dietary deficiency is unlikely. Potassium depletion usually results from severe vomiting and diarrhoea. Some drugs, especially diuretics, also increase potassium losses. Symptoms of deficiency include muscle weakness, vomiting/diarrhoea, mental confusion, and if extreme, heart failure.

Toxicity

Dangerous if renal function is impaired; potassium intake may need to be restricted in people with renal disease.

High intakes (more than 17 g) are acutely toxic and dangerous.

Iron

Necessary for

- Synthesis of haemoglobin which transports oxygen around the body.
- Formation of myoglobin in muscle.
- Enzyme activity.

Principal sources
Dietary iron is present in two forms:

- Haem iron, derived from animal muscle or blood tissue, which is readily absorbed.
- Non-haem iron, an inorganic form of iron, which is less easily absorbed.

Absorption of non-haem iron can be impaired by high intakes of fibre and other plant constituents such as phytates or tannin in tea. It is enhanced by vitamin C.

Haem iron is present in:

Meat especially red meat and liver

Non-haem iron is present in:

Green leafy vegetables
Bread and cereal foods (in the UK, white bread and flour is fortified with iron)
Fortified breakfast cereals
Pulses
Eggs
Dried fruit
Nuts/seeds

Requirements
Dietary iron requirements are difficult to quantify because iron absorption is so variable. On average, only about 15% of the amount consumed is absorbed but this varies according to the form in which it is consumed, the metabolic need for iron and the presence of other dietary components which enhance or hinder its absorption.

Under normal circumstances, the amount of iron lost from the body is small. Although there is continuous turnover of red blood cells, most of the iron present in red blood cells is recycled. Significant iron loss, and thus increased iron requirements, will result from heavy blood loss, i.e. from menstruation, childbirth, surgery, haemorrhage or chronic occult bleeding in the gastrointestinal tract.

Surplus iron in the body is stored in the form of ferritin.

A dietary iron intake of 8.7 mg/day is considered sufficient to meet the needs of adult men. Adolescent males (11–18 years) need to consume more (11.3 mg/day).

Menstruating women and adolescent girls have a particularly high need for dietary iron. The RNI has been set at 14.8 mg/day but it is recognised that even this level of intake may not be sufficient to meet the needs of some individuals with heavy menstrual losses[1].

Deficiency
Inadequate dietary iron intakes results in a reduction in iron stores (and a fall in serum ferritin level) and eventually impairs red blood cell formation causing iron deficiency anaemia characterised by microcytic blood cells and a low concentration of blood haemoglobin.

Iron deficiency is most likely to occur:

- In women with high menstrual losses.
- In pregnant teenagers.
- Following injury or surgery resulting in significant blood loss.
- In gastrointestinal disorders resulting in malabsorption or occult blood loss.
- In people following an unbalanced vegetarian or vegan diet (see Chapter 21).

Excess
There is no risk of iron overdosage from normal foods other than in people with rare metabolic disorders. There is a high risk of toxicity from overdosage with iron supplements, particularly if they are consumed by children.

Zinc

Necessary for

- Enzyme activity in many metabolic pathways.
- Immune function.
- Wound healing.
- Insulin production.
- Growth.

Principal sources

> Meat
> Milk and dairy products
> Bread and cereal products
> Fish and shellfish
> Green leafy vegetables
> Eggs
> Pulses

Zinc absorption is very similar to that of iron; zinc absorption is higher from animal foods, especially meat, than from plant sources and can be impaired by a high dietary content of phytates from cereals and pulses. Iron and zinc also compete for the same absorption sites so a surplus of one can inhibit the absorption of the other. Iron supplementation can trigger zinc deficiency if zinc intake is marginal.

Requirements
There is considerable variability in zinc absorption but it has been estimated that a dietary intake of 9.5 mg/day will cover the requirements of adult men and 7.0 mg/day will be sufficient for most adult women. Adolescent boys and girls also have relatively high dietary requirements (9 mg/day).

Deficiency
Sub-optimal zinc intake may have implications in terms of immune function. Poor healing of leg ulcers and pressure sores in elderly people are sometimes associated with zinc deficiency.
    Deficiency is most likely to occur in:

- Elderly people.
- Children who don't eat meat.
- Vegetarians and vegans.

Toxicity
Isolated supplements of zinc can impair iron absorption (and vice versa – see above) and possibly that of other minerals such as copper. Amounts in excess of 2 g/day will be acutely toxic.

Fluorine (Fluoride)

Necessary for

- Bone and tooth mineralisation.
- Increasing the resistance of the teeth to decay.

Principal sources
Trace amounts of fluoride are present in many foods but significant amounts are provided by:

> Drinking water with a high natural or added level of fluoride
> Fluoride toothpaste
> Fluoride supplements
> Fish

Requirements
Although fluoride is essential, only trace amounts are required. In order to increase the resistance of teeth to decay and protect against dental caries, water fluoride content needs to exceed 1 part per million. If this is not the case, children should be given fluoride supplements.

Deficiency
Low fluoride intakes result in:

- Teeth which are susceptible to decay.
- Lack of bone strength and possibly enhanced risk of osteoporosis in later life.

Excess
Excessive amounts of fluoride are toxic and can result in mottling and crumbling of teeth and changes to the bones (fluorosis). The maximum recommended intake of fluoride for infants and young children is 0.05 mg/kg body weight/day.

Selenium

Necessary for

■ Antioxidant protection.

Selenium is a component of the enzyme glutathione peroxidase which has an important role in protecting intracellular structures against oxidative damage.

Principal sources
Found in a wide variety of foods but important dietary sources are:

Fish and shellfish (the richest source)
Bread and cereals (the main source in the UK diet)
Meat

Requirements
An intake of 1.0 μg/kg body weight/day is thought to be sufficient for most of the population. In adults the RNI has been set at 75 μg/day in men and 60 μg/day in women.

Deficiency
Greater likelihood of oxidative damage. Possible link with some forms of cancer and with the development of coronary heart disease.

Toxicity
High intakes have been shown to result in side effects[1]. The recommended maximum limit of consumption is 6 μg/kg body weight/day. This equates to about 450 μg/day for an average adult man.

Iodine

Necessary for

■ Thyroid function and formation of thyroid hormones (thyroxine and triiodothyronine).

Principal sources
The only natural rich sources of iodine are seafoods but in some countries certain foods, e.g. salt and bread, are fortified with iodine. In the UK milk is an important source of iodine due to iodine levels in animal feeds.

Milk and milk products
Seafood
Iodised salt

Requirements
The minimum requirement for adults is thought to be about 70 μg/day. An intake of 140 μg/day is thought to cover the needs of the vast majority of the adult population.

Deficiency
Thyroid hormones control many metabolic activities and if iodine deficiency inhibits their production, the thyroid gland may enlarge (goitre) in an attempt to produce more. Deficiency of thyroid hormone results in lethargy and low metabolic rate. Goitre resulting from iodine deficiency is extremely rare in the UK.

Toxicity
Not usually a problem although a form of hyperthyroidism can occur with excessively high intakes. The safe upper limit is 17 μg/kg body weight/day (approximately 1 mg/day for an adult).

Copper

Necessary for

■ Constituent of many enzyme systems, including cytochrome oxidase and superoxidase mutase which have key metabolic roles.

Principal sources

Present in trace quantities in many foods

Requirements
These have not been clearly established but 1.2 mg/day is thought to meet the needs of most of the adult population.

Deficiency
In infants, severe copper deficiency can affect bone and blood formation and impair immune function.

In adults, copper deficiency may have a role in the development of cardiovascular disease but further research is required.

Toxicity
High intakes are toxic but this has only been reported in unusual circumstances, e.g. contamination of drinking water.

Manganese

Necessary for

- Component of many enzymes and the activation of others.

Principal sources

Tea

Small quantities are present in many foods.

Requirements
No reference values have been set since deficiency has not been reported. The current average intake of about 4.6 mg/day is thought to be adequate.

Deficiency
Has only been observed under experimental conditions.

Toxicity
Very low. Excess intakes are rapidly excreted.

Chromium

Necessary for

- Insulin function.
- Lipoprotein metabolism.

Principal sources
Because of inadequate analytical techniques prior to 1980, this has been a matter of some confusion. Rich sources of chromium are thought to be:

Brewers' yeast
Meat

Wholegrain cereals
Legumes
Nuts

Highly refined foods may be particularly low in chromium.

Requirements
There is insufficient evidence for these to be accurately determined. A safe and adequate intake for adults is thought to be in excess of 25 μg/day.

Deficiency
Deficiency has been reported on intakes of 6 μg/day but this is unlikely to occur on a normal mixed diet, only on poorly formulated artificial diets (e.g. parenteral feeds).

Toxicity
Unknown at typical levels of consumption. Supplements in excess of 1–2 g/day may cause renal and liver damage.

Molybdenum

Necessary for

- Enzyme function, particularly those involved in DNA metabolism.

Principal sources
Trace amounts are present in many foods.

Requirements
These remain to be determined but safe intakes are believed to be between 50–400 μg/day for adults.

Deficiency
Reported on intakes of 25 μg/day.

Toxicity
High intakes (10–15 mg/day) may affect nucleotide metabolism and copper bioavailability.

Mineral supplements
The absorption and metabolism of minerals are often interrelated so an excessive intake of one (e.g.

iron) can impair the absorption of another (e.g. zinc) and vice versa. Isolated mineral supplements should only be taken when there is a clear clinical or dietary need otherwise a supplement may actually create a deficiency of another nutrient.

As is the case with vitamin supplements, those who tend to buy supplements are often those who least need them.

ANTIOXIDANT NUTRIENTS

These are not a separate category of nutrients but a collection of vitamins and minerals which are of current interest because of their role in the body's defence against cellular damage and the development of disease.

The normal process of oxidative metabolism results in the continuous generation of small numbers of unstable highly reactive molecules called free radicals. In an attempt to find chemical stability, a free radical will attack another molecule which then itself becomes unstable and in turn attacks a neighbouring molecule thus setting up a chain reaction. If unchecked this process can result in extensive cellular damage. The body has a number of antioxidant defence mechanisms to prevent this happening, many of which involve micronutrients – the so-called antioxidant nutrients. Lack of these nutrients may impair the defence mechanisms to such an extent that it may exacerbate the development of some forms of chronic disease, particularly cardiovascular disease (see Chapter 22) and cancer (see Chapter 41). Exposure to environmental pollutants or cigarette smoking also increases free radical production and hence increases the need for antioxidant protection.

Dietary factors which protect against oxidative damage are:

- Vitamin C.
- Vitamin E.
- Beta-carotene (and probably other carotenoids and flavonoids).
- Selenium.

Zinc, copper and manganese and probably other dietary components may also have important roles.

Selenium is important because it is a constituent of enzymes such as superoxide dismutase and glutathione peroxidase which have an important intracellular role in deactivating free radicals. Other minerals may also have a similar function.

Vitamin E and beta-carotene, being fat soluble, act within the lipid layers of cell membranes helping to prevent lipid peroxidation and thus cell membrane damage.

Vitamin C is a powerful scavenger of free radicals in aqueous tissues. It also regenerates vitamin E after it has come into contact with a free radical. Vitamin C may also minimise the pro-oxidant effects of cellular iron.

A co-ordinated response to free radical production will require the presence of all these nutrients. For this reason, isolated supplements of one of them cannot be expected to provide complete antioxidant protection. It should also be borne in mind that there are almost certainly other dietary components with antioxidant properties; some of the beneficial effects of fruit and vegetables may result from as yet unidentified antioxidant components as well as the more obvious ones. Consuming antioxidants in the form of foods may well be more protective than in the form of antioxidant supplements.

REFERENCES

1 Department of Health (1991) *Dietary Reference Values for Food Energy and Nutrients for the United Kingdom*. Report of the COMA Panel on Dietary Reference Values. Report on Health and Social Subjects 41. HMSO, London.
2 Willett, W.C. *et al.* (1993) Intake of trans fatty acids and risk of coronary heart disease among women. *Lancet* 341, 581–5.
3 British Nutrition Foundation (1995) *Trans Fatty Acids*. A Report from the Task Force Committee Report on Trans Fatty Acids. BNF, London.
4 Department of Health (1989) *Dietary Sugars and Human Disease*. Report of the COMA Panel on Dietary Sugars. Report on Health and Social Subjects 37. HMSO, London.
5 Department of Health (1994) *Nutritional Aspects of Cardiovascular Disease*. Report of the COMA Cardiovascular Review Group. Report on Health and Social Subjects 46. HMSO, London.

FURTHER READING

British Nutrition Foundation (1991) *Antioxidant Nutrients in Health and Disease*. Briefing Paper 25. BNF, London.

British Nutrition Foundation (1991) *Non-starch Polysaccharides*. Briefing Paper 22. BNF, London.

Garrow, J.S. & James, W.P.T. (eds) (1993) *Human Nutrition and Dietetics*, 4th edn. Churchill Livingstone, Edinburgh.

Health Education Authority (1990) *Sugars in the Diet*. A briefing paper. HEA, London.

Health Education Authority (1992) *Starch and Dietary Fibre*. A briefing paper. HEA, London.

Health Education Authority (1994) *Dietary Fats*. A briefing paper HEA, London.

Thomas, B. (ed) (1994) *Manual of Dietetic Practice*, 2nd edn. Blackwell Science, Oxford.

2

Dietary Targets

Diet and health are closely related. The human body requires an appropriate mixture of nutrients in order to function properly. It also has considerable ability to adapt to a diet which is not ideal for its needs but there are limits to the extent to which it can do this. Severe or prolonged deficiency of a vital nutrient will impair growth, development or normal function. Prolonged surfeit or imbalance will ultimately have metabolic consequences which increase the risk of disease. Some people will adapt to a poor diet better than others but, since there is no way of identifying those who are most vulnerable, a diet which maximises health and minimises disease risk is important at every stage of life.

Despite the impression that nutritional experts are constantly changing their minds, there is a general consensus as to what sort of diet this should be. Few would now dispute that the average diet in the UK (and most Westernised societies) is too high in fat, sugar and sodium and too low in starchy carbohydrate, fibre, and some vitamins and minerals. Many people consume far more energy (calories) than they require. These factors coupled with others such as an increasingly sedentary lifestyle and smoking have a considerable influence on major health problems such as obesity, heart disease, stroke and some forms of cancer.

THE EXTENT OF THE PROBLEM

The 1991 Health Survey for England, the first in an annual series carried out by the Department of Health and the Office of Population Censuses and Surveys (OPCS), assessed a number of nutrition-related health parameters among a nationally representative sample of 3000 adults[1]. Its findings made gloomy reading. Almost half the population was found to be overweight and a further 13% of men and 15% of women were considered to be obese, figures which were considerably higher than in a similar survey 10 years previously. Over two-thirds of the population had a serum cholesterol level above the desirable level and nearly one-fifth were hypertensive. Most had a level of physical activity below that thought necessary for health. Only 12% of men and 11% of women had none of the main risk factors for cardiovascular disease (smoking, raised blood pressure, raised blood cholesterol and lack of physical activity). Nearly one-third of women showed evidence of low iron stores.

DIETARY TARGETS

In 1992, the Government produced its White Paper *The Health of the Nation* in an attempt to

LIVERPOOL
JOHN MOORES UNIVERSITY
AVRIL ROBARTS LRC
TEL. 0151 231 4022

address these problems[2]. This document set out a number of health related targets (either a reduced incidence of or mortality from certain diseases or a reduced prevalence of lifestyle risk factors such as smoking) to be achieved by the years 2000–2005.

The Health of the Nation identified a number of priority areas for action: coronary heart disease and stroke, cancers, mental health, HIV/AIDS and sexual health, and accidents. A number of task forces were created to devise realistic action plans to meet these targets. Nutrition was identified as being a key part of health promotion and illness prevention via its influences on serum cholesterol levels, obesity, hypertension and bowel disease.

The dietary changes considered necessary to achieve these targets were set out in reports by the Department of Health's Committee on Medical Aspects of Food Policy (COMA)[3,4] and are summarised in Table 2.1. These figures are population targets and are not necessarily what each person should consume. They simply represent changes in dietary composition which if achieved on a population basis would result in a significant improvement in population health. Individuals within the population have varying needs, and a diet of this composition is not necessarily suitable for those who are old, young or ill. Nevertheless most people

would benefit if the composition of their diet shifted in the direction of these targets, i.e. a diet containing less dietary energy in the form of fat, particularly saturated fat, and more in the form of fibre-rich starchy carbohydrate.

Achieving these targets will require considerable changes in the dietary habits of the nation. Although total consumption of fat and saturated fat has slowly declined in recent years, total energy intake has also fallen (largely reflecting our increasingly sedentary lifestyle) so the fall in percentage of energy from fat has hardly changed. *The Dietary and Nutritional Survey of British Adults*[5] showed that only 14% of the population currently consume less than 35% energy from fat and fewer than 3% met the target for saturated fatty acids. Reaching the recommended targets for consumption of fibre and sugars will also require significant dietary change. On average it will necessitate:

- A 50% increase in the consumption of vegetables, fruit, potatoes and bread.
- Full-fat milk, dairy foods and fat spreads being replaced by reduced-fat equivalents.
- Fats rich in saturated fatty acids being replaced by those low in saturates and rich in monounsaturates.

Table 2.1 Recommended composition of the diet of the UK population.

	Current intake[5,6]	Target intake	Necessary change
Total fat	40% energy	35% energy	Decrease (14% reduction)
Saturated fat (% energy)	16% energy	11% energy	Decrease (35% reduction)
Monounsaturated fat (% energy)	15% energy	15% energy	No change
Polyunsaturated fat (% energy)			
n-6 polyunsaturates	7% energy	7% energy	No further increase
Long-chain n-3 polyunsaturates (from fish oils)	0.1g/day	0.2g/day	Intake should be doubled
Trans fatty acids	2% energy	2% energy	No further increase
Total carbohydrate	46% energy	50% energy	Increase (by 9%)
Starches	26% energy	33% energy	Increase (by 27%)
Sugars (non-milk extrinsic sugars)	14% energy	11% energy	Decrease (by 20%)
Protein	14% energy	<15% energy	No change
Fibre (non-starch polysaccharide)	12g/day	18g/day	50% increase
Salt (or equivalent as sodium)	9g (3.6g)	6g (2.4g)	Decrease by one-third

■ The consumption of two portions of fish per week, one of which should be oily fish.

A Nutrition Task Force was created to consider how the *Health of the Nation* targets can be achieved in practice and a national action plan *Eat Well!* was published in 1994[7]. A similar group, the Scottish Diet Action Group, was set up in Scotland. A Physical Activity Task Force was also formed to help tackle the prevention and treatment of obesity.

Dietary guidance for achieving these objectives is discussed in the next chapter (Chapter 3, *Healthy Eating*).

REFERENCES

1 White, A. *et al.* (1993) *Health Survey for England 1991.* HMSO, London.
2 Department of Health (1992) *The Health of the Nation: A Strategy for Health in England.* HMSO, London.
3 Department of Health (1991) *Dietary Reference Values for Food Energy and Nutrients for the United Kingdom.* Report of the COMA Panel on Dietary Reference Values. Report on Health and Social Subjects 41. HMSO, London.
4 Department of Health (1994) *Nutritional Aspects of Cardiovascular Disease.* Report of the COMA Cardiovascular Review Group. Report on Health and Social Subjects 46. HMSO, London.
5 Gregory, J. *et al.* (1990) *The Dietary and Nutritional Survey of British Adults.* HMSO, London.
6 MAFF (1993) *National Food Survey 1992.* HMSO, London.
7 Department of Health (1994) *Eat Well! An action plan from the Nutrition Task Force to achieve the Health of the Nation targets on diet and nutrition.* Available from BAPS, Health Publications Unit, DSS Distribution Centre, Heywood Stores, Manchester Road, Heywood, Lancs OL10 2PZ.

FURTHER READING

Bennett, N. *et al.* (1995) *Health Survey for England 1993.* HMSO, London.
Breeze, E. *et al.* (1994) *Health Survey for England 1992.* HMSO, London.
MAFF (1994) *The Dietary and Nutritional Survey of British Adults – Further Analyses.* HMSO, London.
The Scottish Office Home and Health Department (1993) *The Scottish Diet: Report of a working party to the Chief Medical Officer for Scotland.* The Scottish Office, Edinburgh.

3

Healthy Eating

The general guidelines for a healthy diet have been summarised as:[1]

- Enjoy your food.
- Eat a variety of different foods.
- Eat the right amount to be a healthy weight.
- Eat plenty of foods rich in starch and fibre.
- Don't eat too much fat.
- Don't eat sugary foods too often.
- Look after the vitamins and minerals in your food.
- If you drink alcohol, keep within sensible limits.

These are useful guidelines but on their own are insufficient to help people change their diets. One of the recommendations of the Nutrition Task Force (see Chapter 2), was that a way should be found to translate these nutritional objectives into a form of dietary advice which people can understand. Most people are now aware they should eat 'less fat' and 'more fibre' but many are still unsure what this means in terms of food. Even members of the primary health care team are not always very certain[2,3].

The Nutrition Task Force also felt that the negative image attached to healthy eating needed to be corrected. People tend to regard a healthy diet as a form of penance to be endured from time to time so that they can eat what they like afterwards with a clear conscience. They assume that healthy eating is synonymous with self-denial and means giving up all their favourite foods and replacing them with ones they don't like, can't afford or don't know what to do with (such as beans). An important part of health education is reassuring people that this is not the case.

THE NATIONAL FOOD GUIDE

In order to address these problems, a National Food Guide *The Balance of Good Health* was developed by the Department of Health, the Ministry of Agriculture, Fisheries and Food and the Health Education Authority[4]. After considerable evaluation[5-7], this took the form of a model of a tilted plate with divisions of varying sizes, each representing one of five food groups to show the types and proportions of foods needed to achieve a well-balanced and healthy diet (see Fig. 3.1 and Table 3.1).

The actual amount of foods consumed from each group will obviously vary from person to person. A young active adult will require larger portion sizes than an inactive older person. A 'serving' should therefore be regarded as a relative amount rather than a precisely quantified one. The point is that in relation to the total amount of food eaten, the proportions of different foods consumed should stay the same. The choice of foods within each group can, and should, be varied to increase the likelihood that all essential nutrients will be consumed.

Fundamentally, the National Food Guide is trying to convey two important messages:

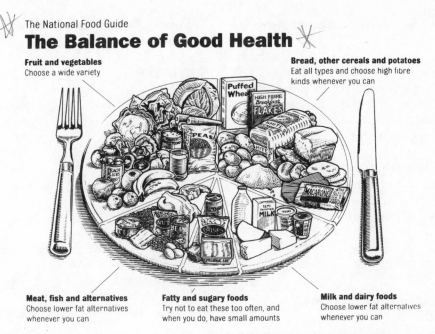

The National Food Guide
The Balance of Good Health

Fruit and vegetables
Choose a wide variety

Bread, other cereals and potatoes
Eat all types and choose high fibre
kinds whenever you can

Meat, fish and alternatives
Choose lower fat alternatives
whenever you can

Fatty and sugary foods
Try not to eat these too often, and
when you do, have small amounts

Milk and dairy foods
Choose lower fat alternatives
whenever you can

Fig. 3.1 The National Food Guide *The Balance of Good Health*. (Reproduced with kind permission of the Health Education Authority.)

Table 3.1 Proportions of foods in a well-balanced, healthy diet.

Food group	Proportion of all food consumed		Approximate number of servings/day
Bread, other cereals and potatoes	About one-third		4–6
Fruit and vegetables	About one-third		5
Milk and dairy foods	About one-third	(up to one-sixth)	3
Meat, fish and alternatives	in total	(up to one-sixth)	2
Fatty and sugary foods		(up to one-twelfth)	Small amounts

(1) It attempts to change the traditional perception that a meal has to be centred around protein-rich foods such as meat, fish, cheese or eggs. Instead starchy foods such as rice, pasta or potatoes should form a much larger proportion of our food intake together with increased amounts of fruit and vegetables.

(2) Foods should not be classified as either 'good' or 'bad'. Healthy eating does not mean that some foods must be eaten and others are banned. It is simply a question of proportion. Over a period of time, some types of foods should be eaten more often, others less so.

The National Food Guide is an important and useful concept for a variety of reasons:

■ It is flexible enough to be applicable to all age groups from toddlers to elderly people.
■ The proportion of food groups stays the same at all levels of energy intake.
■ It does not dictate what people should eat, merely provides guidance on appropriate choices.

- It does not ban specific foods but highlights which should form a smaller proportion of the diet.
- It can be used to assess dietary adequacy. The degree of mismatch between the proportion of food groups in an individual's diet and the recommended proportion indicates the likelihood of nutritional inadequacies or dietary imbalance.
- It can be used as a basis for dietary modification. People can be advised to adjust the proportion of food groups in their diet or alter their choices of foods within a particular group to meet their particular needs.

Food groups in the National Food Guide

The types of foods within each food group and their nutritional significance are discussed below. At first glance, the placement of some foods within a particular group may seem surprising. For example, potatoes form part of the bread/cereals group rather than the fruit/vegetables group; butter is classified as a fatty/sugary food rather than a milk/dairy food. There are sound nutritional or practical reasons for this and these are discussed elsewhere[6].

Composite foods, such as pizza, pies and lasagne, which are comprised of items from several food groups, are more of a problem because they defy neat classification. This can be turned to educational advantage by encouraging people to think about the components of these foods and how they fit into the five food groups. Thus lasagne (which may contain ingredients from all five groups in more or less the recommended proportions) can be seen to be a better choice than an individual meat pie where perhaps only two food groups are represented and the largest component (pastry) is in the fatty/sugary foods group.

Group 1: Bread, other cereals and potatoes

Foods included:

> Bread, rolls, crispbread, muffins, scones, pikelets, chapattis, pitta bread
> Breakfast cereals
> Pasta
> Potatoes
> Rice

Amount to eat:

> About one-third of the total volume of food eaten
> For most people about 4–6 servings/day

This is probably more than people currently consume.

Nutritionally these foods are good sources of:

> Carbohydrate
> Fibre (particularly insoluble fibre)
> B vitamins
> Some calcium and iron

Points to note:

- There is a common misconception that these foods are 'fattening'. In fact the opposite is true – they provide a lot of bulk without too many calories. Their energy content only increases considerably when fat is added to them, e.g. potatoes become chips, or fat is thickly spread on bread.
- Wholemeal bread, brown rice and wholegrain cereals provide the most fibre but increasing the intake of all types of cereal foods will increase fibre consumption.
- Fibre rich cereal foods are less suitable for children or people with small appetites because of their bulk.
- *Bread* Wholemeal bread has a higher content of many vitamins, minerals and trace elements than white bread although to some extent this benefit is offset by decreased absorption as a

result of the higher fibre content. In the UK, white bread and flour are fortified with certain minerals and vitamins and contain significantly more calcium than wholemeal bread/flour. Using thicker slices of bread is a good way of increasing carbohydrate consumption without increasing the amount of fat spread on it.

- *Breakfast cereals* Many are fortified with various micronutrients and can be a valuable dietary source of folate, other B vitamins and iron. Some choices of breakfast cereals are better than others in terms of fibre or sugar content but all breakfast cereals (particularly if consumed with milk) are better than no breakfast at all.
- *Potatoes* Most people think of these as 'vegetables' but in nutritional terms they are more appropriately grouped with other starchy carbohydrate foods. The use of additional fat (e.g. in baked or with mashed potatoes) should be avoided. Chips (but not crisps) are also included in this group because like potatoes (but unlike crisps) they are usually eaten as part of a meal rather than as a snack. They are, however, a high fat choice so overconsumption should be discouraged.

Group 2: Fruit and vegetables

Foods included:

All types of fruit and vegetables (except potatoes – see above)

These can be   fresh
               frozen
               canned
               dried
               juices

Amount to eat:

About one-third of the total volume of food eaten

Aim for a minimum of five portions per day

This is more than most people usually eat.

Nutritionally these foods are good sources of:

Vitamin C
Carotenes and other antioxidants
Folates
Fibre (especially soluble fibre)
Potassium

Points to note:

- In practice most people need to double their intake of fruit and vegetables and consume about 400 g (approximately 1 lb) per day. A useful rule of thumb is five servings a day (excluding potatoes) sometimes referred to in health promotion campaigns as '5-a-day' or 'Take 5'. This is not unrealistic and for example could comprise:
  Two types of vegetables with one main meal
  One vegetable and one portion of fruit with another meal
  A glass of fruit juice with breakfast.
- Both fresh and dried fruit can make useful snacks.
- Yogurt or fromage frais is a good accompaniment to fruit.
- Fruit and vegetables contain virtually no fat unless this is added (e.g. butter added to vegetables; cream added to fruit).
- Water-soluble vitamins such as vitamin C or folates are easily destroyed by heating so vegetables should not be over boiled.

Group 3: Milk and dairy foods

Foods included:

Milk
Cheese
Yogurt
Fromage frais

Amount to eat:

About one-sixth of the total volume of food intake

About 3 servings per day (e.g. $\frac{1}{3}$rd pint of milk, one carton yogurt, small piece (40 g) hard cheese)

Nutritionally these foods are good sources of:

Calcium
Protein
Riboflavin
Vitamins A and D (full fat produce only)

Points to note:

■ Most people should choose reduced-fat or low-fat varieties (e.g. skimmed or semi-skimmed milk, low-fat yogurt). These products contain the same amounts of calcium, protein and riboflavin as their full-fat equivalents but less fat and energy. They will also contain less of the fat-soluble vitamins A and D. Because of this, and their lower energy content, fat-reduced products are not suitable for young children, some elderly people or those who are nutritionally depleted. Children over 2 years can be given semi-skimmed milk provided that they are eating a diverse and adequate diet. Skimmed milk is not suitable for children under 5 years of age
■ Hard and other full-fat cheeses (e.g. Cheshire, Stilton, Brie) have a high fat (and energy) content and should be used with caution by those who need to reduce their energy intake. Conversely, cheese is a valuable food for those who need to increase their energy intake (e.g. chronically ill people with small appetites).
■ Butter and cream, which are almost exclusively comprised of fat, are not included in this grouping.

Group 4: Meat, fish and alternatives

Foods included:

Meat
Poultry
Offal
Fish
Eggs
Liver and kidney
Pulses (beans and lentils)
Nuts

Amount to eat:

Up to about one-sixth of the total volume of food consumed
About 2 servings per day

Nutritionally these foods are good sources of:

Protein
Iron
B vitamins
Zinc
Magnesium

Points to note:

■ These foods are important but should not predominate dietary intake.
■ *Meat (i.e. beef, lamb, pork)* Meat is often incorrectly assumed to be a high fat food. This is only true if meat fat is consumed; the lean part of meat is relatively low in fat but rich in essential nutrients, particularly haem iron. Lean beef or pork only contain about 3 g fat/100 g – a similar level to that in cottage cheese. The misconception about meat has largely arisen because, in food survey data, meat and meat products are usually grouped together and some of the latter do have a very high fat content because they contain considerable amounts of meat fat (e.g. sausages) and sometimes fat from other components such as pastry (e.g. a pork pie). In addition to this, the fat content of meat has declined significantly in recent years as a result of selective breeding techniques; the figures given in many food tables are therefore too high. New figures have recently been produced by MAFF (see references, p. 73).
  Nor is the fat which is present comprised solely of saturated fat; in beef and pork about 50% is in the form of monounsaturated fatty acids. Pork is the most unsaturated meat; lamb the least.
■ *Poultry* This is also subject to misconception, in this case that it is *always* low in fat. The white meat (e.g. breast meat) eaten without the attached skin is relatively low in fat (about 3 g/100 g) but the darker meat (e.g. leg

muscle) has a higher fat content and poultry skin is extremely high in fat. A typical chicken joint eaten with skin can provide over 20g fat.

- *Offal* Liver and kidney are relatively low in fat and rich sources of haem iron. They are also relatively cheap foods but not always popular.
- *Fish* White fish is low in fat (unless fried) and a valuable source of the antioxidant selenium. Oily fish (e.g. herrings, mackerel, pilchards, sardines) contain long-chain n-3 polyunsaturated fatty acids which have antithrombotic and some anti-inflammatory properties. They also are one of the few dietary sources of vitamin D.
- *Eggs* These contain dietary cholesterol but this is not a significant concern unless eggs are consumed in unusually large amounts (several per day) or by people with certain rare lipid disorders. Within the normal range of intake, dietary cholesterol has little effect on blood cholesterol. Eggs should always be well cooked to minimise the risk of salmonella poisoning.
- *Pulses (i.e. beans and lentils)* These can be useful providers of many minerals and trace elements as well as protein. They can be useful to help compensate for a smaller quantity of lean meat being used in a casserole or other composite dish. Baked beans or canned kidney beans are an acceptable and convenient form of pulses for many people.

Group 5: Fatty and sugary foods

Foods included:
Fatty foods

Butter, margarines and fat spreads
Cooking fats and oils
Pastry (e.g. in pies, flans, sausage rolls)
Savoury snacks (e.g. crisps)
Cream
Mayonnaise and salad dressings
Rich sauces and fatty gravies

Sugary foods

Cakes, doughnuts
Biscuits
Puddings, ice cream
Chocolate and confectionery
Non-diet fizzy drinks

Amount to be consumed:

These foods should ideally comprise no more than about one-twelfth of total food intake

This is less than most people usually consume.

Nutrients provided:
These foods are not devoid of nutrients; on the contrary, small amounts of fats and oils are an important source of essential fatty acids. Nor are they 'junk foods' for no such thing exists (only perhaps 'junk' diets). It is wrong to suppose that foods such as crisps, cakes and chocolate, etc., have no nutritional value. Crisps contain vitamin E, cakes contain nutrients derived from ingredients such as flour and eggs, and even chocolate provides some iron. The point is that these foods are not rich sources of these nutrients relative to the amount of energy (often derived from fat) which they provide. Too many of them in a diet will distort the nutritional balance and supplant other foods which are nutritionally much more important. If most of the dietary energy is derived from foods from this group, dietary fat intake will almost certainly be far too high and micronutrient intake undesirably low.

Points to note:

- It is unrealistic to tell people to avoid these foods altogether. They add palatability and convenience to a diet and used sensibly can form part of a balanced healthy diet. The point to emphasise is that these foods should comprise the smallest proportion of the diet and not, as is so often the case, the largest.
- Many of these foods have a high content of salt and *trans* fatty acids.
- *Spreading fats* Butter and margarine (whether hard margarine or polyunsaturated margarine) have the same (high) fat and energy content.

Reduced- or low-fat spreads (sometimes called 'light' or 'extra light') have a significantly lower fat and energy content than 'margarine'. Hard margarine will have a higher content of saturated and *trans* fatty acids than those marketed as high in monounsaturates or polyunsaturates.

The best choice of a fat to spread on bread is a reduced/low-fat spread, and those rich in monounsaturates (e.g. olive oil based) are slightly preferable to those rich in polyunsaturates (e.g. sunflower oil based). Some products have added buttermilk for extra flavour; this does not have any adverse effects on fat content. Some also have a beneficially low sodium content.

■ *Cooking fats* Use of these should be kept to an absolute minimum. Vegetable oils should always be used in preference to lard or dripping. Olive oil is a rich source of monounsaturates; sunflower, safflower and corn oils are rich in n-6 polyunsaturates; rapeseed and soya oils are a richer source of n-3 fatty acids.

Dietary modification using the National Food Guide

national food guide / helps towards

As well as achieving a better overall balance of foods within the diet, health professionals can also use the National Food Guide to make nutritional adjustments by encouraging, or discouraging, the use of particular foods within each food group. For example, in the bread/cereals group, high-fibre choices would be recommended to someone suffering from constipation whereas a child with a small appetite would be encouraged to eat less bulky cereal foods. In the meat, fish and alternatives group, the person at risk of thrombosis might be advised to include oily fish among their choices while someone with a low iron intake may need to be encouraged to include more red meat. Occasionally, some foods may need to be considered as part of another group; an obese person who eats a lot of cheese may be well advised to think of cheese as

being in the fatty/sugary food group rather than a choice from the milk/dairy foods group. The way in which this model can be applied in different age groups and circumstances is discussed throughout this book.

If a specific nutrient (e.g. fat intake) is of particular concern, additional advice concerning food choice and cooking methods may need to be incorporated as appropriate for that individual. Such guidance may include:

Ways of reducing fat intake

■ Avoid frying foods; grill, bake, casserole or steam instead.
■ Use minimal amounts of cooking oil to lubricate cooking pans. Non-stick spray fat is useful for greasing baking trays and tins.
■ Avoid adding fat to cooked foods (e.g. butter/margarine on vegetables or pasta).
■ Remove visible fat from meat and skin from chicken.
■ Drain or skim fat from mince and casseroles.
■ Use low-fat spread instead of butter or margarines.
■ Use reduced-fat milk and dairy produce.
■ Keep hidden sources of fat to a minimum. Particular foods to watch are pastry, pies, biscuits, cakes and meat products. Choose lower fat alternatives when available. Mashed potato toppings can be a good alternative to pastry.
■ If chips are consumed they should be of a low-fat type and oven-baked.

Ways of increasing fibre intake

■ Eat more wholemeal bread or high fibre white bread. Use thicker bread for sandwiches (or rolls).
■ Eat more wholegrain breakfast cereals or those which contain bran or oats.
■ Eat more brown rice or wholewheat pasta.
■ Eat more fresh fruit and vegetables.
■ Use more pulse vegetables (e.g. peas, beans and lentils). Add to casseroles or composite dishes.
■ Use some wholemeal flour in baking: a 50:50 mixture of wholemeal and white flour usually gives good results.

These changes should be introduced gradually; a sudden large increase in fibre consumption can result in distension and flatulence. Additional fluids will also be necessary.

Reducing salt/sodium intake

- Don't add salt to food.
- Use minimum amounts of salt in cooking. Leave it out of recipes altogether (most people will not notice the difference) and at most add only a pinch of salt (rather than a teaspoonful) to vegetable cooking water. Boost flavour by using more herbs, spices, mustard, onion, garlic or lemon juice.
- Use fewer processed convenience foods from cans, jars, packets or cartons. Choose reduced salt versions if available. Use more fresh foods instead.
- Avoid highly salted foods (e.g. cheese, crisps and savoury snacks), salted foods (e.g. salted peanuts), smoked fish, preserved sausage (e.g. salami), yeast extracts.

Other aspects of healthy eating

Cost of a healthy diet

There is continuing debate as to whether a healthy diet costs more than a less healthy diet. It all depends on how the comparison is made. Healthy eating is perceived to be expensive because it is associated with costly foods such as lean meat, fish and fresh fruit. People tend to overlook the fact that other recommended components such as pasta, rice, bread and potatoes are relatively cheap. Healthy food choices need not always incur greater cost: an apple costs no more than a bar of chocolate or a bag of crisps, a glass of milk can be cheaper than a glass of cola, the cheaper plainer breakfast cereals are better choices than more expensive sugar-coated varieties, baked potatoes cost no more than chips. Comparisons of 'healthy' and 'unhealthy' shopping baskets often fail to compare like with like and it is not difficult to devise a mixture of foods which 'prove' the debate about the cost of healthy eating either way.

Most people can eat a healthier diet without spending more on food. To some extent it depends on the starting base. Someone who consumes a lot of cheap meat products, sausages, chips, hard margarine, etc., will find it difficult to make healthy changes without spending more money. But the person who lives mainly on expensive pre-frozen ready meals interspersed with biscuits, savoury snacks and confectionery can almost certainly obtain a better nutrient balance at less cost.

What is undeniable that it is much more difficult for people in low income groups to eat a healthier diet although there are a number of reasons for this apart from the cost of food (see Chapter 19).

REFERENCES

1 Health Education Authority (1993) *Enjoy Healthy Eating.* HEA, London.
2 Francis, J. *et al.* (1989) Would primary health care workers give appropriate dietary advice after cholesterol screening. *British Medical Journal* **298**, 1620–22.
3 Hopper, D. & Barker, M.E. (1995) Dietary advice, nutritional knowledge and attitudes towards nutrition in primary health care. *Journal of Human Nutrition and Dietetics* **8**, 279–86.
4 Health Education Authority (1994) *The Balance of Good Health. Introducing the National Food Guide.* HEA, London.
5 Hunt, P. *et al.* (1995) A National Food Guide for the UK? Background and development. *Journal of Human Nutrition and Dietetics* **8**, 315–22.
6 Gatenby, S.J. *et al.* (1995) The National Food Guide: development of dietetic criteria and nutritional characteristics. *Journal of Human Nutrition and Dietetics* **8**, 323–34.
7 Hunt, P. *et al.* (1995) The format for the National Food Guide: performance and preference studies. *Journal of Human Nutrition and Dietetics* **8**, 335–51.

4

Sensible Drinking

Within a population there is a U-shaped relationship between alcohol consumption and all-cause mortality, those drinking between 8 and 14 units/week having the lowest risk[1]. Moderate consumption of alcohol is associated with a lower risk of death from coronary heart disease (CHD), possibly as a result of beneficial effects on high density lipoprotein (HDL) levels and fibrinolytic factors[2,3]. However, all-cause mortality starts to increase at 21 units/week for men and 14 units/week in women and CHD risk increases considerably in men whose consumption exceeds 40 units/week[1,4]. In the short term, excessive amounts of alcohol can be acutely toxic to the individual as well as potentially dangerous to others as a result of the loss of co-ordination or self-control, and behavioural change which may be of an aggressive or violent nature. In the long term, continued heavy drinking causes liver damage resulting in cirrhosis, pancreatitis and some cancers. Heavy alcohol abuse in pregnancy can cause fetal abnormalities and mental retardation.

RECOMMENDED SENSIBLE DRINKING LIMITS

In the UK, one unit is defined as 8g alcohol and is roughly equivalent to the alcohol present in one measure of spirits, one glass of wine or half a pint of beer (but see below). Until December 1995, the recommended maximum levels of alcohol consumption were 21 units/week for men and 14 units/week for women. The Department of Health now recommends that alcohol guidance should be given in terms of acceptable *daily* intakes rather than as a weekly maximum[5]. It was felt that weekly limits did nothing to discourage bouts of heavy drinking (e.g. all 21 units being consumed on a Saturday night) which clearly pose a health risk yet could still be classified as 'safe'. The new recommended limits are:

Men	3–4 units/day
Women	2–3 units/day

This has been widely interpreted as an increase in the previous limits to 28 units/week for men and 21 units/week for women. Technically this is true, but the main health education message is that people who consistently exceed the new daily limits will be at progressive health risk.

Once ingested, alcohol is rapidly absorbed, particularly if the stomach is empty. Once absorbed it circulates in the blood before being metabolised in the liver to provide energy. It is metabolised more slowly in women which is why they are more susceptible to both the intoxicating effects of alcohol and long-term damage. On average, it takes about an hour for the body to dispose of one unit (8g) of alcohol. Thus, 4 units of alcohol (e.g. 2 pints of beer) will take about 4 hours to clear.

USING THE UNIT SYSTEM

Units are a convenient way of expressing the amount of alcohol in different drinks. One unit of alcohol is approximately equal to:

1 single pub measure of spirits (25 ml)*
1 glass of sherry or fortified wine (75 ml)
1 glass of table wine (100 ml)
Half a pint of standard strength beer, lager or
    cider

*In England and Wales. In Scotland a pub measure will provide $1\frac{1}{4}$ units of alcohol, in Northern Ireland $1\frac{1}{2}$ units.

The unit system is a simple and easy way for people to keep track of their alcohol consumption. There are, however, some pitfalls which may need to be pointed out:

■ *Variation in serving size* The specified measures (e.g. a glass of wine) are those typical of drinks sold in pubs and restaurants. Those dispensed at home may be considerably more generous!

■ *Variation in alcoholic strength* Beers and lagers vary considerably in alcoholic strength and this, coupled with the fact that many are sold in cans containing considerably more than $\frac{1}{2}$ pint, can easily lead someone to underestimate the number of alcohol units consumed. Standard strength beer or lager contains 3.5% alcohol by volume (ABV). Some products have a higher strength than this and extra strong lager or special brews of beer can contain as much as 9% ABV. Some of these may be sold in 440 ml cans, i.e. over $\frac{3}{4}$ pint ($\frac{1}{2}$ pint = 284 ml), so a can of extra strong lager may provide 4 units of alcohol, not as may be assumed, 1 unit. Young adults in particular are likely to make this mistake and not realise that drinking 2–3 cans of such products will have the same effect as drinking 8–12 measures of Scotch.

The alcoholic strength must, by law, be declared on the label of alcoholic drinks and people should be encouraged to look at this information. ABV is sometimes expressed as 'alcohol % vol' or '% vol' but they all mean the same thing.

LOW ALCOHOL DRINKS

These are not always as low in alcohol as may be assumed. Some are virtually alcohol free (0.05% ABV) but most 'low' alcohol beers, lagers and ciders have about one-third of the alcohol content (1.2% ABV) of the standard product. Some low alcohol wines are about half as strong as ordinary table wine. People often assume that all these products have a negligible alcohol content and that it is safe to drive after consuming them; this may not be the case.

REFERENCES

1 Doll, R. *et al.* (1994) Mortality in relation to consumption of alcohol: 13 years' observations on male British doctors. *British Medical Journal* **309**, 911–8.
2 Marmot, M. & Brunner, E. (1991) Alcohol and cardiovascular disease: the status of the U-shaped curve. *British Medical Journal* **303**, 565–8.
3 Hendriks, H.F.J. *et al.* (1994) Effect of moderate dose of alcohol with evening meal on fibrinolytic factors. *British Medical Journal* **308**, 1003–6.
4 Royal Colleges of Physicians, Psychiatrists and General Practitioners (1995) *Alcohol and the Heart in Perspective: Sensible Limits Reaffirmed.* Royal Colleges, London.
5 Department of Health (1995) *Sensible Drinking.* The Report of an Inter-Departmental Working Group. Available from Department of Health, PO Box 410, Wetherby, LS23 7LN.

FURTHER READING

Health Education Authority (1994) *That's the Limit. A guide to sensible drinking*. HEA, London.

Kemm, J. (1993) Editorial: Alcohol and heart disease: the implications of the U-shaped curve. *British Medical Journal* **307**, 1373.

Robertson, I. (1994) Safe drinking. *British Medical Journal* **308**, 346.

Shaper, A.G. (1994) Alcohol intake and mortality. *British Medical Journal* **308**, 589.

5

Assessing Nutritional Requirements

In the UK, requirements for energy and nutrient requirements are detailed in the 1991 Department of Health document *Dietary Reference Values for Food Energy and Nutrients for the United Kingdom*[1]. These recommendations were made after a comprehensive review of available scientific evidence and replace, and in many respects differ from, previous guidance such as the 1979 Recommended Daily Amounts (RDAs). Many other countries produce a similar set of reference figures relevant to their own populations.

DIETARY REFERENCE VALUES (DRVs)

Dietary Reference Values (DRVs) are a vital tool for those involved in the science of nutrition in order to explore the relationships between diet and health or disease. However, dietary reference figures can be, and often are, misused because people misunderstand what these figures really mean. The summary tables of Reference Nutrient Intakes (RNIs) stratified by age and sex are often assumed to show the cut-off points between sufficiency and deficiency, i.e. someone consuming less than the quoted amount has an inadequate intake. In reality, this may not be the case at all because these figures are not intended to be used in this way.

DRVs apply to populations (i.e. groups of people). Among the individuals within a population there will be considerable variability of nutrient

needs so what may be sufficient for one person may be insufficient for another. Like most biological variables (e.g. height), nutrient needs follow the pattern of the normal distribution curve, i.e. the majority of the population cluster around a central point with diminishing proportions extending towards the extreme ends of the normal range. DRVs represent different points on this normal distribution curve.

DRVs are not just a single set of figures but four sets of figures providing guidance on average needs, recommended intakes, minimum needs, and safe levels of intake as appropriate for each nutrient.

Estimated Average Requirement (EAR)

This is the average requirement of a group of people. Many will require more than this amount and many will require less (in the same way that 'average height' in a group of people does not mean everyone is this height; most will be either taller or shorter than the average).

Reference Nutrient Intake (RNI)

This is the amount which meets the needs of virtually everyone in a population except the top 3%

45

who have particularly high requirements. The RNI is therefore *sufficient* for 97% of the population but most people will actually *need* less than this amount.

The RNI is the most familiar DRV figure because it is the one usually quoted as the 'requirement' for a particular nutrient. (The RNI is also equivalent to the older term Recommended Daily Allowance, RDA, which is still used in nutrition labelling.) What the RNI really means is that if a population (e.g. a group of elderly people) is consuming a diet which meets a particular RNI, then the vast majority of those people will be consuming enough of this nutrient for their individual needs. If the mean intake of the group is less than the RNI then an increasing proportion of this population will not be meeting their needs. If an *individual* is consuming a nutrient at the level of the RNI then that person is almost certainly obtaining enough; an individual intake below the RNI does not necessarily mean dietary deficiency because that person's need may well be below this level.

Lower Reference Nutrient Intake (LRNI)

This is the amount which is *only* sufficient for the 3% of the population with particularly low requirements. Most people will actually need more than this amount.

The LRNI is a far better guide to nutritional inadequacy in individuals because there is a high probability that someone consuming a nutrient at or below this level will not be consuming enough for their needs.

Safe intake

This is the amount which is considered to be safe and adequate for most people. The term is used for some micronutrients where there is insufficient data for more precise estimates of requirements to be made.

DRVs should not be regarded as carved in tablets of stone; they are simply the best estimates of likely requirements or appropriate intakes which could be made from the evidence available at the time they were compiled. Some figures may well be modified in due course in the light of new information, in particular for those nutrients whose relationships with disease processes are still being unravelled (e.g. antioxidants) and where optimum requirements for health may be considerably higher than metabolic requirements to prevent deficiency.

ASSESSING INDIVIDUAL NUTRIENT NEEDS

DRVs provide a framework for assessing nutrient requirements but cannot alone specify individual nutrient needs. These will be determined by a number of factors which have to be considered on an individual basis.

DRVs do take some account of the major determinants of nutritional requirements such as:

- *Age* In terms of absolute amounts, infants and children usually require less of a nutrient than an adult. However, in relation to their body size (i.e. requirement per kg of body weight) young humans often require more than older ones. During adolescence, rapid growth may impose exceptional nutrient demands and for a while nutrient requirements may exceed those of adults. After the age of 50, muscle mass and metabolism tend to decline and the requirements for energy and some nutrients decrease.
- *Sex* Men tend to have a larger body frame and greater muscle mass than women so usually therefore have higher energy and nutrient requirements. Women of child-bearing age

have a much higher requirement for iron than men.

■ *Physiological stresses* Pregnancy and lactation impose additional nutrient demands.

However, DRVs can take only partial, or even no, account of some of the other factors affecting nutrient requirements. These include:

■ *Factors affecting nutrient absorption* Not everything consumed is absorbed; over 90% of protein consumed is absorbed but as little as 15% of iron. DRVs do take this into account and quote the amount of a nutrient which needs to be *consumed* to meet physiological needs, not the physiological need itself. Thus the RNI for iron for an adult man is 8.7 mg/day although the actual physiological need for iron is in the region of 1 mg/day.

However, other factors which increase or decrease nutrient absorption can also affect the amount which needs to be consumed to meet requirements.

Nutrient absorption may be *increased* by:

(1) *Other nutrients* e.g. vitamin C intake increases the absorption of non-haem iron.
(2) *Increased physiological need* e.g. the extra need for calcium during pregnancy can usually be met by increased absorption so no *dietary* increment is necessary (see Chapter 12).
(3) *High bioavailability* Nutrients from some foods are absorbed better than others, e.g. calcium in milk is absorbed better than calcium in bread.

Nutrient absorption may be *reduced* by:

(1) *Dietary components which inhibit absorption* e.g. large amounts of insoluble fibre and other plant components, such as phytates or oxalates, may impair the absorption of some minerals and trace elements.
(2) *The presence of other nutrients which compete for the same absorption site* e.g. a high intake of iron may impair the absorption of zinc.

(3) *Lack of enzymes or reduced absorptive capacity in the gastrointestinal tract* e.g. cystic fibrosis, intestinal resection.
(4) *Lack of a second nutrient essential for absorption of the first* e.g. lack of vitamin D will impair the absorption of calcium.

■ *Factors affecting nutrient metabolism* Nutrients do not operate in isolation but as part of a complex web of interconnecting metabolic pathways. The requirement for one nutrient often depends on, or is affected by, the level of intake of another. For example, thiamin requirement (and that of many other B vitamins) depends on total energy intake; vitamin E requirement is related to the intake of polyunsaturated fatty acids.
■ *Factors affecting nutrient excretion* Any factor which alters renal function, e.g. some therapeutic drugs or renal disease, may alter nutrient excretion and so alter nutritional requirements.

Factors affecting individual requirements

In practical terms, factors which may affect individual nutrient needs are:

■ *Metabolic stress* Infection, chronic illness, injury, surgery and convalescence can greatly increase nutrient needs.
■ *Gastrointestinal illness or surgery* These may indirectly increase nutrient needs if they result in impaired nutrient absorption.
■ *Smoking* In addition to the provision of carcinogens, smoking generates the production of high levels of free radicals within the body and therefore increases requirements for antioxidant nutrients, particularly vitamin C.
■ *Use of therapeutic drugs* These can have profound effects on the absorption, utilisation and excretion of nutrients.

■ *Overall dietary balance* A varied, well-balanced diet is much less likely to have nutrient distortions or create metabolic imbalances which may increase demand for a particular nutrient.

■ *The level of physical activity* This is obviously an important determinant of energy requirements and also affects requirements for other nutrients (such as vitamins and minerals) necessary for the metabolic processes which convert food energy into muscular work.

The human organism is above all adaptable and will always attempt to adjust to conditions of surplus or deficit of a particular nutrient by altering its rates of absorption, metabolism or excretion or by mobilising nutrient stores. Ultimately though there is a limit to which it can do this and a sudden increased demand (e.g. through increased physiological or metabolic stress) or decreased availability (e.g. through impaired absorption) can transform borderline sufficiency into inadequacy.

REFERENCES

1 Department of Health (1991) *Dietary Reference Values for Food Energy and Nutrients for the United Kingdom*. Report of the COMA Panel on Dietary Reference Values. Report on Health and Social Subjects 41. HMSO, London.

FURTHER READING

Department of Health (1991) *Dietary Reference Values – A Guide*. HMSO, London.

Health Education Authority (1992) *Scientific Basis of Nutrition Education. A Synopsis of Dietary Reference Values*. HEA, London.

6

Assessing Nutritional Adequacy

There are two main ways in which nutritional adequacy can be assessed:

- *Dietary assessment* – considering whether what people eat is likely to meet their needs.
- *Assessment of nutritional status* – measuring anthropometric or biochemical markers of nutritional adequacy, surplus or deficit.

DIETARY ASSESSMENT

Dietary assessment can be done in several different ways and often more than one approach will be required to provide a broader picture:

- *The dietary record* The subject records everything consumed for a specific length of time (typically 7 days).
- *The dietary recall* The subject remembers and describes everything consumed during a previous period of time (usually 24 hours).
- *The food frequency questionnaire* The subject answers questions about how often particular foods are eaten.
- *The dietary history* By means of questioning (and sometimes food frequency questionnaires and dietary records) a pattern of typical dietary intake, either in the recent or distant past, is built up.

None of these methods is ideal; each has its advantages and disadvantages and it is important to know what these are.

The *dietary record* has the advantage of being an objective measurement at a fixed point in time and not subject to the vagueness or inaccuracy associated with memory or questioning. For this reason the 7-day weighed dietary record is usually the method of choice in dietary surveys. It is, however, only a snapshot in time and does not always give an accurate picture of habitual nutrient intake, particularly that of vitamins and minerals. Despite the advent of sophisticated electronic recording devices, weighed record-keeping is a tedious process for the subject; few people want to have to carry the recording equipment around with them or use it in public eating places. Unweighed food records, where items are described in terms of household measures, are less intrusive but also less accurate. Above all, dietary records have the disadvantage of influencing food intake itself; people may choose foods which are easiest to weigh or describe and few can resist making a few adjustments to make their diet seem more healthy or less greedy.

The *dietary recall* is less likely to suffer from this distortion because it focuses on events which have already happened. Although it is possible for people to invent their previous day's intake, in practice this tends not to happen or is readily detectable because it is surprisingly difficult to lie consistently. The recall method is limited by the fact it only assesses one day's food intake which will not be particularly representative of long-term food habits. It also requires a reasonably good memory so is often less suitable in elderly people.

The *food frequency questionnaire* cannot by itself quantify nutrient intake but it can be a useful way of identifying diets likely to be deficient in certain nutrients, e.g. a low consumption of foods providing calcium or iron. Sometimes the information is used to create an index of dietary quality, e.g. how 'healthy' a diet is. Such indexes are appealing in concept though they are fraught with pitfalls; inappropriate choice of questions will give misleading answers and some questionnaires are susceptible to manipulation – people give the answers which reflect what they feel they ought to do (e.g. 'rarely eat confectionery') rather than what they actually do ('eat some on most days').

The *dietary history* is theoretically ideal because it assesses habitual, i.e. long-term food intake, but in practice, asking people what they 'usually' eat tends to result in vague answers which are difficult to quantify; they too may also be the answers which they feel the questioner wishes to hear. Building in information from food frequency questionnaires and dietary records greatly improves the reliability of the information but this is an extremely time-consuming process.

All these methods require time and dietetic expertise in order to obtain information which is both reliable and interpreted correctly. These commodities are rarely available in the primary care setting. However, aspects of all these methods can be used by primary health care workers to identify dietary imbalances and likely nutritional problems, and to obtain background information which can then be used as a basis for giving dietary advice.

It is nearly always a mistake for the non-dietetic expert to try to calculate nutrient intake in quantified terms. Some of the recently developed user-friendly computer software has made this look deceptively simple. Such programs often generate an impressive-looking output displaying the intake of a vast array of nutrients, perhaps even as a percentage of Dietary Reference Values (DRVs). There is nothing wrong with these programs themselves; the problem is that the accuracy of the output is dependent on the accuracy of the input and the latter may be highly questionable. If the

input is simply a list of foods and drinks consumed the previous day, or even over a few days, this will be neither accurate nor typical enough to say that this represents usual nutrient intake, particularly that of vitamins and minerals (which are often the ones being assessed). As well as being inaccurate, it is also inappropriate to compare individual nutrient intakes to DRVs since these figures (which relate to populations) are not designed to be used in this way (see Chapter 5, *Assessing Nutritional Requirements*). All that is likely to be achieved by this approach is the diagnosis of 'deficiencies' which do not really exist while other genuine inadequacies or dietary imbalances may be missed.

Instead the primary care professional needs to focus on food consumption as a marker of nutrient intake rather than trying to calculate the intake itself. Many of the dietary assessment methods or a combination of them can be adapted for this purpose. The technique employed depends on what one wishes to know. These can be broadly categorised as:

- Assessing general dietary adequacy.
- Identifying dietary or food-related problems.
- Assessing the consumption of specific foods or nutrients.
- Monitoring dietary change.
- Assessing nutritional risk.

Dietary assessment in practice

Assessing general dietary adequacy

The 24-hour recall, i.e. asking someone what they ate 'yesterday', can be a useful starting point for assessing the general quality of the diet. This should be done in a way which avoids leading questions, e.g. 'What did you have for breakfast?' presupposes that breakfast was eaten; 'What was the first thing you had to eat yesterday?' may be more likely to reveal that 'breakfast' was a packet of crisps on the way to school.

This approach can reveal: (1) the usual meal pattern and (2) the types of food consumed.

(1) *The usual meal pattern* e.g. regular meals, the absence of breakfast, prolonged periods without food followed by a large meal, frequent snacking, meals eaten late at night.

The person should be asked whether this pattern is typical of the usual lifestyle. If not, further questioning can establish a more characteristic day's meal pattern.

The likely implications of this meal pattern can then be considered, e.g. late eating at night may be exacerbating heartburn; the person with diabetes will need to alter their diet in a way which avoids long periods without food.

(2) *The types of foods consumed* Important aspects of the dietary pattern to consider include:

   (a) *Are foods from all four major food groups included and in the recommended proportions?* (See Chapter 3, *Healthy Eating*.)

   i.e. *Bread, other cereals and potatoes group* (4–6 servings/day)

   Fruit and vegetables group (5 servings/day)

   Milk and dairy goods group (3 servings/day)

   Meat, fish and alternatives group (2 servings/day)

If an important component of one of these groups is absent (e.g. fresh fruit, meat or milk), gentle enquiry should establish whether this is the norm. If it is, this still may not matter if other foods are consumed which supply equivalent nutrients (see Chapter 3), e.g. a lack of milk matters less if cheese and yogurt are consumed; a lack of fruit may be adequately compensated for by consumption of a wide range of vegetables.

If an entire group is absent, or barely represented, dietary inadequacies are much more likely to exist and this needs to be explored further (see Table 6.1).

   (b) *Are many of these choices high in fat or low in nutrient quality?* For example, are potatoes frequently eaten in the form of chips; are meat products, such as sausages and beefburgers, a predominant component of the meat and alternatives group?

   (c) *Is there a high proportion of foods from the fifth food group, fatty and sugary foods?* If food intake from the above four groups seems less than adequate and a large proportion of the day's food intake can be classified as fatty and sugary foods

Table 6.1 Highlighting dietary inadequacies.

Food group lacking	Diet likely to be low in
Bread, other cereals, potatoes	Dietary fibre (particularly insoluble fibre) Carbohydrate (diet probably either low in energy or high in fat) Iron B vitamins especially thiamin, niacin, folate
Fruit and vegetables	Vitamin C Antioxidant nutrients Dietary fibre (especially soluble fibre)
Milk and dairy foods	Calcium Riboflavin
Meat, fish and alternatives	Iron Zinc Protein B vitamins Omega-3 fatty acids

then the diet is clearly imbalanced and likely to be high in energy and saturated fat.

(d) *Is there a high proportion of convenience foods in the diet?* This can also be a pointer to dietary quality. If virtually everything eaten comes out of a packet, box or can, and very few fresh or unprocessed foods are consumed, the diet is much more likely to be high in fat and sodium content and low in vitamins and minerals.

Identifying dietary or food-related problems

The dietary record/diary can be useful for dietary detective work because it provides a longer term picture of food intake than the 24-hour recall. Weighed records are usually impractical in the primary care setting but descriptive records where people keep a 'dietary diary' of food consumption have many uses. For example:

■ *To explore food intake in children*, particularly when parents report that their child 'doesn't eat'. A food record may reveal that this means the child does not eat many formal meals but consumes a significant amount of food in the form of snacks, sweets and fizzy drinks.

■ *To determine the degree of variety in a diet.* If vitamin and mineral adequacy is of concern, the degree of variety in a diet is a pointer to the likelihood of deficiencies, particularly if the balance of food groups suggests intake may be marginal. If people tend to consume the same foods every day (e.g. lunch is always a cheese sandwich; main meals always contain the same vegetables) micronutrient deficiencies are more likely.

■ *To identify more diffuse relationships between diet and symptoms*, e.g. those caused by food intolerance or factors related to irritable bowel syndrome. Occasionally an obvious dietary culprit can be identified by this means although dietetic expertise will often be needed to identify any genuine relationship (see Chapter 40, *Food Allergy and Intolerance*).

Assessing the consumption of specific foods or nutrients

Food frequency questionnaires, or modifications of them used as a basis for structured questioning, can be used as a way of assessing how often certain foods are consumed. This can be a useful approach if the level of intake of a particular nutrient is of concern, e.g. iron, calcium, zinc, omega-3 fatty acids, vitamin D or folate, particularly if these nutrients are found in foods consumed relatively infrequently, e.g. canned pilchards, liver or spinach.

Monitoring dietary change

Food frequency questionnaires are also useful in health promotion campaigns to monitor dietary change, e.g. a change in the frequency of consumption of fruit and vegetables, use of low-fat spreads, etc.

Attempting to devise an 'index' of dietary quality or healthy eating by applying a scoring system to food frequency consumption data is more hazardous[1,2]. It is surprisingly difficult to devise a system which asks the right questions and assigns an appropriate degree of weight to the answers. In particular, this approach usually fails to take account of different levels of energy intake and the fact that those who eat the most food (but not necessarily the most appropriate diet) also tend to eat more high scoring 'healthy' foods and so appear to consume the healthiest diets. Someone who consumes a lower energy intake but a better balanced diet may have a lower 'healthy eating' score.

Assessing nutritional risk

Identifying factors which may increase the likelihood of nutritional risk can also be an important part of dietary assessment. These may include:

■ *General factors which can affect food intake*
Problems with chewing
Problems with swallowing
Poor appetite
Chronic illness, particularly if gastrointestinal
Poor mobility
Poor food storage facilities

Poor cooking facilities

Low income

■ *Psychological factors which can affect food intake*

Usually eats alone

Depression

Anxiety

Low self-esteem

Recent bereavement

Dementia

■ *Factors which may indicate poor/imbalanced nutrient intake*

Fewer than two meals per day

Fewer than seven hot meals per week

Very few fresh or unprocessed foods in the diet

Lack of dietary variety

Low intake of foods from one or more of the four major food groups

Three or more drinks of beer, spirits or wine every day

Three or more prescribed drugs taken every day

Frequent use of laxatives

Recent weight loss

Recent weight gain

Lists of such indicators can be compiled as a checklist for use with different age groups (e.g. toddlers, elderly people) and can also be a useful screening tool in homogeneous groups of the population.

ASSESSMENT OF NUTRITIONAL STATUS

Nutritional adequacy or imbalance can also be indicated by various anthropometric measurements and indices.

Growth

The progression of growth is an important indicator of dietary adequacy in children. Growth failure affects both skeletal and soft tissues (i.e. height and weight) but weight is more rapidly affected by diet than height. Failure in height progression often reflects long-term nutritional inadequacy.

Growth in children can be monitored by centile charts. These have been derived from measurements derived from large populations and show the distribution of either height or weight (or in infants, head circumference) plotted by age. New Child Growth Standards were published in 1993[3,4] and should now replace the familiar Tanner/Whitehouse standards compiled in the 1950s and 1960s. The latter are out-of-date as a result of the upward shift in the average height and weight of children.

The new charts are based on nine rather than seven centile curves, with additional 0.4th and 99.6th centile lines which have been suggested to be more practical cut-off points for screening purposes than the 3rd or 97th centiles[5]. The new Child Growth Standard centile charts can be purchased at low cost from Harlow Printing Ltd (the address is given at the end of this chapter).

An isolated measurement on a centile chart does not necessarily indicate a great deal. Centile curves simply reflect the pattern of variability in normal growth and it is only a measurement which falls above the 99.6th or below the 0.4th centile which need be a matter of concern. Deviation of growth from a centile line is more indicative of nutritional problems and a growth curve which crosses a centile line between two annual measurements (e.g. crossing from the 25th to the 9th centile) warrants further investigation. A growth curve which crosses a centile line between three annual measurements is an indication for further assessment a year later and subsequent referral if necessary.

Body weight

Body weight, particularly in relation to height, can be an indicator of nutritional status. Low body weight may indicate that a person is in chronic energy deficit and possibly associated nutrient deficit, while excessive body weight usually reflects adiposity although in some cases it can be due to high muscle mass (e.g. those using body-building techniques).

Change in body weight, particularly sudden loss of weight, is a powerful indicator of either underlying illness or dietary change.

Tables giving ranges of weight according to height and, sometimes, body frame size are commonly used in the primary care setting as a way of assessing whether someone is an appropriate weight, although some of these are less useful than others. Tables presenting *average* weight for height can be misleading. These have usually been obtained from life assurance statistics, often from the USA where the population is typically heavier than in the UK. It is possible for someone to be less than average weight but still undesirably overweight. Tables of *ideal* body weight have more value. These have also been derived from morbidity/mortality statistics and show a range of weight associated with lowest morbidity and mortality for a given height.

Adiposity

Body Mass Index (BMI)

BMI is an index calculated from height and weight and is a useful indicator of body fatness. It is calculated from a person's weight (in kg) divided by the squared value of their height (in metres).

$$BMI = \frac{Weight\ (kg)}{Height^2\ (m)}$$

A chart enabling BMI to be estimated from an individual's height and weight is given in Appendix 4.

BMI range indicators are:

<20	Underweight
20–25	Normal range
25–30	Overweight
>30	Obese

There is a U-shaped relationship between BMI and mortality, with the risk rising appreciably above a BMI of about 30 (principally as a result of cardiovascular disease, stroke and diabetes) and also a BMI below 20 (which is often accompanied by neoplastic disease). Current advice is that health risk begins at BMI of 25 although to some extent this may depend on the accompanying level of exercise (see Chapter 25, *Obesity*).

BMI is not a suitable index of fatness in children as its distribution is skewed in this population as a result of the change in body shape in the childhood years. Comparison between the height and weight percentile is more indicative of an inappropriate weight for height (e.g. height on the 50th percentile and weight on the 75th).

BMI is also less useful as a measure of fatness in elderly people as reduced stature caused by bone loss and narrowing intervertebral discs can reduce the validity of the height measurement. There are also practical difficulties in measuring height in disabled or bedbound patients. The demispan (the distance between the sternal notch and the finger roots) is easier to measure and can be used to calculate a similar index to the BMI (see p. 129).

Waist-Hip Ratio (WHR)

BMI indicates the total amount of body fat but where this surplus fat is stored within the body may be more important prognostically. Fat which is stored centrally (i.e. intra-abdominally) is closely associated with problems such as coronary heart disease, stroke and diabetes, gallstones and breast cancer. Fat which is mainly stored peripherally (i.e. subcutaneously in arms and legs) is less associated with metabolic disease and more likely to lead to mechanical problems such as varicose veins and orthopaedic problems. Central obesity is more serious in terms of mortality than peripheral obesity (see Chapter 25).

Fat distribution can easily be assessed by measurement of waist and hip circumference and calculating the ratio between the two. Despite its apparent simplicity, this index has been shown to correlate closely with more sophisticated measurements of body fat distribution made by computerised tomography and magnetic resonance imaging and to have powerful predictive value[6]. This quick and non-invasive method of assessing health risk is ideally suited to primary care. The technique for measuring waist-hip ratio has been standardised by the World Health Organization[7].

$$\text{Waist-Hip Ratio} \atop \text{(WHR)} = \frac{\text{Waist circumference (cm)}}{\text{Hip circumference (cm)}}$$

Obesity accompanied by a high WHR reflects a central fat distribution and is associated with an increased risk of cardiovascular disease. Such people have been colloquially termed 'apples'. Obesity with a low WHR reflects a peripheral fat distribution. These people can be described as 'pears'. People become increasingly 'apple'-shaped with age and with increasing adiposity. Men have a higher WHR than women. A ratio which exceeds 0.9 in men or 0.85 in women is associated with increased risk of metabolic diseases (see Chapter 25, *Obesity*).

Skinfold measurements

Measurement of skinfold thickness reflects body fatness and standard tables exist for the interpretation of skinfold data but this technique is now rarely used in routine clinical work.

Bioelectrical impedance (body composition analysers)

A new technique for assessing the degree of obesity is bioelectrical impedance analysis. This measures the body's resistance or impedance to a small electrical current which can be interpreted to provide an estimate of body water, body fat and fat-free mass. Instruments which measure bioelectrical impedance have recently appeared on the market as a

way of measuring obesity. They are relatively simple to use only requiring the placement of an electrode on the right wrist and foot of a supine subject.

Body composition analysers are useful in the hospital or intensive care setting to monitor hydration status, changes in fluid balance and muscle wasting. In primary care, their use is largely confined to measuring adiposity and it is doubtful whether this method offers any advantage over cheaper alternatives such as BMI or WHR. In addition, there are risk of inaccuracies if:

- The electrodes are not placed correctly.
- The subject has oedema of the limbs or ascites.
- The subject has a full bladder or is sweating excessively.

Biochemical markers of nutritional status

Some biochemical and haematological parameters can be used as indicators of nutritional status although this is a complex subject and their use in this way requires careful interpretation. Readers are referred to other texts for more detailed discussions[8,9,10].

REFERENCES

1 Griffiths, S. *et al.* (1994) Dietary beliefs, practices and attitudes of adults in an inner city population. *Journal of Human Nutrition and Dietetics* 7, 319–34.
2 Davenport, M. *et al.* (1995) Monitoring dietary change in populations and the need for specific food targets: lessons from the North West Thames Regional Health Survey. *Journal of Human Nutrition and Dietetics* 8, 119–28.
3 Child Growth Foundation (1993) *Child Growth Standards.* Child Growth Foundation, London.
4 Freeman, J.V. *et al.* (1995) Cross sectional stature and weight reference curves for the UK, 1990. *Archives of Disease in Childhood* 73, 17–24.

5　Cole, T.J. (1994) Do growth centile charts need a face lift? *British Medical Journal* 308, 641–2.

6　Ashwell, M.A. *et al.* (1985) Obesity: new insight into anthropometric classification of fat distribution shown by computerised tomography. *British Medical Journal* 290, 1692–4.

7　World Health Organization (1989) *Measuring Obesity – Classification and Description of Anthropometric Data*. WHO, Copenhagen.

8　Thomas, B. (ed.) (1994) *Manual of Dietetic Practice*, 2nd edn. Blackwell Science, Oxford.

9　Hoffbrand, A.V. & Pettit, J.E. (1980) *Essential Haematology*. Blackwell Scientific Publications, Oxford.

10　Zilva, J.F. & Pannall, R.P. (1988) *Clinical Chemistry in Diagnosis and Treatment*. Lloyd-Luke, London.

USEFUL ADDRESSES

The new growth centile charts produced by the Child Growth Foundation may be purchased from: Harlow Printing Ltd, Maxwell Street, South Shields, Tyne & Wear NE33 4PU. Tel: 0191 455 4286.

7

Achieving Dietary Change

Persuading people to make permanent changes to their eating habits is difficult. Few people eat for the sole purpose of obtaining nutrients or only as a direct response to hunger. People eat the foods they eat for a variety of reasons – because they like them, because they are available, because they are affordable, because they are convenient, because they provide comfort, because they are given to them. Food habits are deeply ingrained in each person's way of life and changing them is disruptive and stressful.

Nevertheless for many people, dietary change is either essential or advisable and health professionals are increasingly required to help people make the necessary alterations. How they do so greatly affects the likelihood of success. Handing someone a list of dietary instructions is by itself unlikely to be enough. Effective dietary advice requires interaction between adviser and patient/client so that it can be tailored to meet individual needs and circumstances. Achieving dietary change requires more than simply manipulating nutrient intake; ways of achieving behavioural change often need to be considered as well. Good counselling skills will also be vital for success.

A number of factors have to be considered if dietary advice is likely to become dietary practice. The most important of these are discussed below.

MOTIVATION

As with any other significant lifestyle change (such as giving up smoking), people will only make changes if they are personally convinced it is necessary. Simply telling people they *ought* to change is not enough; people will only make that change when they decide for themselves that it is something they really want to do.

In terms of dietary change, motivation will be higher if it is likely to result in symptom relief or prevent the recurrence of disease or a near-fatal event, or if non-compliance has unpleasant consequences (e.g. hypoglycaemia in a diabetic patient on insulin). Motivation will be much lower in those advised to change their eating habits to prevent a disease which may or may not occur at some distant point in the future (e.g. heart disease); the theoretical rewards may seem a poor return for the practical effort involved.

KNOWLEDGE

People can only make the necessary changes if they know how to do so. Guidance must be clear and in terms the individual can understand. Health professionals often overestimate the general public's understanding of nutrition[1]. Telling someone to eat

LIVERPOOL
JOHN MOORES UNIVERSITY
AVRIL ROBARTS LRC
TEL. 0151 231 4022

'less fat' or 'more fibre' is useless if people do not know which foods contain them. Target guidelines such as 'no more than 35% of energy should come from fat' are even more meaningless. People eat food not nutrients and advice must be given in terms of what people eat, not what it contains.

REALISTIC ADVICE

It is important to start from where people are, rather than where one might wish them to be. It is pointless to expect someone who lives on chips and convenience foods to adopt the ideal healthy diet overnight. Change must be gradual and goals must be achievable, e.g. fewer chips or better choices of convenience foods rather than an outright ban. Unachievable goals are bound to lead to non-compliance. For this reason, it is vital that some assessment of what a person usually eats is made before any dietary advice is given.

POSITIVE ADVICE

Dietary advice must be as positive as possible with an emphasis on what people can eat rather than what they cannot. Many people on modified diets feel an acute sense of deprivation, particularly if they have to restrict favourite foods (e.g. cakes, biscuits). Substitution of one type of food for another (e.g. low-fat spread for butter; gluten-free bread for ordinary bread) is easier to accept than replacement with other types of foods (e.g. fruit instead of biscuits).

HELP AND SUPPORT

Significant dietary change requires continuing help and support. Good explanatory literature is often helpful but may not on its own be enough. If a diet is complicated, someone may not have fully understood what is required and may need further explanation. Questions may occur to people some time after the initial discussion. Motivation may fade and need reinforcement. Problems may arise. People should always have a contact point for further advice and many will require regular follow-up.

BARRIERS TO CHANGE

Despite motivating people, educating and supporting them there may still be barriers within individuals which prevent change. These need to be identified and overcome before progress can be made. These may be:

- Concerns about cost.
- Concerns about palatability.
- Lack of cooking skills or facilities.
- Feeling constrained or depressed by having to alter food intake.
- Disruption to the rest of the family.
- External pressures or worries distracting attention from diet.
- Family and social pressures acting against change.
- Fatalistic attitudes to health.

Barriers to change are most likely to be encountered when dietary change involves significant behavioural change (e.g. treatment of obesity) or when the benefits from change are less tangible in the immediate future (e.g. healthy eating). There are many different types of techniques which can be employed to help people identify and overcome the barriers to change and readers are referred to specialised texts for more details of these. For those working in the field of health promotion, the Proschaska and diClemente model of assessing readiness to change can be helpful[2]:

- Pre-contemplation (not even thinking about change/no interest in change).

- Contemplation (thinking about it but no change yet made).
- Decision (realisation that the benefits outweigh the drawbacks).
- Preparation (getting ready for action).
- Action (initiating change).
- Maintenance or relapse. Relapse does not mean total failure, simply that people need to return to the stage of contemplation and try again.

The importance of this model is that it accepts that there is a high probability of failure when people initially try to make a significant lifestyle change (such as altering what they eat) and that this does not mean that the idea should be abandoned but merely reconsidered and then re-applied. People may have to move through the cycle of change and relapse several times before permanent change is achieved.

Using this model for change can also result in more effective use of a health worker's time and resources. If someone is still at the pre-contemplative stage of change, there is no point in providing detailed explanations about the type of changes needed, but it may be possible to help them take a step forward into the phase of contemplation. The person who has relapsed from making change will probably need help in identifying the barriers which have made change difficult, rather than mere repetition of what those changes should be.

HEALTH PROMOTION

Much remains to be learnt about the best strategies for achieving dietary change within the population, and detailed discussion of this subject is beyond the scope of this book. In general terms, dietary education is likely to be more cost-effective if focused on a target group. For example:

- Those at highest risk of a particular disease or deficiency.

- Those who are accessible, e.g. in a particular workplace or school.
- Those whose food habits are still changing, e.g. children.
- Those who are particularly motivated to make dietary changes, e.g. pregnant women.
- Those who wish to change eating habits but lack confidence, knowledge or time.

In practical terms, strategies are likely to be more successful if they are based on participation rather than propaganda. Static posters and leaflets will never achieve as much as an interactive approach such as personal or group discussion or by showing people how changes can be achieved in practice (e.g. cookery classes, supermarket tours) rather than just telling them what to do in theory. Nor should it be forgotten that groups are always comprised of individuals with differing needs, desires, attitudes and circumstances. Ultimately a dietary message always has to have personal relevance if it is to have any impact at all.

REFERENCES

1   Rudat, K. (1992) MORI Research – Attitudes to food, health and nutrition messages among consumers and health professional. In *Making Sense of Food, Nutrition and Communication*, pp. 8–25. Ed. J. Buttriss. National Dairy Council, London.
2   Proschaska, J.O. & diClemente, C.C. (1983) Stages and processes of self-change: towards an integrative model of change. *Jounral of consulting and Clinical Psychoogy* 51, 390–95.

FURTHER READING

Proschaska, J.O. *et al.* (1994) Stages of change and decisional balance for 12 problem behaviours. *Health Psychology* 13, 39–46.
Rollnick, S. *et al.* (1993) Methods of helping patients with behaviour change. *British Medical Journal* 307, 188.
Vickery, C.E. & Hodges, P.A.M. (1986) Counselling strategies for dietary management: expanded possibilities for effective behavioural change. *Journal of the American Dietetic Association* 86, 924–8.

8

Nutritional Support and Supplementation

*NOTE: Specialist products mentioned in this chapter are included merely to illustrate the range which is currently available (in 1996). This information must **not** be regarded as sufficient for prescribing purposes. Similar products do not always have the same clinical indications and new products are constantly being marketed. Prior to their use, up-to-date guidance must be obtained from MIMS, the British National Formulary, dietitians or directly from the manufacturers.*

Although in the UK, many dietary problems result from dietary surplus, a significant proportion of the population can be considered to be seriously undernourished. Chronic illness, surgery and disability can, and often do, result in nutritional depletion because nutritional intake tends to be poor at a time when nutrient requirements are often increased. This may have important consequences. Weight loss does not only result in skeletal muscle wasting and weakness, it can also affect muscle tissue in the heart and chest, impairing cardiac function and increasing the risk of respiratory infections. It is also now well-established that there are close links between nutrition and immune function and that the body adapts to undernutrition by reducing the activity of many physiological systems including the immune system[1]. Several studies have shown that poor nutrition can impair wound healing, increase the risk of infection, delay recovery and increase the risk of mortality from unnecessary complications[2,3,4]. In an era of high-tech medicine, the importance of nutrition is often overlooked.

People in the community who are most at risk of being malnourished are:

- Those recently discharged from hospital after major surgery.
- Those who have had a prolonged stay in hospital (e.g. following hip fracture).
- Those with wasting diseases (e.g. cancer).
- Those with a poor appetite.
- Those who have problems eating (e.g. due to poor dentition) or swallowing.
- Those with malabsorptive disorders.
- Those with any chronic illness which affects dietary intake.
- Those with reduced mobility (e.g. post-hip replacement or fracture).
- Elderly people who are frail or in chronic poor health.
- People with a disability who find it difficult to obtain or prepare food.

Nutritional support is becoming increasingly common in the primary care setting, not only because of the greater recognition of the problems caused by nutritional depletion but also because the trends towards earlier discharge from hospital and the management of many chronic illnesses within the community have resulted in many people requiring nutritional support, sometimes at the level of enteral or parenteral feeding.

In anyone who is undernourished, the primary objective is to increase dietary energy intake. Some of this may need to be in the form of protein but protein supplements alone are rarely appropriate because while energy intake remains inadequate, protein will be used primarily as a fuel source rather than for tissue repair or regeneration. Adequate intakes of vitamins and minerals are also important but micronutrients do not themselves provide energy so vitamin and mineral supplements cannot alone correct undernutrition. Single supplements of vitamins or minerals should only be given when there is a clear clinical need as an unnecessary surplus of one substance can hinder the absorption or metabolism of another and so actually create a nutritional imbalance.

There are progressive levels of nutritional support, depending on clinical need and individual circumstances:

- Those requiring an increased nutrient intake from normal food.
- Those requiring nutrient supplementation in addition to normal food.
- Those requiring partial/total replacement of conventional food by enteral feeding.
- Those needing to be fed by the parenteral route.

INCREASING NUTRIENT INTAKE FROM NORMAL FOOD

Small appetite

It can be difficult to obtain sufficient energy and nutrients if appetite is poor for a prolonged period of time. Dietary measures which may improve the situation are:

- Eating smaller meals at more frequent intervals. Consuming a small meal, snack or nutrient-providing drink every 2–3 hours can significantly improve total daily food intake.
- Encouraging the use of foods which provide a lot of nutrients in a relatively small volume. These include:

- □ Full-cream milk and foods made from it (e.g. custard, milk puddings)
- □ Cheese and full-fat dairy products
- □ Meat
- □ Canned fish
- □ Well-cooked eggs.
- Making foods more energy or nutrient dense without significantly increasing their volume. For example:
  - □ Adding skimmed milk powder to milk to create a fortified milk
  - □ Adding cream, milk or skimmed milk powder to soup
  - □ Adding grated cheese to mashed potato
  - □ Adding butter to vegetables
  - □ Adding glucose powder to soft drinks (glucose is less sweet than table sugar)
  - □ Adding extra sugar, jam, honey or glucose powder to desserts and puddings
  - □ Adding evaporated milk to custard, jelly or milk puddings.
- Concentrating on foods which are particularly liked or fancied. Despite the nutritional advantages of the above suggestions, it is counterproductive to try to persuade people to eat foods which have little appeal.
- Consuming more nutrient-providing drinks, e.g. milk or fruit juice, rather than tea or squash. Powdered nutritional supplements (e.g. Build-up, Complan, Vita) may be helpful.
- Drinking minimal amounts of liquid with meals so that there is more room for food.
- Eating slowly and chewing well so that the stomach does not fill up too quickly.
- Preparing food in advance as much as possible so that appetite is not diminished by the effort of food preparation or prolonged exposure to cooking smells.
- Making use of convenience foods.

Painful or sore mouth

For those who find eating difficult as a result of a painful or sore mouth (e.g. following radiotherapy treatment) helpful advice is:

- Eat foods at moderate temperatures. Very hot or very cold foods will be more painful.
- Eat soft, moist foods, if necessary adding plenty of gravy or custard.
- Milk-based foods and drinks are often soothing.
- Avoid spicy, salty or acid foods.
- Avoid dry, rough foods such as toast, biscuits, crisps, raw apples.
- Drinking liquids may be easier through a straw.

Dry mouth

Helpful measures may include:

- Sipping drinks frequently throughout the day.
- Sucking ice cubes (these can be flavoured with fruit juices) or ice lollies.
- Sucking boiled sweets.
- Ensuring meals are moist by the use of gravy, sauces, custard, evaporated milk, etc.
- Consuming fruit juices or segments derived from grapefruit, pineapple or lemon can help stimulate saliva production.

Artificial saliva preparations are available on prescription.

NUTRIENT SUPPLEMENTATION

Sometimes the above measures are not enough, or simply impractical for those who live alone and find cooking difficult. The use of fortified drinks and sip feed supplements can be enormously beneficial in these circumstances. Supplementation can also be advisable in some people about to undergo major surgery, e.g. hip replacement in an undernourished elderly person.

Powdered nutritional supplements

These are powders which are mixed with milk or water to create a fortified drink or soup. They are not usually prescribable but are readily available in pharmacies and some supermarkets. Savoury varieties may have a high sodium content so may be unsuitable for those with hypertension or kidney/liver disease.

Non-prescribable powdered supplements

Build-up (Nestlé)
Build-up Soup (Nestlé)
Complan – original/sweetened (Heinz)
Complan – chicken (Heinz)
Vita (Boots)

Sip feeds

These usually come in a ready-to-drink form (usually in small boxed cartons with a straw) so that the contents can be sipped over a period of a few hours. Sip feeds are available in a wide variety of flavours; fruit-flavoured ones can be a refreshing change for someone tired of the taste of milky drinks.

These products are ACBS prescribable in the community for disease-related malnutrition and other conditions. Most are nutritionally complete and can, if necessary, be used as the sole source of nourishment. Some are particularly high in energy or protein which may be appropriate in some circumstances. Once opened, contents should be used within 24 hours.

Prescribable sip feeds in ready-to-drink cartons

- *Standard energy content* (1 kcal/ml)
  Ensure (Ross)
  Fresubin (Fresenius)

- *High energy content* (1.5 kcal/ml)
  Entera (Fresenius)
  Ensure Plus (Ross)
  Fortisip (Nutricia)
- *High protein*
  Fortimel (Nutricia)
  Protein Forte (Fresenius)
- *High fibre*
  Fresubin Plus F (Fresenius)
- *Non-milk tasting sip feeds*
  Enlive (Ross)
  Fortijuce (Nutricia)
  Provide (Fresenius)

Enteral feeds used as sip feeds

Some enteral feeding products can also be used as a sip feed eg:

Enrich (Ross)	Nutritionally complete, standard energy
Ensure (Ross)	Nutritionally complete, standard energy/high fibre
Peptamen (Clintec)	Elemental tube feeding product
Paediasure (Ross)	Suitable as a sip feed for children 1–6 years

---

Semi-solid supplements

In addition to drinks, fortified soups and puddings are also available. Semi-solid supplements are prescribable for many disease-related malnourished states and are particularly useful for patients with swallowing difficulties who require semi-solid food:

Formance (Ross)	A semi-solid mousse, high in energy, vitamins and minerals, nutritionally complete.
Fortipudding (Nutricia)	Semi-solid supplement in tub, high protein.
Maxisorb Dessert (SHS)	High protein powdered dessert mix.

Supplements of one or more nutrient

In some people with particularly high energy requirements or special dietetic needs (e.g. cystic fibrosis, fat malabsorption) supplementary sources of one or more nutrients may need to be provided as a way of boosting energy needs in a form which can be tolerated. Dietetic guidance is usually needed on the appropriate use and choice of these products but examples are as follows.

Carbohydrate supplements

Glucose polymers are a readily utilisable source of carbohydrate but without the sweetness of glucose so in powdered form can be added to both sweet or savoury foods. Some are available as flavoured drinks or as a liquid which can be added to drinks.

- *Powders*
  Caloreen (Clintec)
  Maxijul Super Soluble (SHS)
  Maxijul LE (SHS)   (low in electrolytes)
  Polycal (Nutricia)
  Polycose (Ross)
  Vitajoule (Vitaflo)
- *Liquids*
  Calsip (Fresenius)
  Hycal (SmithKline Beecham)
  Maxijul Liquid (SHS)
  Polycal liquid (Nutricia)

Fat supplements

For most purposes, additional energy from fat can be provided in the form of long-chain triglycerides (LCT) but those with fat malabsorption sometimes require fat in the more easily absorbed form of medium-chain triglycerides (MCT).

Calogen (SHS)	LCT fat emulsion
Liquigen (SHS)	50% MCT oil
MCT Oil (Nutricia)	MCT
MCT Oil (Bristol-Myers)	MCT

Fat and carbohydrate supplements

If protein needs to be restricted (e.g. in some forms of renal disease) energy intake may need to be increased with mixtures of fat and glucose polymers:

Duocal Super Soluble (SHS)	Powder
Duocal Liquid (SHS)	Emulsion
MCT Duocal (SHS)	Powder with most fat in the form of MCT
Duobar (SHS)	High energy bar, protein free

Protein supplements

Protein intake can be boosted with supplementary powders providing usually either calcium caseinate or milk proteins. Some products contain smaller quantities of other nutrients or are fortified with vitamins and minerals:

Casilan 90 (Crookes)	Almost exclusively protein
Forceval Protein (Unigreg)	Protein, carbohydrate, vitamins and minerals
Maxipro Super Soluble HBV (SHS)	Mainly protein, some carbohydrate and fat
Promod (Ross)	High protein, some carbohydrate and fat
Protifar (Nutricia)	Almost exclusively protein
Vitapro (Vitaflo)	Almost exclusively protein

ENTERAL FEEDING

Home enteral feeding is becoming increasing common as a result of the trend towards patients being cared for within the community rather than in the hospital setting whenever circumstances permit.

Total enteral nutrition may be necessary where there is:

- Severe anorexia (cancer, AIDS).
- Dysphagia (stroke, motor neurone disease).
- Obstruction or fistulae in the upper gastrointestinal tract.

It may also be used to supplement nutrient intake in cases of severe malabsorption, e.g. short bowel syndrome or where demand for nutrients is particularly high (e.g. cystic fibrosis).

Route of enteral feeding

Enteral feed can be delivered:

- Nasogastrically (by a fine bore tube).
- Directly into the stomach (gastrostomy feeding) or jejunum (jejunostomy feeding).

The nasogastric route is usually used for short-term feeding (for a few weeks). For longer-term feeding, gastrostomy or jejunostomy feeding are preferable because they are more socially acceptable for the patient.

Nasogastric tube feeding

Many ambulant patients can be taught to insert feeding tubes themselves and assemble their infusion for overnight administration or alternatively feed themselves by continuous infusion using a portable pump. They can thus leave hospital and resume a relatively normal life.

Overnight nasogastric feeding can be a particularly useful way of supplementing nutrient intake since it leaves the patient free from equipment during the day. In contrast to belief that it may suppress appetite, it often results in an improvement of food intake during the day.

For those needing continuous feeding, a small lightweight portable pump, such as the Kangaroo K2100 (Sherwood, Davis & Geck), can be fitted into a small back-pack which can then be worn during all normal activities either within or outside the home. This is especially useful for children who have to be enterally fed.

Percutaneous endoscopic gastrostomy (PEG) or jejunostomy feeding

PEG feeding, or a modified version of it, is becoming increasingly popular for long-term nutritional support, particularly in the home setting, as it enables people to go out or see friends without the obvious presence of a feeding tube. The procedure involves the placement of a fine bore polyurethane tube under local anaesthesia into either the duodenum or proximal jejunum.

Most of the considerations of feeding are the same as for those of nasogastric feeding but additionally some care of the stoma site is necessary to prevent tube adhesion and infection. Tube displacement and leakage from catheter junctions are the most common problems; there can also be a small risk of haemorrhage. Patients must be given advice on what to do in such circumstances.

PEG feeding may be contraindicated in patients on steroids, H_2 receptor antagonists or with diabetes because of the increased risk of infection.

Types of enteral feeds

The feeds themselves are prescribable under ACBS arrangements but the associated feeding equipment (tubes, reservoirs and pumps) is not. However, there should be local arrangements to ensure that these are available via an NHS Trust or on loan from manufacturers.

The type of feed used will depend on the patient's nutrient needs and other clinical considerations. Products vary widely in composition to suit different circumstances so one brand of product cannot simply be swapped for another. Factors which may affect feed choice are energy density, non-protein energy:nitrogen ratio, osmolality, electrolyte content, and the type of protein, fat or carbohydrate present which may be relevant to its digestibility or absorption. Some, but not all, enteral feeds are also suitable for sip feed use as well as administration by tube (see 'Sip feeds' above).

Dietetic advice on appropriate choice of feed is essential.

In the past, tube feeding has traditionally been commenced with 'starter' feeds of reduced concentration in an attempt to minimise gastrointestinal problems such as diarrhoea. Research now suggests that this is neither necessary nor beneficial, especially in those with normal gastrointestinal function, and may be unhelpful to those who are critically ill because of the reduced quantities of energy and protein delivered.

Several of the companies producing commercial feeds now offer support services for those on home enteral nutrition, for example providing literature which can be used for training or monitoring home feeding; some also organise home deliveries of supplies and hire of administration pumps.

The main types of feeds are described below.

Whole protein feeds (polymeric feeds)

- *Half-strength feeds* (for low energy requirements)
  Pre-Nutrison (Nutricia)
- *Standard strength*
  Clinifeed 400 (Clintec)
  Enrich (Ross)
  Fresubin Tube Feed (Fresenius)
  Nutrison Standard (Nutricia)
  Osmolite (Ross)
- *High fibre* (these may be more suitable for long-term feeding)
  Ensure (Ross)   1.4 g fibre/100 ml
  Fresubin Isofibre   1.5 g fibre/100 ml
    (Fresenius)
  Fresubin Plus F Muesli   1 g fibre/100 ml
    (Fresenius)
  Jevity (Ross)   1.4 g fibre/100 ml
  Nutrison Fibre (Nutricia) 1.5 g fibre/100 ml
- *High energy* (for high energy requirements or fluid restriction)
  Ensure Plus (Ross)
  Entera (Fresenius)
  Nutrison Energy Plus (Nutricia)
- *High protein*
  Protein Forte (Fresenius)   Standard energy

Clinifeed Protein-Rich   High energy
    (Clintec)
- *General paediatric feeds*
    Nutrison Paediatric Standard (1 kcal/ml)
        (Nutricia)
    Nutrison Paediatric Energy Plus (1.5 kcal/ml)
        (Nutricia)
    Paediasure (Ross)
- *Fat modified* (most/all fat in the form of MCT)
    Liquisorbon MCT (Nutricia)   Liquid
    Triosorbon (Nutricia)   Powder
    Fresubin 750 (Fresenius)   High protein,
                                      high energy

Protein hydrolysate feeds (elemental and peptide formula feeds)

These contain protein which has either been partly digested to peptides and amino acids (peptide formula) or completely hydrolysed to amino acids (elemental formula). Fat may be present as more easily absorbed medium-chain triglycerides (MCT) and carbohydrate in the form of glucose polymers. Some are also enriched with nutrients such as arginine, beta-carotene and omega-3 fatty acids which may be important for immune function. These products tend to be used in people with severe or intractable malabsorption which has not responded to other forms of feeding, or in some types of food intolerance. They are usually more expensive than other feeds and there have been problems with palatability. Some products can be taken as a drink rather than as a tube feed.

- *Semi-elemental/peptide formula*
    Flexical (Bristol Myers)   Powder
    Fresenius OPD (Fresenius)   Liquid
    Perative (Ross)   Liquid
    Pepdite 2+ (SHS)   Powder
    MCT Pepdite 2+ (SHS)   Powder,
                                      contains
                                      MCT
    Peptamen (Clintec)   Liquid, 70% fat
                                      as MCT
    Reabilin (Clintec)   Liquid
    Peptison (Nutricia)   Liquid
    Pepti 2000LF (Nutricia)   Powder/liquid,
                                      low fat

- *Elemental formula*
    Elemental 028 (SHS)   Powder
    Elemental 028   Powder/liquid, higher
        Extra (SHS)   nitrogen, fat and
                                    energy
    MCT Elemental   Powder, contains fat
        028 Extra (SHS)   as MCT
    Emsogen (SHS)   Powder, most fat as
                                MCT

Specialist feeds

Other specialist feeds are available for use in particular circumstances, e.g. advanced HIV disease, liver disease or renal failure. Dietitians will be able to advise on the appropriate use of products.

Problems with enteral feeding

The main hazards of home enteral feeding are as follows.

Regurgitation and pulmonary aspiration

This is most likely to occur in those who are highly dependent or unable to communicate rather than in ambulant patients who can manage the procedure themselves. It is important to check that the rate of infusion is appropriate for the rate of gastric emptying (by aspiration of residual gastric contents). For those who are semi-conscious or have a depressed gag reflex, the head of the bed may need to be raised during infusion.

Bacterial contamination

The risk of contamination has been greatly reduced by the now standard use of sterile commercially produced feeds rather than home-made concoctions of eggs and milk. Nevertheless there is still a risk of contamination if the sterile product has to be reconstituted, decanted or has extra nutrients added to it, or if someone's skin or clothes touch a part of the administration system which comes into contact with the feed. It is vital to avoid contamination during set-up and handling procedures and patients and carers need detailed guidance on these points. Once introduced, any contamination is potentially serious because an enteral feed is an ideal growth medium for bacteria and, once in place, the feed is likely to remain at room temperature for some hours. The newer closed integral feeding systems reduce the risk of external contamination[5,6].

Diarrhoea

Tube feeding can cause a type of diarrhoea which cannot be adequately explained by other causes such as infective agents, antibiotics or poor administration technique. It may be linked with gut motility and may be more of a problem with nasogastric feeding (where gut motility may stay in the fasted state) than with jejunostomy feeding where gut motility follows the normal pattern.

Parenteral nutrition

When it is an option, enteral nutrition is always preferable to parenteral nutrition as it stimulates normal gut function and flora production and maintains gut structure. It is also less likely to lead to complications such as thrombosis and sepsis. Administration of nutrients intravenously may be necessary when there is severe intestinal disease, e.g. short bowel syndrome, obstruction, Crohn's disease, radiation enteritis, and AIDS. Parenteral nutrition may be a temporary measure or a permanent necessity.

Patients are usually given about 2500 kcal (10.5 MJ) energy and 12 g nitrogen as crystalline amino acids in 2500 ml fluid. Energy is provided using glucose and lipid emulsion. Electrolytes, trace elements and vitamins are also added to the mixture. Parenteral feeds are usually supplied pre-mixed in sterile 3-litre bags with the patients adding vitamins and minerals just before infusion. A volume infusion pump is used to ensure a steady rate of flow.

For long-term feeding, the catheter is usually introduced into a major vein such as the subclavian with the tip being advanced to the superior vena cava. Peripheral veins can be used but these tend to thrombose, even when isotonic solutions are used. Recent developments now enable parenteral feeding catheters to be placed percutaneously.

Home parenteral nutrition is becoming increasingly common. This requires considerable commitment and motivation from patients and carers. Apart from having to master the practical aspects such aseptic techniques, there can be practical difficulties such as the size of drip stands and pumps (designed for hospital use not low-ceilinged domestic bedrooms) and the space needed for storage of bulky equipment and solutions or to accommodate necessary items such as a dressing trolley or extra refrigerator. Parenteral nutrition can also be intrusive for the patient, causing problems such as lack of sleep due to the noise of the pump at night (this can affect a partner too) or nocturnal micturition.

Good training of patients and their carers is vital. This should be started while the patient is in hospital under the auspices of a nutrition team and there should be close liaison with the primary care team which will provide home support (e.g. GPs, district nurses and pharmacists). Following discharge from hospital there should be regular follow-ups in the nutrition clinic and the patient should have telephone access to the hospital nutrition team.

Problems with parenteral feeding

Many complications can arise from parenteral feeding and close follow-up and monitoring are essential to avoid or detect these. The most likely problems are:

- *Sepsis* This can be catheter-related with bacteria gaining entry from the skin (this is less likely to happen if the catheter is placed in a skin tunnel). Sepsis is more likely to result from poor aseptic technique when changing the feed.
- *Thrombosis* This can occur at the site of catheter placement, often as a result of the high dextrose content of a feed.
- *Catheter blockage* This may be due to lipid in the feed or a blood clot.

■ *Nutrient imbalance* Electrolyte imbalance, dehydration, vitamin and mineral deficiencies and liver abnormalities can result if feed composition is inappropriate to individual needs.

REFERENCES

1 Chandra, R.K. (1981) Immunocompetence as a functional index of nutritional status. *British Medical Bulletin* **37**, 89–94.
2 Bastow, M.D. *et al.* (1983) Benefits of supplementary tube feeding after fractured neck of feeding: a randomised controlled trial. *British Medical Journal* **287**, 1589–92.
3 Reilly, J.J. *et al.* (1987) Economic impact of malnutrition: A model system for hospitalised patients. *Journal of Parenteral and Enteral Nutrition* **12**, 372–6.
4 Meguid, M.M. *et al.* (1988) IONIP, a criterion of surgical outcome and patient selection for perioperative nutritional support. *British Journal of Clinical Practice* **42**(Suppl), 8–14.
5 Rees, R.G.P. *et al.* (1988) Clinical evaluation of two-litre prepacked enteral diet delivery system: a controlled trial. *Journal of Parenteral and Enteral Nutrition* **12**, 274–77.
6 Patchell, C.J. *et al.* (1994) Bacterial contamination of enteral feeds. *Archives of Disease in Childhood* **70**, 327.

FUTHER READING

British Association for Parenteral and Enteral Nutrition (1994) *Enteral and Parenteral Nutrition in the Community*. A report by a Working Party. BAPEN, Maidenhead.
Chandra, R.K. (1992) Effect of vitamin and trace element supplementation on immune responses and infection in elderly subjects. *Lancet* **340**, 1124–7.
Garrow, J.S. (1994) Starvation in hospital. Editorial and related correspondence. *British Medical Journal* **308**, 934 & 1369.
Grant, A. & Todd, E. (1987) *Enteral and Parenteral Nutrition*, 2nd edn. Blackwell Scientific Publications, Oxford.
Hill, G.L. *et al.* (1977) Malnutrition in hospitalised patients: an unrecognised problem. *Lancet* i, 689–92.
Lennard-Jones, A. (1992) *A Positive Approach to Nutrition as a Treatment. A King's Fund Report*. King's Fund, London.
McWhirter, J.P. & Pennington, C.R. (1994) Incidence and recognition of malnutrition in hospital. *British Medical Journal* **308**, 945.
Taylor, S. & Goodinson-McLaren, S. (1993) *Nutritional Support: A Team Approach* (Clinical Skills Series). Wolfe Publishing Ltd, London.

USEFUL ADDRESSES

British Association for Parenteral and Enteral Nutrition (BAPEN), PO Box 922, Maidenhead, Berks SL6 4SH.

Further details of feeding products and equipment can be obtained from:

The Boots Co. plc, 1 Thane Road West, Nottingham NG2 3AA. Tel: 01602 492900.

Bristol-Myers Squibb Pharmaceuticals Ltd, 141–149 Staines Road, Hounslow, Middx TW3 3JA. Tel: 0181 572 7422.

Clintec Nutrition Ltd, Shaftesbury Court, 18 Chalvey Park, Slough, Berks SL1 2HT. Tel: 01753 550800.

Crookes Healthcare Ltd, PO Box 94, 1 Thane Road West, Nottingham NG2 3AA. Tel: 01602 507431.

Fresenius Ltd, 6–8 Christleton Court, Manor Park, Runcorn, Cheshire WA7 1ST. Tel: 01928 579333.

Merck Biomaterials, 47 Southgate Street, Winchester, Hampshire SO23 9EH. Tel: 01962 877407.

Nestlé *see* Clintec Nutrition Ltd.

Nutricia Clinical Care, Cow & Gate Nutricia Ltd, Whitehorse Business Park, Newmarket Avenue, Trowbridge, Wiltshire BA14 0XQ. Tel: 01225 768381.

Ross Products, a division of Abbott Laboratories Ltd, Abbott House, Norden Road, Maidenhead, Berks SL6 4XE. Tel: 01628 773355. Medical helpline: 0800 252882.

Sherwood, Davis & Geck, Cynamid House, Fareham Road, Gosport, Hampshire PO13 0BR. Tel: 01329 224114/5.

SmithKline Beecham plc, St Georges Avenue, Weybridge, Surrey KT13 0DE. Tel: 01932 822000.

Scientific Hospital Supplies Group UK Ltd (SHS), 100 Wavertree Boulevard, Wavertree Technology Park, Liverpool L7 9PT. SHS helpline/advice line: 0151 228 1992.

Unigreg Ltd, Enterprise House, 181 Garth Road, Morden, Surrey SM4 4LL. Tel: 0181 330 1421.

Vitaflo Ltd, West of Scotland Science Park, Unit 6.12, Kelvin Campus, Glasgow G20 0SP. Freephone: 0800 515174.

9

Food Composition

Most foods are mixtures of nutrients. No food provides every single nutrient which the body requires so it is necessary to eat a mixture of foods in order to meet nutrient needs. The mixture of foods eaten is 'a diet'. Whether this diet is appropriate for health depends on the mixture of nutrients provided by it.

There are two main sources of information about the nutrients present in foods:

- Food tables.
- Food and nutrition labelling.

FOOD TABLES

In the UK, the authoritative source of information on food composition is *McCance and Widdowson's The Composition of Foods* and its various supplements, produced by the Royal Society of Chemistry and the Ministry of Agriculture, Fisheries and Foods[1].

Use of food tables

Despite their accuracy, there are pitfalls associated with the use of food tables if the following aspects are not taken into account:

Not everything consumed is absorbed

Food tables will show whether a nutrient is present in food; they will not show the extent to which it is absorbed.

There is considerable variability in the absorption of nutrients, particularly micronutrients, from different foods. Some are more bioavailable than others, e.g. calcium in milk is more easily absorbed than calcium in green vegetables; haem iron in meat is more easily absorbed than non-haem iron in cereals.

The absorption of some nutrients may be affected by the presence or absence of other dietary components, e.g. phytate inhibits the absorption of zinc; vitamin C enhances the absorption of non-haem iron; calcium depends on vitamin D for its absorption.

Some nutrients may be chemically present in a food but in a form which has very little bioactivity (e.g. some folates or tocopherols). Others may be present in a bound form which makes them physiologically unavailable (e.g. calcium in spinach).

Physiological factors such as pregnancy, lactation or illness can also affect nutrient absorption.

Food tables cannot take account of any of these factors.

Variability in food composition

Figures in food tables are averages derived from analysis of a number of samples. The actual nutrient content of a particular food will be similar to the given figure but not exactly the same. Food composition can be affected by:

- The soil in which plant foods are grown (can markedly affect mineral content).
- Animal feeds (affect the fatty acid content of pork and poultry meat).
- Pasture quality (milk contains more vitamin A in summer than in winter).
- Storage conditions (vitamins can be lost through prolonged storage or exposure to light).
- Degree of ripening (as fruit ripens, its starch content falls and sugar content rises).
- Cooking method (overcooked vegetables lose much of their vitamin C content).
- Cooking practices (e.g. adding salt to water used to cook vegetables).

Food table figures may also become out of date as food composition changes, e.g. the fat content of many types of meat has fallen markedly in recent years and this will not be reflected in older food tables.

The comprehensiveness of a food table affects its accuracy. Abbreviated food tables giving typical figures for combined groups of foods such as 'meat' or 'poultry' can be misleading because the composition of individual foods or components can vary widely from this average, e.g. the fat content of poultry meat can vary four-fold depending on whether it is breast meat alone (3.6 g fat/100 g) or leg meat with skin (16.9 g fat/100 g)[1].

Contribution of a food to nutrient intake

When trying to find out which foods have a high (or perhaps low) content of a particular nutrient, it is tempting to look down the appropriate column in a food table and list the foods which fall into this category. Such a list will certainly be a guide to high (or low) nutrient content per 100 g of these foods. It will not necessarily mean that such foods are good (or poor) sources of this nutrient in a typical diet.

This problem of interpretation arises because foods are not always eaten in 100 g quantities, nor are they eaten the same number of times each day.

The contribution which a food makes to nutrient intake depends on:

- Nutrient content per 100 g (i.e. food table data).
- Quantity consumed (portion size).
- Frequency of consumption (number of portions per day/week/month).

For example, a food table will show that parsley is one of the richest sources of vitamin C in terms of vitamin C content per 100 g. But because a typical portion size of parsley is much smaller than this (perhaps 5 g) and because it is usually consumed infrequently (if at all), it makes a negligible contribution to the vitamin C intake of most people. Conversely, potatoes have a much more modest vitamin C content on a per 100 g basis but are eaten in large portions (e.g. 150 g) and often every day. Potatoes are therefore a much more important source of vitamin C in the average diet than parsley.

This is an important aspect of both dietary assessment and dietary advice. A food with only a moderate content of a nutrient (e.g. folate) but which is eaten frequently (e.g. baked beans) may be a better source of that nutrient than a food with a higher content but which is rarely eaten (e.g. spinach).

FOOD AND NUTRITION LABELLING

Food labelling

Food labels on prepackaged food always provide some information about the nature of the product. In the UK, by law a food label has to state:

What the product is (e.g. yogurt)
Relevant descriptive information (e.g. raspberry)
The ingredients and additives which it contains
Storage and usage instructions

The date by which it should be used

The country of origin (e.g. Made in UK)

The amount contained in the package (weight or volume) (The symbol **e** denotes average quantity, i.e. that individual packages may contain either slightly more or slightly less than this)

The name and address of the manufacturer, packer or seller

Any descriptive information must be accurate and not misleading, e.g. there cannot be a picture of raspberries if the product does not contain actual raspberries but only raspberry flavouring.

Claims

Some products make a nutritional claim of some kind, e.g. low sodium or reduced-fat and the definitions of all such terms are strictly set out in law and enforced by Trading Standards. The term 'reduced' means in comparison with a similar standard product, e.g. a reduced-fat sausage must contain less fat than a standard sausage. It does not necessarily mean that the resultant product contains very little of that particular nutrient (e.g. the fat content of reduced-fat sausages can still be appreciable). 'Low' means that the total amount of nutrient contained must be below a certain level. A product labelled as 'low' in a nutrient will contain less than one which is merely 'reduced'.

It is illegal to claim that a food is capable of preventing, curing or treating human disease unless the food is licensed under the Medicines Act 1968.

Ingredients

The ingredients used to make a food must be listed in descending order of quantity. Thus if water is the first ingredient listed, water is the largest component.

Ingredients lists can be helpful to some people trying to avoid particular foods or food components such as milk or wheat. However, this is not an infallible guide because some food components may be listed in a way which is not immediately obvious, e.g. milk may be described as whey, casein or lacto-globulin. Others may be described in terms which are too vague to be helpful, e.g. 'vegetable oil' may or may not contain soya. Other food components may also be present as part of compound ingredients which do not have to be separately declared (e.g. a pizza may have 'salami' as an ingredient but the individual ingredients of the salami will not be listed). For this reason, an ingredients list should not be taken as proof that a particular dietary component is absent. It can only ascertain that a particular food or food component is present.

Nutrition labelling

Providing nutrition information is at present voluntary – the manufacturer is not obliged to do this although about 75% of prepackaged food does carry nutrition information. The only exception to this is when a nutrition claim is made (see above), so a product claiming to be 'low-fat' must provide nutrition information to support this claim.

If nutrition information is given, it must be given in a prescribed format. Each one of eight specified nutrients must be given (it is not permissible to list some but not others) and they must be listed in a particular order (so fibre, for example, cannot be put at the top of the list). A manufacturer is not allowed to include any other non-specified nutrients even if this would be useful information for the consumer (e.g. *trans* fatty acid content). No visual representation, such as bar charts or diagrams, is allowed.

If nutrition information is given it must comprise:

The content per 100 g or 100 ml of the food of:

Energy (in kJ and kcal)
Protein (g)
Carbohydrate (g)
  of which sugars (g)
Fat (g)
  of which saturates (g)
Sodium (g)
Fibre (g)

Manufacturers also have the option of providing additional information on:

Starch
Polyols (e.g. sorbitol)
Monounsaturates
Polyunsaturates
Cholesterol

Vitamin or mineral content may only be given if a food is deemed to contain 'a significant amount'. This is defined as more than 15% of the Recommended Daily Amount (as defined by EC legislation) per 100 g (or per average serving) of the food. These RDAs are European standards and, confusingly, are not always the same as Dietary Reference Values (DRVs) used in the UK.

Manufacturers have the option of expressing the above information per typical portion of the food consumed but this must be in addition to, not instead of, the per 100 g/100 ml information.

Problems with nutrition labelling information

Nutrition information is expressed per 100 g or per 100 ml of the product

Nutrition information given per 100 g or per 100 ml of the food can be a useful way of comparing like with like, e.g. the fat content of different brands of beefburgers. But because most foods are not eaten in convenient 100 g portions, it is difficult to compare the composition of foods eaten in widely different quantities, e.g. a beefburger (which may weigh 60 g) and a portion of lasagne (which may weigh 300 g).

For this reason, many food producers state the nutrient content per typical serving such as per biscuit or per pie and this is much more helpful to the consumer. However, providing this information is not obligatory and manufacturers are *not* allowed to give per portion data alone. If space on the label is limited, nutrition information will have to be confined to per 100 g data.

People do not always know how to interpret the information

Most people are aware they should be eating 'less fat' or 'more fibre' but have little idea what this means in terms of amounts per day. If a food contains 11 g of fat per serving, is this a little or a lot? Many people have no idea.

It is of course impossible to specify precisely how much of a particular nutrient an individual will need because energy needs, and consequently nutrient requirements, will vary. But in the USA, food labels are allowed to indicate appropriate intakes of fat, protein and carbohydrate on a 'model' diet of 2000 calories and such a system does provide some degree of guidance. If applied to UK dietary targets (see Chapter 2), a model diet of 2000 calories expressed in nutrition labelling format would contain the intakes given in Table 9.1. These are only average targets; people eating more or less than 2000 calories will need proportionally more or less fat, carbohydrate and protein. They do, however, give people some benchmarks of what to aim for.

Different terminology used on food labels and healthy eating recommendations

Some health professionals, and well-informed consumers, can be confused by different terminology used in government healthy eating guidelines and on food labels.

In the UK, official guidance is that people should reduce their salt (sodium chloride) consumption from an average of 9 g/day to 6 g/day. Food labels express the salt content of foods in terms of sodium which is not quantitatively the same. Sodium only comprises 40% of a molecule of salt so the figure on a food label needs to be compared to a recommended maximum intake figure of 2.4 g of sodium, not 6 g of salt.

Table 9.1 Nutrient content of a 'model' diet of 2000 kcal/day.

Food label nutrients	Target intake on 'model' diet of 2000 kcal/day	
Protein	75g	(i.e. up to 15% energy)
Carbohydrate	250g	(i.e. 50% energy)
of which sugars	85g	(i.e. 17% energy*)
Fat	78g	(i.e. 35% energy)
of which saturates	24g	(i.e. 11% energy)
Fibre†	18g	
Sodium‡	2.4g	

Total sugars 'Sugars' on a food label usually means all types of sugars, i.e. intrinsic and milk sugars as well as non-milk extrinsic sugars.
†*Fibre* This figure is the requirement for non-starch polysaccharide. Some fibre figures on food labels also include resistant starch (see below).
‡*Sodium* This figure is equivalent to the target intake of 6g salt/day.

Dietary fibre is another area of confusion. Government guidelines express this as 'non-starch polysaccharide', food labels use the term 'fibre'. Nor is this just a difference in terminology. There are several different methods of fibre analysis and food manufacturers usually, and quite legitimately, use one which measures resistant starch as well as non-starch polysaccharide. This obviously gives a higher figure than a method which measures non-starch polysaccharide alone (which is why they use it). The difference can be substantial, particularly in cereal foods such as wholemeal bread or breakfast cereals which tend to contain a lot of resistant starch. These foods can therefore make it seem easy to meet the target intake of non-starch polysaccharide; in reality the true non-starch polysaccharide content will not be this high.

REFERENCES

1 *McCance and Widdowson's The Composition of Foods*, 5th edn. Ed: Holland, B. *et al.* (1991). Royal Society of Chemistry, Cambridge.
Supplements to *McCance and Widdowson's The Composition of Foods*:
Amino Acid Composition and Fatty Acid Composition, first supplement to the 4th edn. Ed: Paul, A.A. *et al.* (1980). HMSO London/Royal Society of Chemistry, Cambridge.
Immigrant Foods, second supplement to the 4th edn. Ed: Tan, S.P. *et al.* (1985). HMSO London/Royal Society of Chemistry, Cambridge.
Cereals and Cereal Products, third supplement to the 4th edn. Ed: Holland, B. *et al.* (1988). Royal Society of Chemistry, Cambridge.
Milk Products and Eggs, fourth supplement to the 4th edn. Ed: Holland, B. *et al.* (1989). Royal Society of Chemistry, Cambridge.
Vegetables, Herbs and Spices, fifth supplement to the 4th edn. Ed: Holland, B. *et al.* (1991). Royal Society of Chemistry, Cambridge.
Fruit and Nuts, first supplement to the 5th edn. Ed: Holland, B. *et al.* (1992). Royal Society of Chemistry, Cambridge.
Vegetable Dishes, second supplement to the 5th edn. Ed: Holland, B. *et al.* (1992). Royal Society of Chemistry, Cambridge.
Meat, Poultry and Game. Ed. Chan, W. *et al.* (1995). Royal Society of Chemistry, Cambridge.

FURTHER READING

British Nutrition Foundation (1993) *Nutrition Labelling*. Briefing Paper No 21. BNF, London.
Davies, J. & Dickerson, J. (1991) *Nutrient Content of Food Portions*. Royal Society of Chemistry, Cambridge.
MAFF/Crawley, H. (1994) *Food Portion Sizes*, 2nd edn. HMSO, London.
MAFF (1991) *Understanding Food Labels*. A Foodsense guide from the Food Safety Directorate. Reference no. PB0553. Available free (see Appendix 1).

10

Food Additives and Sweeteners

FOOD ADDITIVES

In recent years there has been a lot of concern among the general public about food additives, much of which is misplaced. Many people believe themselves or their children to be 'allergic' to food additives. While a few people are sensitive to particular additives, the prevalence of genuine intolerance may be as low as 0.01%, i.e. about 1 person in 10000[1,2]. The most common sensitivity is probably to the irritant effect of sulphite preservatives, particularly in some asthmatic people (see 'Asthma' in Chapter 40).

Food additives are always present in food for a good reason, either to protect it from microbial spoilage, retard rancidity, keep its structure intact or make it look and taste acceptable. Without food additives, many of the manufactured foods we take for granted (e.g. margarines and spreads) could not exist.

All food additives undergo stringent safety evaluation before being permitted for use. Those which satisfy safety criteria laid down by the European Union are given an 'E' number to denote which type of additive it is and that it has been approved for use throughout the European Union. The vast majority of the 300 or so food additives permitted for use in the UK have now been given E number status. The only exceptions are flavouring compounds which have yet to be classified because there are so many of them (about 3500). As individual flavouring compounds are used in such minute concentrations (sometimes several thousand times less than the amounts of other types of additives) and most are copies of flavours found naturally in foods, they are not thought to pose any health hazard.

Some food additives are synthetic compounds but many are found in nature and some are extracted from plant or animal material, e.g. E160 is beta-carotene, the yellow pigment in carrots and other vegetables; E162 is betanin, the purple pigment in beetroot. Some food additives are also vitamins, e.g. E306 is vitamin E; E300 is ascorbic acid (vitamin C) and E101 is riboflavin (a B group vitamin).

If an additive is added to food, its presence and function must be declared in the ingredients list on the food label. Because of the bad publicity given to E numbers, many are now declared by their chemical name rather than by their E number. As it is impractical to list flavourings separately, the presence of these in foods in indicated simply by the word 'Flavouring(s)'.

The main classifications of the E number system are as follows.

Colours (E100–E180)

Many people assume that there is no justification for adding colour additives to foods. It is true

74

that in some food products they have been used to create an unnecessary level of colour, for example there is no need for some orange drinks to be quite such a virulent orange. But without restitution of some colour, many manufactured foods (particularly margarines, fat spreads, canned fruits and vegetables) would be a dirty grey colour in appearance. Although this would not affect their taste, most of us would find it difficult to eat such foods. Visual appearance has a profound effect on taste perception; if something looks unpleasant it tends to taste unpleasant.

The food colours which have caused most concern are the yellow/red azo dyes, all of which have E numbers between E102 and E130. Tartrazine (E102) is the most reactive of these substances and can cause problems for a small number of people. There is, however, no evidence that it causes widespread hyperactivity in children (see 'Hyperactivity' in Chapter 40). Nevertheless as a result of the bad publicity given to these additives, their use in foods has been dramatically curtailed and many are being replaced by plant pigments such as annatto (E160b) or curcumin (E100) which is extracted from the spice turmeric.

Preservatives (E200–E283)

These prevent spoilage by bacteria, moulds and other organisms thus helping to reduce the risk of food poisoning and extending the storage life of foods. Food preservation has been practised for centuries by, for example, salting, smoking or adding vinegar to foods. Modern preservatives do the same job but in a way which is less intrusive in terms of flavour.

The main types of preservatives are:

Sorbates	E200–E203
Benzoates	E210–E219
Sulphur dioxide and sulphites	E220–E228
Nitrites/nitrates	E249–E252
Propionates	E280–E283

Some people are sensitive to the irritant effects of sulphur dioxide (present either in its own right or liberated from sulphite additives).

Antioxidants (E300–E322)

These may be added to fats and oils to prevent rancidity. They should not be confused with dietary antioxidants necessary to prevent peroxidation in cellular tissues (see p. 29), although the processes of rancidity and peroxidation are very similar and some antioxidant additives are in fact antioxidant nutrients. Antioxidant additives include:

Ascorbic acid (vitamin C) and ascorbates	E300–E304
Tocopherols (vitamin E) and derivatives	E306–E309
Gallates	E310–E312
Butylated hydroxyanisole (BHA)	E320
Butylated hydroxytoluene (BHT)	E321
Lecithins	E322

BHA and BHT are not permitted for use in foods produced specifically for children.

Lecithins can be derived from egg or soya which may be relevant to those who are allergic to these foods (see Chapter 40, *Food Allergy and Intolerance*).

Emulsifiers and stabilisers (E400–E499)

These influence the texture of a food and the stability of its structure, e.g. they prevent the separation of oil-based and water-based ingredients.

Alginates	E400–E405
Agar	E406

Carrageenan	E407
Gums (e.g. locust bean, guar)	E410–E415
Pectins	E440
Celluloses	E460–E466
Fatty acid derivatives	E470–E483

Few problems have been associated with the use of emulsifiers and stabilisers. However, many of those which are fatty acid derivatives are extracted from animal fats so foods containing them may be avoided by strict vegetarians and vegans (see Chapter 21). In practice, this means the exclusion of a considerable number of manufactured foods.

Other functions

Other additives (usually with E numbers in the 300s or 500s) may be used to perform a variety of functions such as regulating acidity, holding moisture, preventing a food sticking to its wrapping or acting as a propellant. None of these is known to cause specific problems.

SWEETENERS

Most sweeteners are also food additives and, if added to manufactured foods, their presence must be declared on food labels. However, unlike other additives, sweeteners can also be regarded as food products because the consumer can use them directly as a sugar-substitute in foods. It is in this context that they are considered here.

Sugar-substitute sweeteners can be divided into two types: those which have no significant nutritional value (non-nutritive or intense sweeteners) and those which do provide energy (nutritive or bulk sweeteners).

Non-nutritive sweeteners
(intense sweeteners)

These compounds are all intensely sweet and so are only required in minute amounts to provide the equivalent sweetness of sugar. They are widely used in low sugar or low energy products (e.g. 'diet' drinks or yogurts) and are available as table-top sweeteners in either liquid or tablet form.

Those which are most commonly used are:

Saccharine
Aspartame
Acesulfame-K

These are often used in combination in order to give the best flavour balance. Other compounds such as neohesperidine, dihydrochalcone and thaumatin are also used by the food industry and cyclamate was added to the list of permitted sweeteners in January 1996.

- *Saccharine* This is a synthetic substance 300–500 times sweeter than sugar. It has a pronounced aftertaste and becomes very bitter on heating so cannot be added to something before it is cooked, only afterwards when the food is cool.
- *Aspartame* This is derived from two amino acids and is about 160 times sweeter than sugar. It has the closest taste to sugar but is unstable to heat and warm storage conditions. It is metabolised to the amino acid phenylalanine so is contraindicated in those with phenylketonuria.
- *Acesulfame-K* This is a synthetic substance 130–200 times sweeter than sucrose. It is an organic salt which is not digested. It has a synergistic effect with other sweeteners and is often used in combination with aspartame and saccharine. It is the most stable of all the intense sweeteners and less likely to decompose on heating but does have a slight aftertaste.

All intense sweeteners are calorie-free and a useful alternative to sugar in drinks and to sweeten cold or precooked foods, particularly for people with diabetes. People on weight-reducing diets may also find them helpful but the benefit in terms of calorie intake should not be overestimated. The energy saving from a cup of coffee with a sweetener instead of two teaspoons of sugar is only 40 kcal. Intense sweeteners do not provide the bulk or properties of sugar so cannot be used for baking (e.g. to make cakes).

No intense sweetener may be used in foods specially prepared for babies or young children.

Nutritive sweeteners
(bulk sweeteners)

These comprise:

- Polyols
  - Sorbitol
  - Lactitol
  - Maltitol
  - Xylitol
  - Mannitol
  - Isomalt
- Fructose
- Hydrogenated glucose syrup

Unlike intense sweeteners, these provide bulk and some of the technical properties of sugar so can be used in baked products. However, most also have an appreciable energy content, and there are a number of other disadvantages which limit their usefulness.

- *Polyols* These are sugar alcohols, i.e. not true sugars but related to them. Polyols have a lower energy content than sucrose (2.4 kcal/g versus 4 kcal/g) but are also less sweet, so need to be consumed in larger quantities for equivalent sweetness. This obviously negates any advantage in terms of energy reduction and makes

them unsuitable as a sugar substitute for those who are overweight.

The main disadvantage of polyols is that they are poorly absorbed and can cause osmotic diarrhoea. Some people, especially children, are very sensitive to this effect. For this reason, the maximum recommended intake is 50 g total polyols/day.

Because polyols have little direct effect on blood glucose or insulin levels, they have in the past been used as an alternative to sucrose by people with diabetes and in diabetic foods. This is now considered to be of little benefit and because of their attendant disadvantages in terms of energy content and side effects polyols, or products containing them, are no longer recommended for use by diabetic patients (see Chapter 27).

Most polyols are non-cariogenic and isomalt, xylitol and maltitol are often used as a constituent of sugar-free chewing gums and sweets.

- *Fructose* Fructose is not, in legislative terms, a 'sweetener' because it is an ordinary carbohydrate (and one of the two constituents of the sucrose molecule). It is slightly sweeter than sucrose and, because its metabolism is not dependent on insulin, it has been used as an alternative sweetener by people with diabetes. However, as with polyols, this is no longer recommended (see Chapter 27).

  Because it is an ordinary carbohydrate, fructose has the same energy content as any other sugar (4 kcal/g) so offers no advantage to those who are overweight.

  Large amounts of fructose do have the capacity to cause osmotic diarrhoea in some people, especially children.

- *Hydrogenated glucose syrup* This is a commercially-used sweetener comprised of modified glucose units which are broken down in the gut to sorbitol and glucose. It is less cariogenic than sucrose but also less sweet. It has the same energy content. It offers no advantage to slimmers or people with diabetes.

Sugar substitutes

These are combinations of ordinary table sugar mixed with one or more intense sweeteners such as aspartame and acesulfame-K. They are promoted for use on cereals, in drinks and cold desserts. Most are unsuitable for baking. In terms of a teaspoon of sugar, they offer a calorie saving of between 50 and 90% but in practice this will only represent a small daily energy saving (the energy contribution from sugar added to drinks is, in terms of total energy intake, normally quite small). Use of intense sweeteners alone, or simply not adding any sugar at all, are better alternatives for those who are overweight. Sugar substitutes are unsuitable for people with diabetes.

REFERENCES

1 Young, E. *et al.* (1987) The prevalence of reactions to food additives in a survey population. *Journal of the Royal College of Physicians* 21, 241–7.
2 Young, E. *et al.* (1994) A population study of food intolerance. *Lancet* 343, 1127–30.

FURTHER READING

Hanssen, M. (1987) *E for Additives*. Thorsons, Northamptomshire.
MAFF (1991) *About Food Additives*. A Foodsense guide from the Food Safety Directorate. Reference no. PB0552. Available free (see Appendix 1).

11

Food Safety

Food poisoning is a serious health concern because it can have fatal consequences in vulnerable groups and its prevalence has risen considerably in recent years[1,2]. Many of these cases result from incorrect preparation or storage of food within the home.

Food poisoning may be caused by bacteria, bacterial toxins, viruses, mycotoxins from moulds and fungi, chemical toxins (e.g. undercooked kidney beans) and protozoa. These often result in gastrointestinal illness but this is not always the case. The main types of symptoms and some of their causes are:

- *Gastrointestinal symptoms:*
  Salmonella
  Campylobacter
  Staphylococci (e.g. *Staph. aureus*)
  Escherichia coli (the rare variant *E. coli 0157*, occasionally present in undercooked red meat, can have fatal consequences due to internal bleeding and renal damage)
  Clostridium perfringens
  Shigella
  Enteroviruses, rotaviruses, parvoviruses
- *Flu-like symptoms:*
  Listeria (symptoms can progress to meningitis and septicaemia and also cause brain damage in an unborn child)
  Toxoplasmosis
- *Neurological symptoms:*

  Clostridium botulinum (extremely rare but can cause paralysis of respiratory and other muscles with fatal consequences)
  Neurotoxins present in some types of raw beans

Types of food poisoning which are of greatest concern are considered below.

Salmonellosis

Salmonella poisoning is of concern because its prevalence is rising and new strains of salmonella are appearing, some of them antibiotic resistant. Salmonellosis is a notifiable disease in Europe and North America. The symptoms usually occur 12–36 hours after infection and include severe abdominal pain, diarrhoea and fever, sometimes accompanied by nausea and vomiting. Its consequences may be fatal in vulnerable groups such as young children or elderly people.

There are about 700 different types of salmonella bacteria found in animals and birds but the main source of infection in man is from *Salmonella enteritidis* phage type 4, present in raw or undercooked poultry and eggs. Despite stringent measures to reduce the prevalence of the organism in poultry flocks, a 1991 survey found that 1 in 880 British eggs on sale to the public was contaminated with *Salmonella enteritidis*[3]. Although this is a small percentage, when it is considered that several million eggs are sold every day, it still represents a considerable risk of infection if those which are contaminated are eaten raw or lightly cooked.

Most cases of salmonella poisoning are avoidable if recommended guidance on the safe storage, handling and cooking of food is observed.

Campylobacter infection

This usually causes severe diarrhoea which can be bloodstained, together with milder nausea, vomiting and fever. The symptoms usually appear within 16–18 hours of infection. The organism can be present in raw meat and poultry and also unpasteurised milk. A major source of infection is from household pets; 50% of dogs and cats excrete campylobacter in their faeces and, if their fur becomes contaminated, the organism can be passed to humans when the animal is stroked.

Listeriosis

Listeriosis is less common than other types of food poisoning but its consequences in pregnant women can be devastating. It typically causes flu-like symptoms rather than vomiting or diarrhoea, and results from infection with *Listeria monocytogenes*. This is an unusual organism because it has the ability to multiply rapidly at refrigeration temperatures. The rise in listeriosis during the 1980s arose partly from the increasing use of cook–chill foods and ready meals which were then inadequately reheated (which destroys the organism) or from pre-prepared foods which are eaten cold (e.g. paté, pre-packed salads). Unpasteurised milk and products made from it, such as mould-ripened or blue-veined cheeses, can also be a significant source. Listeriosis is a considerable hazard in those who are pregnant because it is likely to

cause spontaneous abortion or mental retardation in the fetus. It can also have serious consequences in young infants, elderly people and those with suppressed immune systems.

Staphylococcal infection

Symptoms usually appear fairly rapidly after infection (within 1–6 hours) and are usually those of profuse vomiting, sometimes with later diarrhoea. It nearly always results from human contamination as a result of poor food handling procedures and is most likely to occur from eating cold foods prepared in advance, e.g. cream filled cakes, potato salad or sandwiches. Alternatively, staphylococci may contaminate and incubate in cooked food left in a warm place (particularly soups, gravies and casseroles). Subsequent reheating may not render it safe. Unlike many other forms of food poisoning, staphylococcal-related symptoms are caused by bacterial toxins rather than the organisms themselves. These toxins are not destroyed by heat.

FOOD SAFETY GUIDANCE

The vast majority of cases of food poisoning could be prevented if correct food storage and handling procedures were observed.

■ *General principles*
  □ Protect food from contamination.
  □ Use it within a safe period.
  □ If food needs to be cooked, cook it thoroughly.
  □ Keep food cold or hot, not 'warm'.
■ *Buying food*
  □ Buy food from hygienic, reputable outlets.
  □ Check that the 'Use by' date is still valid.

- Avoid food with damaged packaging or in badly dented cans.
- Avoid dirty or cracked eggs.
- Take chilled or frozen food home as soon as possible. Use an insulated bag or box in hot weather.
- **Food preparation**
  - Keep kitchen surfaces clean.
  - Wash hands thoroughly before handling food.
  - Wash hands, chopping boards and utensils after preparing raw meat.
  - Use clean tea towels and wiping cloths.
  - Keep pets away from food or kitchen surfaces.
  - Keep pets' feeding dishes separate from those used by the household.
  - Use rubber gloves to handle cat litter trays.
- **Food storage**
  - Keep the fridge clean and free from drips, spills and decaying bits of vegetable matter.
  - Keep different types of foods, e.g. vegetables, raw meat, cooked foods, dairy products, separate from each other.
  - In the fridge, store cooked or pre-prepared foods above raw meats and vegetables.
  - Ensure that the juices from raw meat or defrosting foods cannot drip on to other foods.
  - Use a thermometer to check that the fridge is below 5°C and the freezer below −18°C.
  - Never refreeze thawed food.
  - Buy fresh eggs in small quantities at a time and keep in the fridge.
  - Do not eat food after the 'Use by' date*.
  - Eat opened jars, vacuum packs or cartons within the recommended times.

*Foods which deteriorate quickly (e.g. chilled convenience foods, packaged ham) will have a 'Use by' date. After this date the food should be regarded as unfit to eat. Foods which last longer (e.g. biscuits, breakfast cereals) have a 'Best before' date. After this date, the food may not be harmful but its flavour and texture will begin to deteriorate.

- **Food cooking**
  - Defrost poultry or meat thoroughly before cooking.
  - Check that poultry or large joints of meat are cooked right through (use a meat thermometer or pierce the thickest part with a skewer – the juices should run clear).
  - Follow manufacturer's instructions for the reheating of precooked chilled or frozen foods (e.g. pies, flans, ready meals). Ensure they are piping hot before being consumed.
  - Observe standing time for microwaved food to ensure the heat distribution is even.
  - Cook eggs until the yolk is set; never use raw egg in mayonnaises or desserts.
  - Cooked food should not be left for more than 1 hour before being refrigerated or frozen.
  - Do not reheat food more than once.
  - Never keep cooked food in the fridge for more than 1–2 days before it is eaten.

REFERENCES
1 Richmond, M. (1990) *Microbiological Safety of Food*. Part 1. Report of the Committee on the Microbiological Safety of Food (The Richmond report). HMSO, London.
2 Richmond, M. (1991) *Microbiological Safety of Food*. Part 2. Report of the Committee on the Microbiological Safety of Food (The Richmond report). HMSO, London.
3 Advisory Committee on the Microbiological Safety of Food (1993) *Report on Salmonella in Eggs*. HMSO, London.

FURTHER READING
MAFF (1991) *Food Safety*. A Foodsense guide from the Food Safety Directorate. Reference no. PB0551. Available free (see Appendix 1).

PART 2

Diet and People

12

Pregnancy

Dietary advice for pregnant women has changed considerably in recent years as the relationship between maternal nutrition and fetal health has become more clearly understood. In the past dietary guidance has focused mainly on the need to protect the mother from the nutritional costs of pregnancy, particularly in the later stages. It is now known that dietary factors can also affect the fetus, particularly in the very earliest stages of pregnancy, possibly even before it commences. There is also growing evidence that nutritional influences during fetal life may have long-lasting consequences in terms of health in later adult life[1,2].

The implications of nutrition on fetal and maternal health change as pregnancy progresses. Prior to the formation of the placenta, an embryo is directly exposed to the maternal blood circulation and hence can be influenced by an excess or deficiency of nutrients or by the presence of any other toxic or teratogenic substances. As the placenta develops, it has an increasing ability to prevent potentially harmful substances reaching the embryo, but until this protective mechanism is in place, the developing embryo is very vulnerable to external influences, including dietary ones.

As pregnancy progresses, the nutritional needs of the fetus take increasing priority over those of the mother. In the early weeks, a number of adaptive mechanisms occur in the mother to help meet the fetal demand for nutrients – maternal absorption of vitamins and minerals is increased and their excretion reduced, protein and energy metabolism become more efficient and nutrient stores are mobilised. By about 20 weeks, the demand for extra nutrients is high but the placenta has also become increasingly adept at extracting the required nutrients from the maternal circulation; at this stage it is the mother, rather than the fetus, who will suffer from any dietary inadequacies.

NUTRITIONAL CONSIDERATIONS

Traditionally, nutrient requirements for pregnancy have been based on the calculated nutritional cost of pregnancy resulting from the creation of new tissues. It is now realised that these apparent needs are not necessarily true physiological needs because of the sophisticated adaptive mechanisms which the body employs to maximise its nutritional resources.

For this reason, the Reference Nutrient Intakes (RNIs) given for pregnancy can at first appear to be puzzling because there is no recommended increase in the consumption of minerals such as calcium and iron despite the high demand for them during pregnancy. In contrast, increased intakes of nutrients such as thiamin, riboflavin and vitamin A are recommended even though dietary deficiencies of these nutrients are not generally thought to be a problem and, in the case of vitamin A, excessive intake may even be hazardous. The reason for these apparent anomalies is that the RNIs are not stating the increased nutrient requirements for pregnancy *per se*, but only the increased requirements which cannot be met by biological adaptation during pregnancy. In addition, RNI figures are the amounts deemed to be sufficient for the population as a whole; most individuals within this population will actually need far less (see Chapter 5, *Assessing Nutritional Requirements*).

RNI figures therefore reflect the nutrient needs of pregnant women in general; they cannot be applied to every individual pregnant woman because individual nutrient needs will vary. What matters in the individual is whether the diet being consumed has any obvious imbalances or deficiencies and hence is less likely to meet the probable nutrient needs.

Energy

The theoretical energy cost of a pregnancy is about 60000 kcal (about an extra 200 kcal/day) but few women need to increase their energy intake by this amount, nor for the whole of their pregnancy. In early pregnancy, energy requirements do not increase at all and when they do rise tend to be offset by reduced activity and adaptive changes in energy metabolism. Dietary Reference Values (DRVs) suggest that on average, pregnant women require an additional 200 kcal/day in the last trimester of pregnancy only. In practice the metabolic and behavioural response to pregnancy is so variable that energy requirements cannot be predicted in an individual at all.

Rather than attempting to quantify energy requirements in terms of calories, individual energy needs can best be gauged by body weight and weight gain. Someone who is underweight at the start of pregnancy may well have low nutrient reserves and so an increased food and energy intake may be advisable. In someone of normal weight, the need for additional energy is likely to be much less. In those who are overweight or obese, energy intake rarely needs to be increased at all and it is dietary quality which needs to be addressed.

Table 12.1 Desirable weight gain targets during pregnancy.

Pre-pregnancy weight	Desirable weight gain
Normal weight	9 kg
Overweight	7.5 kg
Underweight	13.5 kg

The degree of weight gain is important because it can affect both maternal and fetal health. Excessive weight gain increases the risk of pre-eclampsia and gestational diabetes and also the likelihood of maternal obesity if the excess fat stores are not lost after the baby is born. Poor weight gain, particularly in someone who is underweight at the start of pregnancy, is more likely to result in an infant of low birthweight and further depletion of maternal nutrient stores.

On average a pregnant woman gains 10–12 kg during pregnancy but a uniform figure for recommended weight gain is no longer thought to be appropriate. Those who are underweight at the start of pregnancy should gain more than average while those who are obese should gain less. Desirable weight gain targets are shown in Table 12.1.

Those who gain weight very rapidly, or commence pregnancy at an excessive weight, should not go on a strict diet because this inevitably restricts the intake of essential micronutrients. Instead people should adjust the proportions of foods obtained from the different food groups – fewer fatty and sugary foods but more from other groups, particularly fruit and vegetables.

Protein

There is an increased requirement for protein during pregnancy as a result of the creation of new tissues. However, in this country it is rarely necessary for a pregnant woman to consume extra protein since average intakes are usually well above the likely requirements. People who may have in-adequate protein intakes are:

- Vegans who do not obtain an appropriate mix-ture of amino acids (see Chapter 21).
- Those on diets of low nutrient quality (e.g. women living in deprived socioeconomic circumstances).

Folate

Folic acid is essential for cell division and is an important nutrient throughout pregnancy. Chronic folate deficiency in pregnancy results in megaloblastic anaemia and supplementation to prevent this remains an important preventative measure.

More recently it has been established that folate may be of crucial importance in early pregnancy. An inadequate supply of folate at the the time of neural tube closure (about 28 days after con-ception) has been shown to increase the risk of neural tube defects (NTD) such as spina bifida, and folate supplementation has been shown to result in a dramatic fall in the incidence of NTD recurrence[3,4].

As a result of these findings, an Expert Advisory Group from the Department of Health has issued recommendations on folate intake and pregnancy[5]. Because folate exerts its crucial influence at such an early stage of pregnancy, the need for additional folate may occur before a woman realises she is pregnant. The Expert Group therefore advises that all women who are, or are *intending to become* preg-nant, should consume an appropriate intake of folate. Since many pregnancies are unplanned (and such pregnancies are even less likely to be diag-nosed at an early stage) some health professionals feel that all sexually active women of child-bearing age should take steps to ensure they consume suffi-cient folate.

Parents who have already had one child with NTD, or if either one themselves had a NTD, have a 10-fold increase in the risk of having a second affected child. Women in this group are recom-mended to take a much higher level of folate sup-plementation, based on the amount shown to be protective in clinical trials.

The recommended levels of folate supplementa-tion are:

- *Women with no history of NTD* should con-sume an additional $400\,\mu g$ (0.4 mg) folate/day either in the form of folate-rich foods or a sup-plement. Ideally this should commence before conception and be continued for the first 12 weeks of pregnancy.
- *Women with a history of NTD* should be pre-scribed a 5 mg supplement of folate, ideally be-fore conception and continued for the first 12 weeks of pregnancy. This level of supplemen-tation is not recommended for all women be-cause of the rare but serious complications which may occur in those who are either B_{12} deficient (where high doses of folic acid may precipitate sub-acute combined degeneration of the spinal cord) or on anticonvulsant therapy (where high doses of folic acid may interfere with drug control).

The current average dietary intake of folate is about $200\,\mu g$ (0.2 mg)/day[6]. The recommendation to consume an additional $400\,\mu g$/day (i.e. $600\,\mu g$ in total) means that the usual dietary intake of folate has to be trebled. While in theory it is possible to achieve this by eating more folate-containing foods (green leafy vegetables, beans, pulses, fortified bread and breakfast cereals and some fruits) in practice this is not easy. Folate-rich foods are not always popular or consumed very frequently and, since folate is easily destroyed by heating, it is also questionable how much folate remains in foods such as well-boiled green vegeta-bles by the time they reach a dinner plate. In women who eat a well-balanced healthy diet, particularly one containing fortified cereal foods, folate intake may be adequate. For most women, folate supplements are a sensible precaution.

If supplements are used, it is important that preparations containing an appropriate dose of folic acid are used. Some multivitamin supplements have a low folate content and there are considerable dangers from overdosage of other vitamins if several tablets are taken in order to obtain the required amount of folate.

Recent surveys suggests there is still poor awareness among women of the importance of folate in early pregnancy[7,8]. Most either fail to increase folate intake at all or do so at a stage when it is too late to be protective. Preconception advice clinics have an important educational role but these will not reach people who have an unplanned pregnancy. A government-funded campaign to heighten awareness was started at the beginning of 1996.

It is important to realise that folate supplementation will not prevent *all* cases of NTD occurrence or recurrence. Supplementation trials suggest that it fails to protect a small proportion of women, possibly those with an inborn defect of folic acid metabolism.

Iron

Extra iron is required in pregnancy for expansion of red cell mass, development of the fetus and placenta and as a reserve for blood loss during delivery. However, in normal circumstances these needs can be met from increased intestinal absorption, reduced iron losses due to cessation of menstruation and mobilisation of maternal iron stores and so no dietary increase is necessary.

For this and other reasons, the need for routine iron supplementation during pregnancy has been questioned. The assumption that additional iron is necessary has largely arisen because of the observed fall in haemoglobin level which occurs as pregnancy progresses. However, in most cases this is not anaemia (when there will also be a reduction in red cell size) but simply a dilution effect resulting from the plasma volume expanding more than the red cell mass. Unnecessary iron supplementation may be unwise as, apart from causing gastrointestinal side effects, it can impair the absorption of other vital minerals, particularly zinc.

Nevertheless, iron status is an important aspect to consider in someone who is pregnant. The increased needs for iron can only be met in conditions of iron sufficiency; a person who starts pregnancy with a low iron intake and inadequate iron stores may well be unable to meet these needs. Genuine anaemia can impair fetal growth and increase the risk of low birthweight and premature delivery as well as resulting in chronic ill-health for the mother. People who are most likely to have low iron stores and hence need either dietary guidance or iron supplementation are those with:

- Chronic low dietary intake of iron (see p. 25).
- Haemoglobin level <12g/dl in *early* pregnancy.
- Serum ferritin level below 25 μg/l at the start of pregnancy.
- History of anaemia.
- History of heavy menstrual blood loss.
- Short interval since a previous pregnancy.
- High parity.
- Multiple pregnancy.
- Clinical factors affecting iron absorption (e.g. malabsorptive states).

Calcium

Calcium requirements double during pregnancy, and are particularly high in the last 10 weeks when calcium is being laid down in the fetal skeleton. Surprisingly though, no dietary increase is thought necessary because of the adaptive changes which occur in calcium absorption and metabolism. Nevertheless, as in the case with iron, the increased needs can only be met if calcium intake and calcium stores are sufficient in the first place; those in whom these may be inadequate are:

- Those who consume little or no milk or dairy products.
- Teenage mothers who are themselves still laying down calcium.

Vitamin D

Vitamin D requirements are normally met from skin synthesis following exposure to sunlight. In pregnancy, this source may not be adequate to meet the increased needs and hence ensure adequate absorption of calcium. Since vitamin D is not widely present in foods, a supplement of $10\,\mu g$/day is recommended. This is particularly important for women with least exposure to sunlight, e.g. Asian mothers and women living in northern Britain.

Vitamin C

Intake should be increased in order to help increase the absorption of non-haem iron.

OTHER DIETARY ASPECTS

Alcohol

Excessive alcohol consumption is hazardous at any stage of pregnancy and alcohol abuse can result in fetal alcohol syndrome characterised by mental and physical retardation. However, whether there is any hazard from 'sensible' drinking is less clear. The most likely period of risk is in the early stages of pregnancy and it is probably wise to avoid alcohol completely throughout the first trimester. However once embryogenesis is complete, there is no evidence that the occasional drink causes any harm.

Vitamin A

Vitamin A is an important nutrient during pregnancy but excessive intakes are known to cause foetal abnormalities in experimental animals. The dose response effect in humans is less certain but there is some evidence that intakes in excess of $6000\,\mu g$/day may increase the risk of deformities[9]. In recent years it has become apparent that liver and foods made from it, such as paté, contain extremely high quantities of vitamin A, over twice as much as that indicated in official food tables. This is thought to result from the high content of vitamin A in animal feedstuffs which then becomes concentrated in animal liver. Liver has in the past often been recommended to pregnant women because it is a good source of iron; current government advice is that it should be avoided completely[10].

Vitamin A supplements (or multivitamin supplements containing it) should also not be taken during pregnancy, especially during the early stages, unless this is medically indicated. Sufficient vitamin A to meet the needs of pregnancy can be obtained from a normal healthy diet which contains foods such as margarine, dairy foods, vegetables and fruit.

Food hygiene

In pregnancy there are particular risks from certain food-borne infections:

- Listeriosis.
- Salmonellosis.
- Toxoplasmosis.

Listeriosis
Listeriosis, caused by the bacterium *Listeria monocytogenes*, can result in miscarriage or still-birth, and pregnant women are advised to avoid

foods which are the most likely source of listeria organisms. These are:

Unpasteurised milk (from cows, goats or sheep)
Cheeses made from unpasteurised milk (typically fermented or cultured cheeses such as Brie, Camembert or blue-veined varieties)
Paté.

Precooked foods such as flans, pies and ready meals can also be a source of listeria if they are not thoroughly reheated before being consumed.

Salmonellosis

Salmonella infection can result in severe gastroenteritis. The most likely source of salmonella is raw egg consumed either via home-made mayonnaise or desserts. Pregnant women should ensure any eggs they buy are fresh, stored in the fridge and cooked thoroughly (until the yolk is set) before being consumed.

Toxoplasmosis

This is an infection resulting from a parasite found in cats' faeces, soil, raw meat and unpasteurised milk. In pregnancy it can result in severe fetal abnormalities including mental retardation and blindness. Preventative measures are largely those of good food hygiene concerning the safe handling, storage and prevention of contamination of food (see Chapter 11, *Food Safety*).

DIETARY GUIDANCE FOR PREGNANCY

Pre-conception

- Think carefully about diet and start to make healthy eating changes.
- Increase folic acid intake either by a daily supplement of 400 μg (0.4mg/day) or by increasing the consumption of folate-rich foods, especially fortified bread and breakfast cereals.

- If overweight, reduce the consumption of fatty and sugary foods and eat more foods from the fruit/vegetables and bread/cereals groups.
- If underweight, ensure that the diet is of good nutritional quality by consuming a variety of foods from all four major food groups.
- Avoid liver and all products made from it.
- Avoid excessive amounts of alcohol.
- Address other lifestyle factors (e.g. stop smoking, take more exercise).

Pregnancy
General measures throughout pregnancy

- Eat a varied balanced diet based on healthy eating guidelines.
- Eat regular meals including breakfast.
- Eat to appetite unless excessive weight gain starts to occur; if it does, reduce consumption of fatty and sugary foods.
- Avoid liver and products containing it.
- Avoid excessive amounts of alcohol.
- Observe strict food hygiene.
- Vitamin D supplements are advisable for those exposed to little sunlight.

Additional advice during various stages of pregnancy
First trimester

- Continue to take folate supplements until the twelfth week of pregnancy.
- If the quantity of food consumed is reduced as a result of nausea or sickness, ensure that the foods which are consumed are of good nutritional quality.
- Avoid rapid weight gain at this stage.
- Avoidance of alcohol is probably wise.

Second and third trimesters

- Maintain a diet of high nutrient quality (particularly in respect of iron, calcium, folate, vitamin D and vitamin C) by ensuring the diet contains an appropriate balance of foods from the four main food groups (see Table 12.2).
- Excessive weight gain should be curtailed only by restriction of fatty and sugary foods, not those from the groups in Table 12.2.

Table 12.2 An appropriate balance of foods for the second and third trimesters of pregnancy.

Food group	Servings per day
Bread, cereals, rice, pasta and potatoes	4–6
Fruit and vegetables	5
Milk and dairy products	2–3
Meat, fish, eggs, pulses	2

■ If constipation is a problem, intake of fluid and insoluble fibre (wholegrain varieties of bread and cereals, and fibrous vegetables) should be increased.

■ Heartburn can be alleviated by smaller, more frequent meals, avoidance of rich or fatty foods and avoidance of eating late in the evening.

REFERENCES

1 Barker, D.J.P. *et al.* (1993a) Fetal nutrition and cardiovascular disease in adult life. *Lancet* i, 938–41.
2 Barker, D.J.P. *et al.* (1993b) Type 2 (non-insulin dependent) diabetes mellitus, hypertension and hyperlipidaemia (syndrome X): relation to fetal growth. *Diabetologia* **36**, 62–7.
3 Laurence, K.M. *et al.* (1981) Double-blind randomised controlled trial of folate treatment before conception to prevent recurrence of neural tube defects. *British Medical Journal* **282**, 1509–11.
4 Medical Research Council Vitamin Study Research Group (1991) Prevention of neural tube defects: results of the Medical Research Council Vitamin study. *Lancet* ii, 131–7.
5 Department of Health Expert Advisory Group (1992) *Folic Acid and the Prevention of Neural Tube Defects*. Department of Health, London.
6 Gregory, J. *et al.* (1990) *The Dietary and Nutritional Survey of British Adults*. HMSO, London.
7 Consumers' Association (1993) *Report of the Survey of Folic Acid Awareness*. Consumers' Association, London.
8 Sutcliffe, M. *et al.* (1994) Prevention of neural tube defects. *Lancet* **344**, 1174.
9 Martinez-Frias, M.L., & Salvador, J. (1990) Epidemiological aspects of prenatal exposure to high doses of vitamin A in Spain. *European Journal of Epidemiology* **6**, 118–23.
10 Chief Medical Officer & Chief Nursing Officer (1993) *Vitamin A and Pregnancy*. PL/CMO (93)15, PL/CNO (93)7. Department of Health, London.

FURTHER READING

British Nutrition Foundation (1994) *Nutrition in Pregnancy*. Briefing Paper. BNF, London.
Central Office of Information/Department of Health (1993) *Pregnancy, Folic Acid and You: Reducing the Risk of Spina Bifida*. Available from BAPS, Health Publication Unit, DSS Distribution Centre, Heywood Stores, Manchester Road, Heywood, Lancashire OL10 2PZ.
Department of Health (1992) *While You Are Pregnant: Safe Eating and How to Avoid Infection from Food and Animals*. Department of Health, London.
National Dairy Council (1994) *Maternal and Fetal Nutrition*. Fact File 11. National Dairy Council, London.

USEFUL ADDRESSES

Association for Spina Bifida and Hydrocephalus (ASBAH), ASBAH House, 42 Park Road, Peterborough PE1 2UQ. Tel: 01733 555988.
National Childbirth Trust (NCT), Alexandra House, Oldham Terrace, London W3 6NH. Tel: 0181 992 8637.

13

Infants

The quality of nutrition in infancy and early childhood can have profound consequences. An inadequate or imbalanced diet not only affects growth and development in the early years but may also influence the susceptibility to diseases such as coronary heart disease in later life[1].

Two factors are of central relevance to the nutritional needs of infants:

(1) As a result of the rapid rate of growth and development, requirements for energy and nutrients are relatively high. Compared with an adult, infants have a higher requirement per kg body weight for energy, protein, iron and calcium.
(2) Many body systems are still immature, particularly gastrointestinal, renal and immune function. Inappropriate feeding can therefore result in problems caused by inadequate digestion, poor absorption, impaired excretion or infection.

Nature has designed the ideal product to meet these needs in the form of breast milk.

BREAST FEEDING

Without question, breast milk is the best source of nutrition for newborn infants for the following reasons:

- It has the ideal nutritional composition for young humans.
- It is easily digested.
- Many micronutrients are more easily absorbed from breast milk.
- It contains the long-chain fatty acids known to be essential for brain development.
- It contains immunoglobulins and other components which protect against infection.
- It contains factors which may promote growth.
- It helps colonisation of the intestine with appropriate microbes important in the suppression of pathogens.
- Its nutritional composition adapts during the course of a feed and in line with the development of the infant.
- It is bacteriologically safe.
- There is no risk of solute overload from an inappropriate formulation.
- It has a low allergenic potential.

Breast feeding also has advantages for the mother:

- It promotes bonding between mother and child.
- It is convenient.
- It helps reduce adipose tissue stored during pregnancy.
- There are no worries about whether it is the right composition.

Prevalence of breast feeding

Despite these clear advantages and the recommendation that breast milk should be the sole source of nutrition at the start of life[2], the prevalence of breast feeding in the UK is still low. A 1990 survey of infant feeding practices[3] showed that:

■ Fewer than two-thirds (64%) of infants were breast fed at birth.

■ Only half (51%) were breast fed for more than 2 weeks.

■ Just over one-third (39%) were breast fed for 6 weeks.

■ Only one-quarter (25%) were still being breast fed at 4 months.

There were also marked differences in the prevalence of breast feeding between different socio-economic groups: 90% of mothers in class 1 started breast feeding but fewer than 50% in classes IV and V. Women who were most likely to breast feed were:

■ First time mothers.

■ Mothers educated beyond the age of 18.

■ Older mothers (first child after the age of 25).

■ Mothers living in the south-east of England.

■ Mothers whose husbands are non-manual workers.

It has been estimated considerable savings could be made in terms of reduced hospital admissions for gastroenteritis if all babies were breast fed during the first year of life[4]. The *Health of the Nation* target is that by the year 2000, 75% of infants are breast fed at birth and 50% are still breast fed at the age of 6 weeks.

Factors affecting the prevalence of breast feeding

The reasons why the overall prevalence is so low and why so many mothers abandon breast feeding is not well understood but it is important that these issues are addressed if the *Health of the Nation* targets are to be achieved. Some of the relevant factors may be as follows.

Reasons for not starting breast feeding

■ It is considered to be embarrassing.

■ It is perceived as a 'middle-class' thing to do.

■ Formula feeds are thought to be more 'scientific' or better.

■ With a bottle feed it is easier to see how much the infant is consuming.

■ Advice from family and friends.

■ Previous failure at breast feeding (many do not attempt it a second time).

Reasons for discontinuing breast feeding

■ Lack of encouragement in the early stages when breast feeding can be uncomfortable.

■ Failure to establish a good supply of milk, often as a result of the use of complementary dextrose or formula feeds in the initial post-partum period or due to poor advice concerning feeding technique or frequency.

■ The infant has to be fed by other people (often because of an early return to work). Using a formula milk is easier than expressing breast milk to be given from a bottle.

■ 'Insufficient milk'. This is a commonly cited reason, particularly when the infant is about 6 weeks old. The child may be fractious, the mother is tired, and well-meaning relatives or health professionals suggest that the infant is hungry and needs complementary feeds of either dextrose or formula milk. This advice is nearly always disastrous. Breast milk, operates on a 'supply and demand' basis. If the infant is not receiving enough milk it is because it is not being fed often enough or for long enough. Increased consumption of milk will result in an increased supply. In contrast, supplementary feeds will make the situation worse; demand for breast milk will decline and milk production will decline as well. The use of a formula feed then becomes inevitable.

■ 'Poor weight gain'. This is often perceived rather than real. New mothers tend to compare their infant's progress with those of others born at about the same time. If everyone else's child seems larger or heavier, the inexperienced mother often concludes that her own must be underfed.

Promoting breast feeding

Education

The benefits of breast feeding need to be promoted early in pregnancy; most mothers decide how they will feed their infants long before delivery and do not change their minds subsequently[5]. Even this may not be soon enough; attitudes towards infant feeding may be formed long before pregnancy occurs and it may be vital that education begins during the school years via National Curriculum or GCSE courses.

It is also important that expectant mothers are given realistic advice about the practicalities of breast feeding. It takes time for breast feeding to become established and in the early post-partum period it can be a frustrating, uncomfortable, even painful process. If people are not aware of this, the reality comes as an unpleasant surprise and they tend to conclude that breast feeding is difficult and they are no good at it anyway. People need to know that:

■ Everyone is capable of breast feeding.
■ The early drawbacks don't last long.

■ Once established, breast feeding is easy and enjoyable.
■ The benefits for both mother and child are enormous.

While every encouragement should be given to breast feeding, women must not be bullied into doing so, nor made to feel guilty and inadequate if they do not. There may be many factors influencing a mother's choice of infant feeding and the decision made by the mother must be respected. What matters is that the mother is able to make an *informed* choice about the method of infant feeding. The role of the health professional is to ensure that mothers understand the significance of the options available and that their decision is not being affected by unnecessary fears or incorrect beliefs.

Establishing breast feeding

To help establish breast feeding, infants should be put to the breast as soon as possible after the birth. The suckling instinct is particularly strong immediately in the newborn.

To begin with, when breast feeding is still a learning process for both mother and child, infants should be suckled on demand but for only a few minutes each side to prevent nipple soreness. At this stage, breast feeding is less important as a source of nutrients but invaluable for the antibodies contained in colostrum produced in the post-partum period. After the third or fourth day, full milk is produced (often with temporary problems of breast tenderness and engorgement) and gradually feeding will become fully established. Infants should always be fed on demand and for as they long as they wish. No extra fluids (water, dextrose solutions or formula feeds) should be given.

The hindmilk contains more fat, energy and essential nutrients than the foremilk and as the infant grows it is important that they receive the hindmilk in order to meet nutrient needs. One breast should be emptied completely before feeding starts on the other side.

Ideally, breast feeding should be the sole source of nutrition until weaning, after which it should decline gradually and cease altogether at about the age of one year. If breast feeding ceases before the age of one year, formula milk rather than unmodified cows' milk should be used as a drink.

Providing advice and support

Breast feeding mothers should have access to advice and support from health professionals and it is vital that the information given is consistent. If the GP, midwife and health visitor all give different advice, the mother is bound to end up confused and anxious. Local infant feeding policies are a helpful way of ensuring that everyone gives the same messages.

Breast feeding counsellors from organisations such as the National Childbirth Trust are also a valuable source of support. Vulnerable mothers from lower socio-economic groups and from varying cultural backgrounds may need particular encouragement to make contact with these groups.

Diet and lactation

Milk production is an energy intensive process requiring on average an additional 500 kcal/day. Much of this can be derived from the adipose stores laid down during pregnancy but many women find that their appetite increases and, so long as weight does not actually increase, they should be encouraged to respond to this by eating more.

It is, however, important that appetite is satisfied with foods of high nutrient quality, not fatty and sugary foods alone. Requirements for protein, calcium, folate, vitamin C and vitamin A increase significantly during lactation and increments of some other vitamins and trace elements are also recommended. This necessitates a balanced intake of foods from all the four major food groups and those from the milk/dairy foods and meat/fish/pulses groups should be particularly encouraged.

Sufficient fluid intake is also vital. All lactating mothers should be encouraged to drink more liquid than usual and not to ignore thirst. Caffeine (from tea, coffee, cola drinks) and alcohol are excreted in breast milk so excessive quantities should be avoided.

Contraindications to breast feeding

HIV infection

HIV positive mothers can transmit the infection to infants via breast milk. The practice is therefore discouraged in the UK (though not necessarily in developing countries where the health risk from contaminated water used to make formula feeds or malnutrition is considered greater than the risk from HIV)[6].

Therapeutic drugs

Many drugs can be excreted in breast milk so must always be used with caution. If a drug contraindicated during breast feeding is only needed for a short period, breast feeding can be temporarily discontinued (breast milk being expressed and discarded during this time) and then restarted. A chronic need for drugs such as cytotoxics or some anti-epileptics usually precludes breast feeding.

FORMULA FEEDING

Bottle feeding will always be a necessary or preferred option for some mothers. Formula milk cannot match the immunological and other benefits of breast milk but its nutritional composition is as close to breast milk as possible. There are two types of formula milks for normal infants:

- Whey-dominant
- Casein-dominant

Each is derived from cows' milk but in whey-dominant formulas the milk protein has been modified to make it more closely resemble that found in breast milk. Whey-based milks have a casein:whey ratio of 40:60; in casein-dominant milks the ratio is 80:20. Whey-dominant milks, being more similar to human milk, are the preferred choice from birth onwards or if breast feeding is discontinued and these are usually marketed as 'first' milks. Casein-dominant milks are supposed to be more suitable for older or more hungry babies although the energy content of casein milks is no different from that of whey milks so there is no obvious nutritional advantage. It may be, however, that the type of curds formed in the stomach from casein take longer to digest than those from whey and hence leave a baby feeling more satisfied.

Recently it has been questioned whether most formula milks meet the needs for the long-chain fatty acids which are essential for brain and neural development, in particular arachidonic acid and docosahexaenoic acid (DHA)[7]. Although these can be synthesised from other fatty acids (linoleic and alpha-linolenic acids) the enzymes necessary to do this are not thought to be active until an infant is a few months old. There is therefore doubt as to whether a young infant can synthesise sufficient arachidonic acid and DHA for its needs, particularly at a time of rapid brain growth. It may be relevant that breast milk itself does contain arachidonic acid and DHA and currently (April 1996) one manufacturer also adds them to its formula milks. However, most infant formulas only contain the precursors for making these substances, not the end products themselves. This subject remains an area of active research.

Types of formula milks

■ Whey-dominant

Milupa	Aptamil with Milupan*
Cow & Gate	Nutrilon Premium
Farley's	First Milk
Wyeth	SMA Gold
Boots	Formula 1

*Contains added arachidonic acid and docosahexaenoic acid

■ Casein-dominant

Milupa	Milumil
Cow & Gate	Nutrilon Plus
Farley's	Second Milk
Wyeth	SMA White
Boots	Formula 2

Unmodified milks (cows', goats', sheep) or ordinary soya milks must never be given to infants under the age of 12 months.

Practical aspects of bottle feeding

Quantity
On average, infants consume about 120–200 ml/kg body weight/day. However, some babies will require more, some less and mothers should not become too obsessed by the amount taken. Infants who are basically content and growing normally are receiving enough.

Reconstitution
It is important that powdered feeds are reconstituted correctly. Studies of infant feeding practices suggest that many feeds are more concentrated than they should be, either because mothers inadvertently compress extra milk powder into the measuring spoon or because they deliberately add a little extra on the grounds that this is bound to be beneficial. In practice this will only create thirst and possibly solute overload and increase the risk of obesity. Cartons of infant formula in a ready-to-feed form eliminate this problem but are much more expensive.

Reheating
Bottles of infant feed should not be warmed in a microwave oven as the heating process can be very uneven, causing hot spots which can scald the baby's mouth.

Teat hole size
This has to be just right. If too large, fluid will gush out of the bottle making the infant choke. If too

small, the infant has to suck hard to obtain the contents and will either get exhausted before enough has been consumed, or swallow too much air and develop wind. Milk should steadily drip out when the bottle is inverted.

Hygiene

Bacterial contamination of milk is a major cause of gastroenteritis in bottle fed infants. It is vital that all feeding equipment is properly sterilised, that feeds are made up hygienically and that made-up milk is stored correctly. Microwave ovens are not a suitable way of sterilising bottles as air bubbles can be trapped preventing total sterilisation.

Fluid

Unlike breast fed infants, those fed formula milks can get thirsty so should be offered cooled boiled water from time to time, particularly in hot weather. Fruit-based drinks are not necessary and may encourage the development of nursing bottle caries.

General aspects

- Nothing should ever be added to a bottle feed, e.g. cereals or rusk.
- Infants should not be left to sleep with a bottle in their mouth.
- With modern infant formulas, additional vitamins are not necessary.

Follow-on milks

These are formula milks designed to meet the nutritional needs of infants between the ages of 6 and 12 months, particularly for that of iron. The need for a dietary source of iron becomes increasingly important around the age of 4–6 months due to the combination of rapid growth and depletion of the iron stores present at birth. This stage of a child's life normally coincides with weaning and in theory a child's iron needs can be met from non-milk dietary sources. In practice, this is not always the

case as infants may not initially be offered or consume sufficient quantities of iron-containing foods. In these circumstances, follow-on milks are useful.

Follow-on formula milks

Cow & Gate	Step-up
SMA	Progress
Milupa	Forward
Farley's	Follow-on milk
Boots	Milk drink

Pre-term infants

Pre-term infants have a greater immaturity of the digestive system and often have feeding difficulties. Breast milk is considered to be the ideal source of nutrition because of its protective factors and high digestibility. The mother's milk can be administered nasogastrically if suckl-ing is not possible. Sometimes a combination of breast milk and breast milk fortifiers (so boosting the content of energy, protein, vitamins and minerals) is used. Breast milk fortifiers are:

Cow & Gate	Nutriprem
Mead Johnson	Enfamil
Milupa	Eoprotein

Pre-term infant formula feeds are also available. These contain a higher concentration of nutrients than standard formula milks to compensate for the reduced volume of feed which can be consumed. It may be important that these formulas contain the long-chain fatty acids arachidonic acid and docosahexaenoic acid (DHA) which are essential for brain and neural development. At this stage of infant development, these fatty acids would normally be supplied by placental transfer since the enzymes capable of making them do not mature until early infancy. A dietary source is therefore almost certainly necessary. At present, some pre-term formulas do contain long-chain fatty acids and others may well do so in the future.

LIVERPOOL
JOHN MOORES UNIVERSITY
AVRIL ROBARTS LRC
TEL. 0151 231 4022

Pre-term formula milks

Cow & Gate	Nutriprem LBW
Milupa	Prematil with Milupan
Farleys	Osterprem
SMA	SMA low birthweight formula

Infant formulas which are intermediate between low birthweight and standard infant formulas are:

| Cow & Gate | Nutriprem 2 |
| Farley | Premcare |

Specialist infant formula milks

Soya infant formulas

Soya infant formulas are not recommended for general use because their content of non-milk sugars may increase the risk of dental caries. It used to be thought that they were less allergenic than formulas containing cows' milk protein and that they may help prevent atopic diseases such as eczema or asthma, but there is little evidence that this is the case. At best, they may only delay its appearance. There is no evidence that soya-based formulas milks prevent colic.

Soya infant formula should only be used for:

- Cases of proven intolerance to cows' milk protein, lactose, sucrose or galactose.
- Vegan infants.

Some infants who are intolerant to cows' milk protein are also sensitive to soya protein; in these circumstances a protein hydrolysate infant formula will be necessary.

Soya infant formulas have a high aluminium content and are not suitable for pre-term infants or those with impaired renal function.

Ordinary soya-based drinks sold in some health food shops and supermarkets are not the same as soya infant formulas and are *not* suitable for use for infants or children below the age of 5 years, having too low a content of energy, vitamins and minerals.

Soya-based infant formulas are:

Abbott	Isomil
Cow & Gate	Infasoy
Farley	Ostersoy
Mead Johnson	Prosobee
SMA	Wysoy

Dietetic advice should be sought concerning the use of protein hydrolysate and other specialised infant feeding formulas necessary for severe intolerance or malabsorption.

INFANT FEEDING PROBLEMS

Colic

Colic causes episodes of acute abdominal pain in an otherwise fit baby, typically between the ages of 6 and 12 weeks and often in the early evening. It is thought to be a consequence of intestinal immaturity; the complex movements of peristalsis are not co-ordinated properly and pockets of gas and air can build up which then trigger intense contractions of the intestinal wall.

Colic tends to be more common in bottle fed infants, possibly because this method of feeding results in ingestion of larger quantities of air. Mothers of breast fed infants with colic have sometimes been advised to avoid cows' milk and dairy products but there is little scientific evidence that this is beneficial to the infant and it is highly likely to be detrimental to the mother as a result of the reduced calcium intake.

Prevention should focus on minimising the amount of air swallowed via feeding (e.g. relieving wind during and at the end of a feed, and checking teat hole size if bottle fed). Gentle stomach massage after a feed (rubbing in a circular motion close to the navel in widening circles with increasing pressure) can also be effective. If the problem persists, dimethicone can help disperse gas trapped in the stomach. Antispasmodics can prescribed for infants over the age of 6 months.

Poor weight gain

A slow rate of growth is not necessarily a cause for concern; the infant may simply be genetically small. Nevertheless the following factors should be considered, particularly if the infants seems discontent or unwell:

- Inadequate nutrient intake, e.g.
    Poor breastfeeding technique
    Ignorance (formula made up incorrectly)
    Neglect
    Inability to feed correctly (e.g. cleft palate).
- Inadequate absorption (food intolerance or gastrointestinal disease).
- Inadequate utilisation (metabolic disorder or nutrient deficiency).

Excessive weight gain

This is rarely a problem in the infant which is exclusively breast fed. Bottle fed infants often do grow more rapidly and, if weight gain is excessive, the amount of formula given and especially its dilution should be checked. If these seem appropriate, no further action is necessary at this stage as the surplus weight may well disappear when the infant starts to become more active. Weight should be reviewed after a few months.

Diarrhoea and/or vomiting

These are always serious in an infant because of the life-threatening dehydration and electrolyte depletion which can occur. The combination of vomiting and diarrhoea is a more serious threat than diarrhoea alone. Gastrointestinal infections are more likely to occur in bottle fed than breast fed infants because of the greater potential for feed contamination and the lower immunological protection.

If these occur, feeding should be stopped and electrolyte replacement fluids substituted until the acute symptoms disappear. Feeds should then be reintroduced gradually, formula feeds being made up at reduced strength (quarter-strength initially, then half-strength). Hygiene procedures should be reviewed with the mothers of bottle fed infants.

WEANING

Weaning has two objectives:

(1) To meet the demand for nutrients and energy needed for growth which can no longer be supplied by milk alone.
(2) To accustom the infant to a wide variety of tastes and textures and lay the foundations of healthy eating habits.

Mothers often lack confidence about the weaning process feeling unsure when to start, what to give or whether they are doing it properly. Some find that the type of advice given by health professionals is too vague and theoretical, for example stressing the importance of iron but not explaining which foods contain it. Mothers also tend to worry unnecessarily about some aspects of the diet especially 'additives' not realising that nutritional adequacy is far more important. Misconceptions about sugar are also common; it is often assumed that fruit juice is better than other sweetened drinks because the sugar is put there by nature not a food manufacturer. In reality, it can be just as damaging to teeth.

Weaning is a gradual process and its progression is dependent upon physical development. The co-ordination skills required to take food off a spoon, transfer it to the back of the mouth and then swallow it are quite sophisticated. The process of chewing and later the use of hands and then cutlery to bring food to the mouth are also physical skills which have to be learnt. The ease with which infants adapt to weaning also varies. Some children will happily accept whatever is offered, others will spit anything unfamiliar straight across the kitchen. Different infants will therefore adapt to weaning at different rates. The priority for parents is not to become over-anxious about the whole process. Infants are quite capable of sensing parental concerns and may interpret these signals as meaning that this new experience of feeding is a threat, not a pleasure.

Initially, while the infant is still learning the new techniques required, the amounts of food consumed will be small and its nutritional significance negligible. Milk will still be the nutritional mainstay of the diet. Gradually an increased quantity and greater variety of foods will be consumed and nutritional reliance on milk will lessen.

A comprehensive report *Weaning and the Weaning Diet* was published by the Department of Health in 1994[8] and the following weaning guidance is based on its recommendations.

Nutritional aspects of weaning

Weaning is a time of nutritional vulnerability because increasing requirements for many nutrients coincide with the gradual depletion of nutrient stores present at birth. Important aspects of the diet are considered below.

Energy
Without sufficient energy, protein and other nutrients cannot be utilised properly and the child cannot grow. Because appetite is still small, this energy needs to be provided in a relatively concentrated form. Foods which are reduced in fat (e.g. skimmed milk) are not therefore appropriate for this age group. Similarly too many fibre-rich foods (e.g. wholegrain cereals) will fill the child up before it has consumed sufficient nutrients.

Sugars are an important source of energy at this age but most should still be derived from milk and those present in fruit and vegetables. Unnecessary use of added or extrinsic sugars (e.g. table sugars, sweetened foods or fruit juices) must be avoided because of the risk of dental caries but this needs to be kept in perspective. In practice, many of the so-called intrinsic forms of sugar (e.g. whole fruit) will be given to an infant in an extrinsic form (fruit is likely to be stewed and puréed). Adding small amounts of sugar to achieve an acceptable palatability (e.g. if puréed fruit has a sour taste) is not therefore a matter for concern – a purée derived from riper (hence sweeter) fruit will have a similar composition. What matters is that the infant is not encouraged to indulge the natural preference for sweetness by being offered excessively sweet foods or sweetened foods or drinks between mealtimes.

Minerals and vitamins
Dietary variety is important to ensure that all essential minerals, trace elements and vitamins are provided. Those which require particular consideration are:

- *Iron* Iron content is a particularly important aspect of the weaning diet because the iron stores present at birth will be virtually exhausted but the need for iron is still increasing. Iron deficiency anaemia is common in this age group, and can have serious, possibly irreversible, consequences in terms of mental development. Foods rich in haem iron (red meat) should be encouraged in preference to non-haem sources (cereals, pulses and vegetables) which are less well absorbed and may also contain phytates. Follow-on milks and fortified weaning foods can make a valuable contribution to dietary iron intakes.
- *Zinc* Zinc deficiency may impair growth and intakes may be inadequate if meat, its major source, is not included in the diet at this stage.
- *Sodium (salt)* Infants are very inefficient at excreting sodium and salt should never be added to a weaning food.
- *Vitamin D* This is an important nutrient at this stage because of its role in the utilisation of calcium. Deficiency is a risk between the age of 6 and 12 months because requirements are high

(due to rapid bone growth) but provision may be low (infants tend to be protected from sunlight so skin synthesis is minimal). Formula milk is supplemented with vitamin D but breast fed infants should be given a supplement (as A,D,C drops) from the age of 6 months. Many commercial weaning foods contain supplementary vitamin D.

■ *Vitamin C* High intakes of vitamin C will improve the absorption of non-haem iron. While fruit and vegetable consumption remains low, welfare vitamin drops and many commercial infant foods will ensure an adequate supply.

Fluid

Before 6 months, no additional drinks are needed in breast fed infants and formula fed infants only need additional water.

After the age of 6 months, diluted fruit juices and baby drinks can be given as part of a meal. Between meals, drinks should be confined to breast or formula milk or water. Infants should be encouraged to drink from a cup at the age of 6 months and discouraged from feeding from a bottle after one year. Infants must never be left with a bottle or feeding reservoir containing a sugar-containing drink.

From the age of one year, pasteurised cows' milk can be used as a main drink. Cows' milk can, however, be added to foods after the age of 6 months.

Goats' or sheep's milk are not suitable for infants under the age of 1 year. If they are then introduced at this stage, they must be pasteurised or boiled.

Tea is unsuitable as a drink for young children because its tannin content interferes with iron absorption.

Practical aspects of weaning

When to start weaning

Weaning should start:

■ Not earlier than 4 months.
■ Not later than 6 months.

Before the age of 4 months, weaning can be hazardous because:

■ The gastrointestinal tract is immature: digestive enzyme production is not fully developed and the gut wall is more permeable to some of the foreign proteins introduced with food thus increasing the risk of allergic reaction.
■ The kidney is immature: it may not be able to eliminate surplus electrolytes via urine.
■ Neuromuscular co-ordination may not have reached the stage whereby food can be swallowed without choking.

It is clear that many mothers ignore this advice, particularly those who are young and in lower socio-economic groups. The 1992 survey of the diets of British infants[9] found that almost one-quarter of mothers introduced solids to their babies at 0–2 months of age, usually because they believed that milk wasn't enough or because the baby was waking at night.

After the age of 6 months, some form of additional nutrient supply is essential to meet increased needs. Indications that a child is ready to try solid food are:

■ If the infant still seems hungry after a milk feed, even if the quantity has been increased.
■ If more feeds are being demanded.
■ If an infant who normally sleeps through the night starts to wake again.

How to start weaning

Suitable foods The first foods to be offered should be:

   Non-wheat cereals (e.g. baby rice)
   Vegetables
   Non-citrus fruit

Cows' milk should not be added to foods such as breakfast cereals until the age of 6 months or given as a drink until the age of 1 year. From the age of 4 months, cows' milk can be used in the form of cheese-based sauces, custard or yogurt.

Foods containing wheat, eggs and citrus fruits should not be introduced before the age of 6 months because these can provoke allergic reactions. It is no longer thought necessary to introduce foods one at a time unless there is a history of atopic disease.

Foods which are high in salt, sugar and fibre or those where the fat content has been reduced (e.g. skimmed milk, reduced-fat dairy products) are unsuitable.

Infants should not be given whole or chopped nuts because of the risk of choking and their toxicity if inhaled.

Consistency　This should be thin and smooth at first so that the baby can develop a sucking reflex to take food from a spoon. Gradually food can progress to being more textured (scrambled or minced) and then chopped. From the age of 6 months, finger foods are important for feeding development. To reduce the risk of choking, these should initially be foods which soften in the mouth (e.g. bread); harder finger foods (pieces of apple or carrot) should only be given when the child is more competent. Children must never be left unsupervised with finger foods. All mothers should be taught emergency procedures for choking.

Commercially prepared weaning foods　Although not essential, most mothers use commercially produced weaning foods at some stage during the weaning process because they are so convenient. Ordinary family food may not be suitable for the infant because it contains too much sugar, salt or other seasonings or it may not be ready at the time the infant needs to be fed. It is also frustrating to spend time preparing a special purée for the infant only for it to be rejected at the first mouthful.

In the early stages of weaning, the dried products reconstituted with boiling water are very convenient because they can be made up in very small quantities so avoiding waste. Jars with ready-to-use contents are useful when the child consumes larger quantities and a family meal is either not suitable, not yet ready or the child needs feeding away from home. Junior foods, for babies from around 7 months, are textured with small, soft pieces of food to encourage chewing.

Foods produced specifically for infants have to conform with strict regulations governing their composition and safety. They are not allowed to contain artificial colourings, flavourings or preservatives and many are fortified with iron, other minerals and vitamins. They are, however, relatively expensive and mothers should not be encouraged to rely on them exclusively as their bland taste may discourage the infant from trying normal household foods.

Timetable for weaning

This varies according to the needs and development of the infant but general guidelines are:

Stage 1　　4–6 months
Initially:
　Aim:　To get the infant used to the idea of the spoon, rather than to provide nourishment.
　Frequency:　Once a day, after (or during) one feed.
　Quantity:　Initially 1, then 1–2 teaspoons.
　Suitable foods:
　　Baby rice
　　Puréed vegetables cooked without salt (e.g. potato, carrot)
　　Puréed non-citrus fruit (e.g. apple, pear, banana)
　Milk feeds:　No change.
Gradual progression to:
　Aim:　Introducing new tastes and providing some nourishment.
　Frequency:　After 2, then after 3 feeds per day.
　Quantity:　Dictated by appetite.
　Suitable foods:　Baby rice (or cereal) at one meal only
　　Wider variety of puréed vegetables
　　Wider variety of puréed non-citrus fruit
　　Puréed meat, chicken, fish or liver
　　Puréed pulses (e.g. split lentils)
　　Custard, yogurt
　Milk feeds:　Usual number.

Stage 2   6–9 months

Aim: To lessen the dependence on milk as a source of nourishment.

Frequency: 3–5 times per day. Solids should be given before the milk feed.

Quantity: More substantial servings.

New foods to try:
   Cows' milk for mixing cereals
   Cauliflower/macaroni cheese
   Rice pudding
   Wheat-containing cereals
   Dairy foods (yogurt, fromage frais, cottage cheese)
   Eggs (well-cooked)
   Citrus fruits
   More family foods without added salt, sugar or spices

Texture: Can be less smooth, e.g. mashed, minced or scrambled and then chopped.

Introduce: Soft finger foods, e.g. bread, pitta bread, banana, orange segments. Harder finger foods (carrot, apple) as competence improves.

Milk feeds: Being reduced.

Stage 3   9–12 months

Aim: Learning to chew and feed themselves.

Frequency: A regular meal pattern.

Quantity: As dictated by appetite.

Suitable foods: Normal family food, mashed or chopped as necessary.

Milk feeds: Usually only one before bedtime.

After the age of one year, an infant should be consuming a varied balanced diet containing suitable choices from all four main food groups (bread/cereals, fruit/vegetables, milk and dairy foods, meat and alternatives). Full-fat cows' milk can replace formula or breast milk at this stage.

General aspects of weaning

Other points which may need to be emphasised to mothers are summarised below.

Rate of progress

- Infants vary in their rate of development; let the child dictate the pace.
- Don't become over-anxious; all children are weaned eventually.
- Offer a variety of foods of a suitable consistency for the child's stage of development.
- If a food does not seem to be wanted, don't force it. Try another time.
- Never add solids to bottle feeds; it doesn't help the learning process and can cause choking.

Food hygiene

- Wash hands before preparing food and ensure all equipment is clean.
- Never reheat left-over food.
- Discard any remaining contents from jars.

Food preparation

- Make sure that the food offered is not too hot. If it has been heated in a microwave oven, stir well to ensure that the heat distribution is even.
- Do not add salt to any food.
- Only add sugar at a level which is essential for palatability.
- When eggs are introduced, these should be cooked until the yolk is set.

Special considerations

Vegan and vegetarian infants (see also Chapter 21)

A vegan weaning diet will be deficient in riboflavin (obtained mainly from dairy products) and in B_{12} (found only in animal foods). Vegan infants should be given supplements of these vitamins in addition to A, C and D drops and these should be continued until the age of 5 years.

Both vegan and vegetarian infants are at risk of iron deficiency. Commercial weaning foods fortified with iron are probably essential for these infants. A source of vitamin C (e.g. fruit or fruit juice) should be included with every meal to facilitate absorption of non-haem iron.

Family history of atopy (see also Chapter 40)

Breast feeding should be encouraged for at least 6 months in those with family history of atopy or gluten enteropathy. Weaning should not start before 4 months and the infant should not be given any of the most allergenic foods such as cows' milk, wheat, eggs or fish before the age of 6 months at the earliest. Those requiring dietary modification should receive qualified dietetic advice.

Dental caries (see also Chapter 28)

This is a particular problem among socially deprived families and is often associated with the use of honey-coated dummies and infants being left with bottles of sweetened drinks. These practices should be strongly discouraged.

Other important measures to prevent dental decay in infants are:

- Establish a teeth cleaning habit with fluoride toothpaste as soon as the teeth erupt.
- From the age of 6 months, fluoride supplements should be given to infants in areas of low water fluoride content.
- Discourage the use of feeding bottles after the age of 1 year.
- The frequency of consumption of sugar-containing foods and drinks should be kept to a minimum.

REFERENCES

1 Barker, D.J.P. (ed.) (1992) *Fetal and Infant Origins of Adult Disease*. British Medical Journal, London.
2 Department of Health and Social Security (1988) *Present Day Practice in Infant Feeding*. Third Report. COMA Report on Health and Social Subjects 32. HMSO, London.
3 White, A. *et al.* (1992) *Infant Feeding 1990*. Office of Population, Censuses and Surveys. HMSO, London.
4 Waterston, L.T. & Davies, J. (1993) Could hospitals do more to encourage breastfeeding? *British Medical Journal* (Editorial) 307, 1437.
5 Hally M.R. *et al.* (1984) Factors influencing the feeding of first born infants. *Acta Paediatrica Scandinavic* 73, 33–9.
6 World Health Organization (1992) *Consensus Statement from WHO/UNICEF Consultation on HIV Transmission and Breastfeeding*. WHO, Geneva.
7 Farquharson, J. *et al.* (1992) Infant cerebral cortex phospholipid fatty acid composition and diet. *Lancet* 340, 810–13.
8 Department of Health (1994) *Weaning and the Weaning Diet*. COMA Report on Health and Social Subjects 45. HMSO, London.
9 Mills, A. & Tyler, H. (1992) *Food and Nutrient Intakes of British Infants Aged 6–12 Months*. A Survey from the Ministry of Agriculture, Fisheries and Food. HMSO, London.

FURTHER READING

Forsyth, J.S., Ogston, S,A., Clark, A., Florey, C. du V. & Howie, P-W. (1993) Relation between early introduction of solid food to infants and their weight and illnesses during the first two years of life. *British Medical Journal* 306, 1572.
Health Education Authority (1994) *From Milk to Mixed Feeding*. HEA, London.
Hyde, L . (1994) Knowledge of basic infant nutrition amongst community health professionals. *Maternal and Child Health* 1, 27–32.
Lucas, A., Morley, R., Cole, T.J., Lister, G. & Leeson-Payne, C. (1992) Breast milk and subsequent intelligence quotient in children born preterm. *Lancet* 339, 261–4.
Mitton, S.G. (1994) What are the indications for prescribing soya milk for infants? *British Medical Journal* 308, 266.

USEFUL ADDRESSES

Association of Breastfeeding Mothers, 26 Holmshaw Close, Sydenham, London SE26 4TH. Tel: 0181 778 4769.
La Lèche League, Po Box BM 3424, London WC1N 3XX. Tel: 0171 242 1278.
National Childbirth Trust (NCT), Alexandra House, Oldham Terrace, Acton, London W3 6HN. Tel: 0181 992 8637.

14

Toddlers and Pre-school Children

Children in this age group have:

- High energy and nutrient requirements relative to their size.
- Small stomachs so cannot consume large quantities of food at a time.
- Variable appetite due to fluctuations in growth rate and activity level.

Much of their food intake therefore needs to be of high nutrient quality, i.e. providing vitamins and minerals as well as sources of energy. It also needs to be consumed in small quantities at regular intervals. A meal pattern of several small meals and between-meal snacks is often far more appropriate than two or three large meals per day.

At the same time, the foundations of the eating pattern in later life are being laid down. Specific food preferences will change over the years but attitudes to eating – which types of foods which are considered 'normal' and whether meals are regarded as social occasions or just something eaten while watching television – will be moulded during the early years. Mealtimes are also an important time to communicate and interact with young children. Good eating habits enhance communication skills and language development; delayed speech and poor eating habits often co-exist.

NUTRITIONAL CONSIDERATIONS

Adult healthy eating principles should not be applied too zealously in terms of nutritional composition; if the diet is too low in fat and high in fibre, children will be unable to eat sufficient of it to obtain all the energy and nutrients they need. However, children do need to consume a varied diet comprised of foods from all four of the healthy eating food groups in order to obtain sufficient minerals and vitamins to meet their needs. Nutrients of particular importance in this age group are:

Iron
Calcium
Vitamin C
Vitamin D

A comprehensive report of the diet and nutritional status of children between the ages of $1\frac{1}{2}$ and $4\frac{1}{2}$ was published in 1995 as part of the Department of Health/MAFF National Diet and Nutrition Survey Programme[1]. It found that, in terms of energy and overall nutrient intake, children of this age group are generally well-nourished, are taller, heavier but not fatter than those of 25 years ago. It did, however, highlight some specific concerns. Although most children consumed adequate energy for their needs, a considerable proportion of this energy was derived from foods such as biscuits, crisps, confectionery and sugar-containing drinks. As a result, many children consumed intakes of non-milk extrinsic sugars and sodium which greatly exceeded recommended levels while overall nutritional quality in terms of mineral and vitamin content tended to be low. These trends tended to be more marked in children from lower socio-economic groups.

Inadequate iron intake was highlighted as being of particular concern. Average iron intakes were low; 1 in 12 children was found to be anaemic (blood haemoglobin below 11 g/l). This prevalence level rose to 1 in 8 in those between the ages of $1\frac{1}{2}$ and $2\frac{1}{2}$ years. Anaemia in early childhood is a serious health risk because it can cause irreversible delay in psychomotor development. Low iron status at this age often results from a chronic dietary iron shortage dating from the weaning period.

A high prevalence of dental decay was also evident[2]. Overall, 1 in 6 pre-school children was found to have some dental decay, a figure which increased throughout the age group and was closely linked with the frequency of consumption of sugar-containing foods.

DIETARY GUIDANCE

Both assessment of dietary adequacy and advice on food consumption should be based on considerations of food choice. An adequate diet is likely to be one containing a selection of foods from all four of the major food groups; a diet where there is a noticeable lack of foods from one or more of these groups or a heavy reliance on foods from the fifth group, fatty and sugary foods, is more likely to be imbalanced.

Food choice

Bread, other cereals and potatoes: 4 or more servings per day

- Suitable choices: bread, potatoes, pasta, rice and breakfast cereals.
- Some of these choices can be wholemeal or wholegrain varieties but not too many or the diet will be too filling for the child's appetite.

Fruit and vegetables group: 4 or more servings per day

- Suitable choices: a wide variety of either fresh, frozen or canned products.
- Green vegetables can be encouraged but are often actively disliked. This does not matter if other choices from this group are included.
- Fruit juices can damaging to teeth as a result of their acidity and sugar content; they should be consumed with meals rather than in-between.

Milk and dairy foods group: 2–3 servings per day

- Suitable choices: full-fat milk, cheese, yogurt, fromage frais.
- The average toddler obtains about two-thirds of its calcium intake from milk and milk products. If these foods are excluded (e.g. due to milk intolerance or veganism) specialist dietetic help is needed to ensure that alternative sources of calcium are provided.
- Children who dislike milk as a drink will often consume it in an alternative form, e.g. as custard, in a pudding or as a flavoured milk drink. If not, products such as yogurt, cheese, or fromage frais may be acceptable.
- Pre-school children should be given full-fat rather than reduced-fat dairy products because of their higher energy density and content of fat-soluble vitamins. If parents prefer, or the child is putting on too much weight, semi-skimmed milk can be included after the age of

2 if the child has a good appetite and eats a wide variety of foods.

Meat, fish and alternatives group: 1–2 servings per day

- Suitable choices: minced beef/lamb/pork, fish fingers, poultry, liver, baked beans, eggs.
- Children who consume no red meat or offal are at risk of iron deficiency because these foods are such a concentrated source of haem iron. Non-haem iron in cereal foods and green vegetables is much less well absorbed and, since consumption of these foods is rarely high in this age group, it is difficult to meet the high iron needs from these foods alone. Non-meat eaters should be encouraged to eat fortified white bread and breakfast cereals and to consume a source of vitamin C (fruit or fruit juice) with every meal. Iron supplementation may need to be considered. Expert dietetic advice may be necessary.

Fatty and sugary foods group

- The dietary content of foods such as cakes, biscuits, crisps, sweets, chocolate and sugar-containing drinks has to be watched. These foods need not be excluded altogether, indeed such advice would be regarded as totally impractical by most parents. What is important is that consumption of these foods is not so high that they displace more important foods or, as happens in some cases, that the diet is *entirely* comprised of fatty/sugary foods and high fat choices from other groups such as sausages and chips.
- Reducing the *frequency* of consumption of sugar-containing foods and drinks is an important preventative measure for dental caries. In particular the use of sweetened drinks between meals should be avoided; milk or water are always preferable alternatives.

General dietary aspects

- Food should be offered about 5–6 times per day in the form of both family meals and between-meal snacks.
- Eating should be seen as fun and enjoyable.
- Dietary quality is more important than dietary quantity.
- A variety of foods from all four major food groups should be encouraged. Undue reliance on fatty and sugary foods should be avoided.
- Between-meal snacks should not be confined to biscuits or crisps. Fruit, yogurt or a sandwich are better alternatives most of the time.
- Between-meal drinks should either be milk or water.
- The *frequency* of consumption of sugar-containing drinks and sweets should be closely watched. Sugary foods and drinks (including fruit juices) should ideally only be consumed at mealtimes.
- Vitamin drops providing vitamins A, D and C should be given until the age of 2 years and preferably until the age of 5.

DIET-RELATED PROBLEMS

Faddy eating

Children of this age group are notoriously fickle about what they eat. Various types of foods, such as eggs, meat or green vegetables, may be refused and some children voluntarily restrict themselves to a very small number of foods. While not ideal, this does not always matter very much in nutritional terms. No specific food is essential to health and alternatives from the same general food group will provide similar nutrients. A diet which may seem bizarre and restrictive can sometimes be surprisingly nutritionally adequate; for example, a child who will only eat liver sausage sandwiches, bananas and yogurt is in fact consuming foods from all four of the major food groups. If the child seems healthy, active and is growing well, there is little to worry about. Nutritional intake is only likely to be severely imbalanced if:

■ An entire food group is virtually excluded (e.g. most fruit and vegetables).
■ A major source of a particular nutrient for this age group is excluded, e.g. meat (iron and zinc) or milk (calcium).
■ The child consumes a disproportionately high quantity of foods from the fatty and sugary foods group.

Alternative food choices (or if necessary supplements) to redress this imbalance can be suggested. New foods may be accepted more readily when the child is particularly hungry. Improving the type of snacks offered between meals (e.g. a sandwich rather than crisps; a drink of milk rather than orange squash) can make a significant difference to dietary quality.

Pre-school children's eating habits often improve dramatically once they come into contact with other children and see the types of foods which they enjoy. Starting play-group or nursery education also means they tend to expend more energy and hence are hungrier at mealtimes.

Poor appetite

Rather than having specific likes and dislikes, some children seem generally disinterested in food. Mothers may report that their child 'doesn't eat anything at all'. The possibility of a physical or psychological cause for poor appetite should always be considered, particularly in those who seem listless and unwell. In the apparently healthy child, disinterest in food may result from:

■ *Normal variation in appetite.* Children grow in spurts rather than continuously so it is only

to be expected that food intake will increase during phases of active growth and decrease in between these periods.
■ *The child eats more than the parent realises.* 'Eating very little' may in fact mean eating very little at main meals; the parent simply may not realise how much energy and nutrients are obtained from snacks and drinks at other times. A dietary record of everything consumed by the child over a period of one week can reveal whether the child genuinely eats very little or just very little of what the parent considers to be 'proper' food.
■ *Timing of snacks.* Snacks consumed close to mealtimes will obviously suppress the amount of food consumed.
■ *Fluid consumption.* Fluid, especially fizzy drinks, consumed just before or at the beginning of a meal will create a feeling of satiety and so reduce food intake. Drinks should be provided towards the end of or after a meal.
■ *Food presentation.* Small children can be overwhelmed by an enormous mound of food on a plate. Small portions of attractively presented food on a small plate will be much more appealing.

Food refusal

Some children use food refusal as a weapon for asserting independence or to gain attention. Every meal can turn into a battle of wills with the mother becoming increasingly desperate to find a way of persuading the child to eat and the child being equally determined to resist and thoroughly enjoying the sense of power.

Persuasion and bribery are useless in this situation and always counterproductive. Instead parents have to give the child the impression that they simply don't care whether the child eats or not (acting skills may be required). A child is unable to use food refusal as a weapon if other people refuse to join in the battle. A selection of food should be offered and if refused should be removed without comment and no alternatives offered. To begin with, this will be difficult; it is so much easier to produce a pacifying biscuit than listen to a raging hungry toddler. Nevertheless this strategy of calm acceptance always resolves the situation and usually quite quickly. Once a child learns that no other food will be forthcoming other than that produced at mealtimes, they will eat because at this age they have no other means of obtaining food for themselves (unless a biscuit tin is kept within reach). No child of this age voluntarily starves itself to death.

Overweight and obesity

Obesity is quite rare in this age group but some toddlers can be considered to be overweight. Strict dieting is never appropriate although excessive consumption of foods such as crisps, biscuits and sweets should be curtailed and any sugar-containing drinks replaced by low calorie versions. Sensible varied eating and plenty of physical activity should be encouraged and children allowed to 'grow into' their weight.

Poor growth, underweight and failure to thrive

The diagnosis of failure to thrive is important because it may lead to permanent damage or developmental delay and may indicate neglect and abuse. Weight and/or height on or below the 0.4th centile (see 'Growth' in Chapter 6) is suggestive of failure to thrive and should always be investigated but it does not always mean that something is wrong, the child may simply be one of those at the extreme end of the normal range. An organic cause is more likely if children seem listless, have frequent infections or symptoms suggestive of malabsorption and this obviously needs to be followed

up. Progression of weight or height veering off or crossing a centile curve also suggests a physical or perhaps psychological cause.

If an underweight child seems otherwise healthy, the possibility of a dietary explanation should be considered; an inadequate energy intake is the most common cause. In this age group this is most likely to result from:

- Food refusal by the child due to parent/child conflict.
- Food restriction by the parent due to perceived hazards or undesirability of certain foods or parental diagnosis of 'allergy' in the child.
- Inadequate food provision either as a result of ignorance or deliberate child neglect.

Toddler diarrhoea

Episodes of diarrhoea which do not appear to be associated with infection may have a dietary cause. The most common culprit is large quantities of fruit or fruit juice. The immature gut is inefficient at absorbing fructose and a large load of this in the gut can cause an osmotic diarrhoea. Large quantities of ordinary sugar (i.e. sucrose), which is digested in the gut to fructose and glucose, can have the same effect.

Food intolerance (see also Chapter 40)

Those with a genuine food intolerance, e.g. milk intolerance or coeliac disease, are at high risk of nutrient deficiency and require expert guidance from a dietitian. Serious nutrient imbalances can result from parental diagnosis of food intolerance and food exclusion.

REFERENCES

1   OPCS (1995) *National Diet and Nutrition Survey: children aged 1½ to 4½ years. Volume 1: Report of the diet and nutrition survey.* HMSO, London.
2   OPCS (1995) *National Diet and Nutrition Survey: children aged 1½ to 4½ years. Volume 2: Report of the dental survey.* HMSO, London.

FURTHER READING

Batchelor, J. & Kerslake, A. (1990) *Failure to Find Failure to Thrive: the case for improving screening, prevention and treatment in primary care.* Whiting and Birch Ltd.

Marcovitch, H. (1994) Failure to thrive. *British Medical Journal* **308**, 35.
Payne, J.A. & Bolton, N.R. (1992a) Nutrient intake and growth in preschool children. I Comparison of energy intake and sources of energy with growth. *Journal of Human Nutrition and Dietetics* **5**, 287–98.
Payne, J.A. & Bolton, N.R. (1992b) Nutrient intake and growth in preschool children. II Intake of minerals and vitamins. *Journal of Human Nutrition and Dietetics* **5**, 299–304.

USEFUL ADDRESSES

The new growth centile charts produced by the Child Growth Foundation (see 'Growth' in Chapter 6) may be purchased from: Harlow Printing Ltd, Maxwell Street, South Shields, Tyne & Wear NE33 4PU. Tel: 0191 455 4286.

15

School-aged Children

Children of school age have increasing freedom of choice over what they eat. More meals will be consumed outside the home (e.g. at school or at friends' homes), many children will be allowed to select food for themselves, and food choices will be increasingly affected by outside influences such as peer pressure and advertising. To begin with these influences can be beneficial and the faddy child will usually eat a much more varied diet; as the years progress, these factors may be less helpful if food choice increasingly favours items of poor nutrient quality.

NUTRITIONAL CONSIDERATIONS

Although growth velocity is slower than in infancy and early childhood, school-aged children still have relatively higher nutrient needs and smaller appetites than adults. A diet of high nutrient density (i.e. rich in essential nutrients per 1000 kcal energy) remains important.

The 1989 Department of Health survey on *The Diets of British Schoolchildren*[1] suggested that many children fail to consume such a diet. Although in general children eat sufficient energy for their needs and sometimes too much, intake of fat and sugars tends to be high and intake of essential micronutrients tends to be low. These trends become more apparent as socio-economic circumstances decline. Girls are at greater risk of micronutrient deficiencies than boys because intake of minerals and vitamins is closely associated with total energy intake and in general girls eat less than boys.

Particular nutritional concerns were:

- *Fat* About 75% of children had a fat intake which exceeded the adult target of 35% of dietary energy.
- *Sugars* As might be expected, consumption of sugars was considerably higher than recommended levels. Average consumption was 123 g/day which represented 23% of dietary energy. Although the total level of sugar consumption has not changed much in the last decade, what has changed is that the proportion of sugars derived from milk has declined while that from extrinsic sources, such as sugary foods, drinks and confectionery, has increased. The high frequency of consumption of sugar-containing foods in some children greatly increases the risk of dental caries.
- *Iron* As many as 1 in 3 girls had an iron intake which was almost certainly insufficient for their needs (i.e. below the Lower Reference Nutrient Intake). The risk of low iron status and anaemia is high, especially once girls reach menarche.
- *Calcium* Girls tend to drink less milk than boys and about 1 in 4 girls had low calcium intakes. This may have implications for bone growth and the risk of osteoporosis in later life (see Chapter 36).

■ *Folate* This is an important nutrient for growth but intakes were low in many children, especially those who do not consume breakfast cereals or many vegetables.

Intakes of other vitamins, such as riboflavin and vitamin A, magnesium and zinc also tended to be lower than would seem desirable.

The reason for these imbalances is not hard to find. Although useful foods such as bread and milk do feature in children diets, a large proportion of their dietary energy is derived from chips, biscuits, meat products, cakes and puddings, i.e. foods of relatively low nutrient density. Consumption of important sources of micronutrients, such as fruit and vegetables, tends to be low.

DIETARY GUIDANCE

There are practical difficulties in translating dietary guidelines into acceptable diets for children. Healthy eating guidance must, above all, be pragmatic. It may be ideal that a child eats no chips or chocolate but it is rarely realistic. Wholemeal bread may be a better choice than white bread but a sandwich made from any type of bread is a better snack than a bar of chocolate. Sugar-coated breakfast cereals may not be the ideal choice nutritionally but such a cereal consumed with milk is far preferable to no breakfast at all. It is always better to work with children's preferences than against them; changes should be introduced gradually and at a pace which the child will accept.

Food choice

Children will not necessarily prefer or need to consume the same foods as adults but their diets should be comprised of foods from the same healthy eating food groupings.

Bread, other cereals and potatoes group: 4 or more servings per day

Consumption of these foods should be encouraged as they are important providers of complex carbohydrate, fibre, B vitamins and some calcium and iron. Foods which are usually popular are: bread and rolls, breakfast cereals, pasta, rice, pizza, mashed and baked potatoes. Chips can be an occasional choice but preferably not the predominant one.

Wholemeal or wholegrain varieties of these foods can be encouraged but not excessively so, particularly in children at the younger end of the age range or who have a small appetite. It is far more important that children consume plenty of foods from this group than that all the foods consumed are 'healthy' choices.

Fruit and vegetables group: 4 or more servings per day

These are essential providers of vitamin C and other micronutrients, such as carotenes and folate, and most children consume far too little from this food group. Vegetables, especially green leafy vegetables and salad, are often disliked by this age group in which case it is better to find acceptable alternatives rather than to make an issue over 'eating up greens'. Diced or grated vegetables may be accepted as part of composite dishes such as pasta sauce, cottage pie, casseroles, soups or home-made hamburgers. The crunchy texture of stir-fried vegetables often appeals more than the traditionally boiled versions. Brightly coloured vegetables such as sweetcorn and peas tend to be more appealing than a heap of boiled cabbage.

Fresh fruit is ideal as a snack or dessert but there are other alternatives for those who refuse to eat an apple or a banana. Canned fruit (preferably in juice rather than syrup) may be enjoyed on its own, with custard or yogurt or mixed with jelly on a sponge flan base. Frozen fruit is also useful as a basis for desserts or mousses. Dried fruits, e.g. currants or raisins, are often acceptable as a snack. Drinks of fruit juice with meals should be encouraged as this will assist iron absorption as well as providing additional vitamin C. Fruit juice should be avoided between meals as the combination of its acidity and sugar content gives it a high cariogenic potential (see Chapter 28).

Milk and dairy foods group: 3–4 servings per day

(A glass of milk or carton of yogurt or approximately 30 g of cheese counts as one serving.)

These foods are vital as a source of calcium, riboflavin and protein. From the age of 5, skimmed or semi-skimmed milk and reduced-fat dairy products may be used. If children do not like milk on its own, it may be acceptable as a flavoured drink or in the form of custard, sauces, or soups. If not, the following should be encouraged:

Cubes of cheese (or individual portions of mini-cheeses)
Grated cheese (in sauces, as a topping on pizzas, toast or savoury dishes, in sandwiches, filled baked potatoes or added to mashed potato)
Yogurt (if disliked on its own is sometimes acceptable mixed with fruit purées)
Fromage frais
Cheese spread
Home-made ice cream containing milk

In children who consume very few of these foods, calcium intake can be boosted by foods such as white bread (fortified with calcium in the UK), canned fish such as pilchards or sardines, or green leafy vegetables. If consumption of milk and dairy foods is excluded altogether (e.g. milk intolerance, veganism) expert dietetic help should be sought.

Meat, fish and alternatives group: 1–2 servings per day

This group provides protein, iron, zinc and many B vitamins, especially B_{12}. Red meat or liver should be encouraged at least once a week because the bioavailability of iron and zinc is so much better from these foods than from other sources. Children who eat little or no meat must have a good iron intake from cereal and vegetable foods plus a high intake of vitamin C with meals if they are to meet their nutritional needs.

Chicken, turkey and fish (both white fish, such as fish fingers or fishcakes, and canned fish, such as pilchards or tuna) are also valuable foods although they are relatively low in iron.

Meat products such as burgers and sausages are popular with children but should be occasional choices rather than eaten every day. Reduced-fat versions are preferable.

Pulses such as peas and baked beans are liked by most children.

Fatty and sugary foods group

Inevitably foods such as crisps, cakes, biscuits, sweets and chocolate will be present in most children's diets. The important message to get across is that these foods can be part of the diet but should not be the mainstay of it nor, on their own, a substitute for a meal.

Advice concerning sugar-containing foods and drinks should focus on minimising the *frequency* of consumption more than the total amount since it is this factor more than the total amount consumed which is more relevant to the development of dental caries (see Chapter 28). It is also important that parents are encouraged to promote suitable alternatives to sugar-rich foods, i.e. more starchy carbohydrate foods such as bread or potatoes and more fruit and vegetables. If children simply eat more crisps and chips to compensate for fewer sweets and biscuits, the nutritional benefits will be negligible.

The consumption of savoury snack foods should not be at such a level that it displaces more important foods such as fruit and yogurt from the diet or reduces the appetite for a main meal.

Meal pattern

Breakfast is important. Not only can it make a valuable contribution to the daily intake of nutrients, particularly if it is comprised of breakfast cereal and milk (or bread/toast plus a drink of milk) but it is less likely to result in hunger later in the morning causing either poor concentration during lessons or a perceived need for snacks such as crisps or chocolate.

Children should be encouraged to sit down and eat at least one meal a day in the company of other people rather than continually eating snacks while on the move or in front of the television.

OTHER DIETARY ASPECTS

Vitamin and mineral supplements

Despite the fact micronutrient intakes tend to be low, widespread supplementation is not the answer (although it may be necessary in some individual cases).

The claim made a few years ago, that vitamins and mineral deficiencies in children impaired some aspects of non-verbal intelligence and that supplementation improved performance, led to high sales of certain vitamin and mineral supplements. Other carefully controlled studies have failed to repeat this finding and there is no evidence that, in general, such a measure is either necessary or beneficial[2]. Most parents who buy such supplements are those from higher income groups whose children are least in need of them and vitamin and mineral supplements certainly cannot boost the intelligence of those whose nutrient intake is already adequate. If money is short, purchase of supplements can place an unnecessary strain on the household finances. Above all, these products tend to foster the idea that an unhealthy, unbalanced diet is acceptable as long as supplements are taken and so do little to encourage the type of healthy eating pattern necessary for long-term health.

There are, however, sub-groups of children, particularly those from low income groups or deprived backgrounds, whose intake of some micronutrients is of concern[3]. It is well-established that anaemia can impair intellectual development in the early years and it is not unlikely that prolonged deficiencies of other nutrients have adverse

effects; iron, zinc and thiamin all have important effects on cognitive function. In such cases, every effort should be made to improve the quality and meal pattern of the diet. Supplements may be necessary if this cannot be achieved or if dietary intake is clearly deficient.

Nutrition education in schools

Attitudes to food and healthy eating will be influenced by understanding and experience gained at school. Children need to be taught what good nutrition means and why it is important, particularly in respect of their long-term health. They also need to know how to put it into practice by being given the opportunity to cook food, taste unfamiliar foods and make sensible food choices.

The British Nutrition Foundation, in conjunction with the Ministry of Agriculture, Fisheries and Food and the Department of Health, has produced an innovative teaching programme *Food – A Fact of Life* for use in schools[4]. This provides a framework for food and nutrition education at all levels (Key Stages 1, 2 and 3) of the National Curriculum together with resource material for both teachers and pupils.

School meals

Since the 1980 Education Act, schools are no longer obliged to provide meals for all children, only for those entitled to free school meals. Where meals are provided they no longer have to comply with the nutritional standards laid down in 1941, nor do they have to be sold at a statutory price. The majority of schools still provide meals of some kind (usually set meals in primary schools and a cash-cafeteria system in secondary schools) although fewer than half of all school children now consume school meals compared to about two-thirds of children 15 years ago[5]. The introduction of competitive tendering for school meals services in 1988 has not always assisted nutritional quality. While children are now more likely to be offered popular foods, such foods are often those which are least suitable choices on a daily basis (e.g. chips and burgers).

Although current school meals are not ideal they are important. For some children, the school meal is the only main meal of the day. About 1 in 6 secondary school children have nothing to eat before leaving for school and 1 in 10 do not have a cooked meal in the evening[6]. For some primary school children, the school meal is the only time they sit down and eat with other people; many will also be introduced to foods they would not be offered at home. Children receiving free school meals (often the most nutritionally deprived groups) are particularly dependent on the school meal as a source of vitamin C and other micronutrients[1].

It is not easy for those providing school meals to achieve a balance between what parents and contract purchasers wish to be provided (meat, potatoes, vegetables, salad, and fruit) and what the consumers themselves would prefer (pizzas, burgers, chips, sausage rolls and fizzy drinks). If 'healthy' food is provided and uptake is low, the service becomes financially unviable. The best school meals find a balance between the two. The schools themselves can also increase the benefits from school meals by:

- Providing children with guidance on sensible food choice.
- Making dining areas a pleasant environment in which to eat and chat with friends.
- Offering a breakfast service as well as lunch.
- Providing snacks such as sandwiches, filled rolls, fruit and milk drinks rather than confectionery and soft drinks.

In many areas of the country there are now local initiatives to improve the quality and uptake of school meals. A school-based nutrition policy can help develop consistency between what is taught about healthy eating in the classroom and what is available in the school dining area, tuck shop and

vending machines. The most successful of these policies are those which involve the children themselves in their construction[7]. The School Meals Campaign, launched in 1992 and which now has government support, can offer advice and help to those wishing to improve the quality of local school meals services.

DIET-RELATED PROBLEMS

Overweight and obesity (see also Chapter 25)

Overweight in children needs to be taken seriously. The overweight child can rapidly become the obese child who, in the short term, is likely to be a victim of taunting and teasing and, in the long term, is at risk of serious health problems.

It is important to identify the factors which have led to the above average weight gain:

- *Family history* Obese parents are more likely to have an obese child. Although there is a genetic susceptibility to obesity, this does not mean, as many parents believe, that obesity in their family is inevitable and nothing can be done about it. Very often, the inappropriate eating habits which enable obesity to develop in a parent are also those of the child.
- *Obesity history* The child who has been overweight since infancy will be more difficult to treat than those where the problem is more recent. In the latter case, possible psychological reasons for a sudden weight increase should be explored, e.g. comfort eating caused by a family break-up or bullying at school.
- *Dietary history* It is difficult to obtain meaningful dietary information from the parents of an obese child because they tend to give the answers that they think the health professional wants to hear, i.e. that the child rarely eats chips, sweets and only the occasional biscuit.

Even parents of normal weight children seem wracked by guilt at having to admit that their child eats these types of foods at all; the parents of an obese child are even more sensitive to the possible shortcomings in their child's diet. Prior to dietary enquiry it must be explained to the parents that their child's overweight results from an imbalance between energy consumed and energy required rather than the fact that their child (like most children) eats foods such as sweets. The weight problem can only be corrected if the reasons for this mismatch are identified. Once parents have this perspective they are more likely to provide accurate information.

A dietary record of the child's food intake for a week is useful, not to try to calculate calorie intake (which will almost certainly be underestimated) but to ascertain the typical meal pattern and the overall balance of foods from different food groups in the diet. This information can then be used as the basis for recommending dietary adjustments. Advice may not even be necessary; the act of writing everything down can make some parents realise just how much their child consumes in the form of unnecessary soft drinks and snacks.

■ *Activity level* Many overweight children dislike school sporting activities because of the associated teasing by their peers, but nevertheless for most children it is a compulsory part of school life. Asking children what they do outside school hours may give a better indication of their physical activity level. Those who do not mention playing football, swimming, going horse-riding or to dancing classes, or belonging to cubs, guides, etc., are likely to be spending more of their leisure time in front of the TV.

Strict dieting is never appropriate in this age group because a drastically reduced energy intake will also reduce intake of micronutrients to undesirably low levels. Serious obesity in a child should be referred to a dietitian. Moderate overweight can be managed within the primary care setting by encouraging a better dietary balance from the four major groups and a lower consumption of fatty and sugary foods. This should stop further weight increase and enable children to 'grow into' their weight. Parental support is essential; if being fat is regarded as the norm in a particular family and no-one is particularly concerned about it, then dietary advice is likely to be ignored.

Overweight in children resulting from comfort eating will not be resolved until the underlying emotional problems are tackled.

Underweight

In any child who is underweight three possibilities must be considered:

(1) The presence of a medical problem affecting appetite, absorption or metabolism.
(2) An inadequate nutrient intake.
(3) That nothing is wrong; the child may simply be at the extreme end of the normal distribution curve.

In the absence of obvious signs or symptoms of disease, a nutritional explanation should be explored, particularly if the rate of growth has crossed a centile curve (see 'Growth' in Chapter 6). Dietary inadequacy may result from:

■ *Poor appetite* – resulting from anxiety (bullying, family tensions), abuse or neglect, or too much fluid prior to or with meals.
■ *Food restriction by the child* – using food refusal as a means of gaining attention, slimming due to peer pressure or imitation of a parent, or anorexia nervosa.
■ *Food restriction by the parent* – for moral or 'health' reasons.
■ *Lack of dietary energy* – inadequate food provision due to ignorance, poverty or neglect.

■ *Lack of one or more nutrients* – poor food choice or provision.

Management of underweight depends on its cause. Many parents can be reassured that there is no fundamental problem. Poor eating habits due to unbalanced food groups or poor meal patterns can usually be resolved by explanation and education. Psychosocial eating problems resulting from tensions within the family can sometimes be ameliorated by appropriate discussion and counselling. Severe behavioural disturbance or signs of obsessive slimming, or concerns about child neglect or abuse require expert referral.

Dental caries (see also Chapter 28)

The most important preventative measures in children are:

■ Regular use of fluoride toothpaste and good oral hygiene.
■ Reducing the frequency of consumption of sugar-containing foods, particularly between meals.
■ Regular dental check-ups.

Vegetarianism/veganism (see also Chapter 21)

Inappropriate vegetarian diets can be low in energy and micronutrients, especially iron and zinc, and can impair growth and health. It is vital that vegan children (who exclude all foods of animal origin including milk) consume alternative sources of calcium and vitamin B_{12}.

Food intolerance (see also Chapter 40)

In this age group suspected food intolerance should always be referred to a dietitian as the risk of deficiencies from food exclusion is high. Parentally diagnosed cases of 'allergy' should also receive expert attention as this often results in children being given distorted diets of poor nutrient content, particularly if important foods such as milk or bread are excluded.

REFERENCES

1 Department of Health (1989) *The Diets of British Schoolchildren.* COMA Report on Health and Social Subjects 36. HMSO, London.
2 Crombie, I.K. *et al.* (1990) Effect of vitamin and mineral supplementation on verbal and non-verbal reasoning of schoolchildren. *Lancet* 335, 744–7.
3 Nelson, M. (1992) Vitamin and mineral supplementation and academic performance in schoolchildren. *Proceedings of the Nutrition Society.* 51, 303–13.
4 British Nutrition Foundation *Food – A Fact of Life.* A nutrition education programme for use in schools. British Nutrition Foundation, London.
5 The Gardner Merchant School Meals Survey (1990) Details from: Gardner Merchant Ltd, Stonehill Green, Westlea, Swindon, Wiltshire SN5 7UD.
6 Balding, J. (1988) *Young People in 1987.* Health Education Authority Schools Health Education Unit, Exeter.
7 Harvey, J. & Passmore, S. (1994) *School Nutrition Action Groups: A New Policy for Managing Food and Nutrition in Schools.* Birmingham Health Education Unit in association with The Meat and Livestock Commission. Details from: Health Education Unit, Martineau Centre, 74 Balden Road, Harborne, Birmingham B32 2EH.

FURTHER READING

Caroline Walker Trust (1992) *Nutritional Guidelines for School Meals.* The Caroline Walker Trust, London. Details from: School Meals, PO Box 7, London W3 6XJ.

Health Education Authority (1995) *Diet and Health in School Age Children*. A Briefing Paper prepared by Anne Coles and Sheila Turner. HEA, London.

RESOURCES

Video *Healthy Eating for Children* by Jayne Wolliner SRD.
    This is designed for parents and child carers but is suitable for use by health professionals for group work to stimulate discussion. Details from: Axiom One Ltd, 26 Lupus Street, London SW1V 3DZ. Tel: 0171 821 9157.

USEFUL ADDRESSES

The School Meals Campaign, PO Box 402, London WC1H 9TZ. Tel: 0171 383 7638.

The new growth centile charts produced by the Child Growth Foundation (see, 'Growth' in Chapter 6) may be purchased from: Harlow Printing Ltd, Maxwell Street, South Shields, Tyne & Wear NE33 4PU. Tel: 0191 455 4286.

16

Adolescents and Young Adults

Adolescence is a period of transition and this applies to eating habits too. Teenagers have increasing control over what and when they eat. Experimentation with new foods, food patterns or type of foods is common. Most eat less food at home with the family and more outside in the company of friends. Regular meals may be replaced by a pattern of 'grazing' – snacks and fast foods eaten throughout the day in accordance with hunger and availability.

This age group is notoriously unreceptive to healthy eating advice. Many are well aware of what they should be eating; most choose to disregard it. Peer pressure is high and fashions for particular foods or diets are common; many adopt vegetarianism or start slimming. A few develop an obsessional interest in food leading to anorexia nervosa or bulimia.

NUTRITIONAL CONSIDERATIONS

Adolescence is a time of rapid growth and the primary dietary need is for energy. A finicky child may be transformed into a teenager with a voracious appetite for anything and everything.

Ideally, the proportion of this dietary energy supplied by fat and carbohydrate should comply with healthy eating recommendations. In practice, dietary surveys on this age group show that this is usually not the case; average consumption of fat and sugars is high while that of carbohydrate and fibre is low[1,2]. While undesirable, in the short term such a diet will probably not do much harm. The problems arise if a diet of this type persists into adulthood thus increasing health risks in later life.

Teenagers' diets are also often of low nutrient density, i.e. providing a low level of vitamins and minerals relative to their energy content. Overt nutritional deficiencies are rare and most likely to be seen in those who deliberately manipulate their dietary intake, ironically often on the grounds of 'health'. Marginal deficiencies which may have health implications in later life may however be more common, especially in people from low income groups, or who have low educational attainment or are unemployed. Nutrients of particular concern are:

- *Calcium* About 45% of adult skeletal mass is formed during adolescence. Bones grow in length and once this process is completed calcium is laid down to maximise bone strength. Peak bone mass is reached between the ages of 20 and 30; after this age, bone mass declines. The higher the level of peak bone mass achieved, the lower the risk of osteoporosis in later life (see Chapter 36). Calcium is thus of vital importance in this age group but it seems likely that in many young people, particularly girls, this need is not being met[3].
- *Iron* Signs of iron deficiency are not uncommon among adolescents, particularly girls who tend to have a lower dietary intake of iron than

boys but have higher iron requirements. The prevalence of anaemia in adolescent girls has been found to be in the region of 10% and at least as many again have been found to have low iron stores[4]. The problem is more common in disadvantaged groups, such as those on low incomes, and also in teenage girls who are vegetarians or on slimming diets in whom the prevalence of iron deficiency may be as high as 25%.

Because of the high iron needs of teenage girls, and because red meat is normally the largest contributor to iron intake (almost 20%) in this age group[5], dietary exclusion of meat necessitates measures to ensure adequate iron intake from other sources. In the teenage diet, breakfast cereals, bread and potatoes (including chips) are likely to be important sources of iron.

■ *Other micronutrients* Intakes of other micronutrients such as zinc, copper, thiamin, riboflavin and B$_6$ have also been shown to be generally low in teenagers[2].

DIETARY GUIDANCE

Teenagers are rarely impressed by arguments that they should eat a healthy diet in order to protect themselves against heart disease or osteoporosis in later life; most simply cannot envisage themselves ever being that old. Appealing to vanity can be more successful; if teenagers think a healthy lifestyle means looking leaner, fitter, and more attractive they may be more interested.

Food choice

As with other age groups, teenagers should be encouraged to consume a variety of foods from all four major food groups.

Bread, other cereals and potatoes group: 4–6 or more servings per day

Foods such as bread, pasta, rice, baked potatoes should be used as much as possible to satisfy hunger.

Fruit and vegetables group: 5 servings per day

Some teenagers include very few of these foods in their diet. Consumption of fresh fruit, fruit juice, salad or other vegetables should be encouraged, especially in those who do not consume meat and so need to maximise their absorption of non-haem iron.

Milk and dairy foods group: 4 or more servings per day

In this age group it is almost impossible to meet the high requirement for calcium if plenty of these foods are not consumed. Reduced-fat versions are preferable in health terms and provide the same amount of calcium as full-fat products.

Meat, fish and alternatives group: 2–3 servings per day

Some meat, poultry, fish, eggs, beans or pulses should be eaten every day. Meat products with a high fat content (sausages, burgers) should feature less often. If no red meat is consumed at all, alternative sources of iron must be considered (see p. 145).

Fatty and sugary foods group

A diet comprised mainly of fry-ups, cola, crisps and chocolate bars is not a good idea. Most teenagers will not be prepared to forego these foods nor is it necessary to suggest that they should do so, although they can be encouraged to choose reduced-fat and low sugar versions where possible. The main point to emphasis is that these foods should be an adjunct to foods from the four main food groups, not a total substitute for them.

OTHER DIETARY ASPECTS

Additional points to make are:

■ *The importance of breakfast* For many teenagers and young adults, breakfast is either nothing at all or a bag of crisps or chocolate bar on the way to college or work. Teenagers who regularly consume breakfast comprised of a cereal food (breakfast cereal or bread) and milk have a demonstrably higher intake of micronutrients such as riboflavin, folate and calcium[6]. Breakfast also lessens the desire for a succession of fat and sugar-rich snacks later in the morning.

■ *The importance of eating some fresh food every day* Not everything consumed should come out of a packet, box or can.

■ *Physical exercise* Regular exercise is important for fitness and also has a vital part to play in maximising bone mass since bones, like muscles, increase their strength when they are worked. Acquiring the exercise habit in the teenage years increases the likelihood of regular exercise in the adult years.

■ *Alcohol* Guidance on the sensible use of alcohol is very important for this age group. In particular they need guidance on how to assess the alcoholic strength of any drinks they consume (see Chapter 4, *Sensible Drinking*). The rule of thumb guidance that one unit of alcohol is contained in half a pint of beer or one glass of wine or one measure of spirits is often misinterpreted. Many teenagers assume this to mean that any can of beer or lager contains one unit of alcohol. This can be a considerable underestimate. Some of the canned products which are fashionable among young people contain considerably more than half a pint and have a much higher alcoholic strength than standard beer. One 440 ml can of extra strong (9%) lager may provide 4 of units alcohol, so 3 or 4 cans are equivalent to 12–16 single measures of Scotch.

Low alcohol drinks are not always as low in alcohol as people imagine; some are virtually alcohol-free but others have between one-third and one-quarter of the usual strength.

Many teenagers/young adults are not only novice drinkers but also novice drivers. Mistakes resulting from inexperience are likely to happen in either area. Mistakes made in both areas simultaneously are particularly likely to have lethal consequences.

DIET-RELATED PROBLEMS

Overweight and slimming

About 8% of teenagers are, by normal criteria, overweight. However, about 25% of teenage girls consider themselves to be overweight and well over 50% admit to dieting in the recent past, a prevalence which may rise to 75% in the later teenage years[7]. Many are therefore making unnecessary reductions in energy intake and this has been shown to have a significant impact on the intake of many important micronutrients, particularly calcium, iron and many B vitamins[8]. This is of considerable concern.

Boys appear to be less likely to want to lose weight and many are more preoccupied with trying to increase their physique. Those who do want to lose weight tend to prefer to increase their exercise levels rather than diet.

Teenagers who do need to lose weight, or those who are determined to do so, should be discouraged from dieting by skipping meals or following the latest fad diet advocating a restricted and often bizarre choice of foods. Sensible slimming advice should focus on adjustment of the proportion of food groups (i.e. more from the bread/cereals and fruit and vegetable groups; fewer from the sugary/fatty foods group and adequate amounts of low or reduced-fat components of the milk/dairy foods and meat/fish groups).

LIVERPOOL
JOHN MOORES UNIVERSITY
AVRIL ROBARTS LRC
TEL. 0151 231 4022

Anorexia nervosa/bulimia
(see also Chapter 26)

Only a small proportion of teenage dieting progresses to anorexia nervosa or bulimia but most eating disorders originate with slimming. The factors which lead to a desire for moderate weight loss becoming an obsession with body size and shape and distorted perception of body image are complex, and are usually due to underlying emotional or psychological disturbance. The consequences of eating disorders are serious and often fatal, and it vital that signs of their development are picked up at an early stage. Psychiatric and dietetic referral is essential.

Acne

Contrary to popular belief, there is little scientific evidence that acne is related to a high consumption of fatty or sugary foods. It has simply been assumed that because these are typical features of teenagers they must be causally linked. Hormonal factors and skin hygiene are more important determinants of acne.

Vegetarianism
(see also Chapter 21)

Teenage vegetarianism can be a problem because in this age group it so often results in a nutritionally inadequate diet. This need not be the case and teenagers who take the trouble to find out about and follow recommended vegetarian dietary guidelines will not be nutritionally at risk. More typically though, teenagers simply stop eating meat and fail to consider what needs to be eaten instead. Most assume that other foods such as cheese, eggs or yogurt are an adequate substitute for meat. In terms of protein they are, but in terms of minerals, especially iron and zinc, they are not and other dietary adjustments must be made to ensure that these nutrients are provided. If this does not happen, teenage girls are likely to enter their adult child-bearing years in a state of chronic iron deficit.

Family conflicts over vegetarianism sometimes need to be defused. Many teenagers are highly committed to the moral principle behind vegetarianism and parental hostility will not make them alter what may be strongly held views. Parents should respect their teenager's point of view and encourage them to obtain sensible dietary guidance and make it possible for it to be followed. The teenager needs to accept that others have the right to a different opinion from their own and that the views of one person should not be allowed to dominate the household.

REFERENCES

1 Crawley, H. (1993) The energy, nutrient and food intakes of teenagers aged 16–17 years in Britain. *British Journal of Nutrition* 70, 15–26.
2 Bull, N.L. (1985) Dietary habits of 15 to 25 year olds. Report of a survey conducted for the Ministry of Agriculture, Fisheries and Food. *Human Nutrition: Applied Nutrition* **39A**, Supplement 1, 1–68.
3 Department of Health (1989) *The Diets of British Schoolchildren.* COMA Report on Health and Social Subjects 36. HMSO, London.
4 Nelson, M., White, J. & Rhodes, C. (1993) Haemoglobin, ferritin and iron intakes in British children aged 12–14 years: a preliminary investigation. *British Journal of Nutrition* 70, 147–55.
5 Moynihan, P.J. *et al.* (1994) Dietary sources of iron in English adolescents. *Journal of Human Nutrition and Dietetics* 7, 225–30.
6 Crawley, H. (1993) The role of breakfast cereals in the diets of 16–17 year old teenagers in Britain. *Journal of Human Nutrition and Dietetics* 6, 205–16.
7 Balding, J. (1988) *Young People in 1987.* Health Education Authority Schools Health Education Unit, Exeter.
8 Crawley, H. & Shergill-Bonner, R. (1995) The nutrient and food intakes of 16–17 year old female dieters. *Journal of Human Nutrition and Dietetics* 8, 25–34.

FURTHER READING

Health Education Authority (1994) *That's The Limit. A Guide to Sensible Drinking.* HEA, London.
National Dairy Council (1995) *Nutrition and Teenagers.* Fact File 5 (revised edition). NDC, London.

17

Elderly People

The UK has an increasingly ageing population. Thirty years ago, about 1 in 8 of the population was aged 65 years or over. Currently, this figure is about 1 in 6. In thirty years time, it is estimated that it will have risen to 1 in 4[1].

However, the 9 million 'elderly people' in the UK are a diverse group. Some are as fit and active as people many years younger, others are frail and require a high level of care. This needs to be taken into account when dietary recommendations are being applied.

NUTRITIONAL CONSIDERATIONS

Dietary aims in this age group are:

- To maintain health and fitness with advancing years.
- To support the most frail and vulnerable.

In terms of nutritional objectives, elderly people can be broadly categorised as:

- 'Young elderly' people   65–74 years
- 'Older elderly' people   75 years or above
  This older group contains a sub-group of 'Frail elderly' people.

Young elderly people may have at least 20 years of active life ahead of them and promoting health and fitness is the priority. In the older group, the objective is to attain good quality of life, maintaining health for as long as possible and minimising the effects of chronic disability and illness.

Nutritional needs and problems of elderly people were discussed in detail in the 1992 Department of Health's COMA report *The Nutrition of Elderly People*[1]. This concluded that, in general, healthy eating guidelines are as relevant to older people as to younger adults. In terms of dietary composition, it recommended that elderly people should also consume more energy in the form of carbohydrate and less as fat, and that non-milk extrinsic sugars should not comprise more than 10% of energy intake. However, these guidelines need to be applied with an element of commonsense. Healthy eating objectives are important in younger elderly people and remain relevant in anyone remaining fit and active. They should not be applied too zealously in those who are frail or ill; in such people a 'healthy diet' may have quite a different composition.

Energy

The requirement for energy tends to decline with advancing years, particularly if people become less active. However, the requirement for protein, vitamins and minerals is unchanged. This means that even if energy intake falls, the intake of these other nutrients needs to stay the same. The diet therefore needs to be nutrient dense, i.e. contain foods which are rich in essential nutrients rather than those which supply mainly energy alone.

nutrient absorption and can cause intestinal obstruction.

Fat

Plasma cholesterol level remains a predictor of coronary heart disease at least up to the age of 70 years and possibly beyond[2]. Advice to reduce consumption of total and saturated fat is therefore reasonable advice for 'younger' elderly people. Above the age of 75, fat restriction is less likely to be beneficial since the atherosclerotic effects of a high cholesterol level will already have occurred. In this age group it is probably more important to concentrate on reducing the risk of thrombosis, e.g. by increasing the consumption of the fatty acids found in fish oils.

Fat restriction is not appropriate in those who, for reasons of illness or frailty, have a small appetite.

Fibre/non-starch polysaccharide

Fibre, particularly insoluble fibre, is an important dietary constituent in this age group who have a high prevalence of constipation and are at high risk of more serious bowel disorders. Consumption of cereal foods, and fruit and vegetables should be encouraged. Wholegrain or wholemeal varieties of cereals are the best sources of insoluble fibre but people with small appetites should not consume too many of these foods because their bulkiness tends to compromise the intake of other foods and nutrients. Excessively high fibre intakes, particularly of phytate-containing cereals, will also impair the absorption of some minerals and trace elements and this may have a significant effect in someone whose intake of these nutrients is already low. Raw bran is not a suitable source of fibre because it impairs

Sugars

Many elderly people have a high sugar intake. Whether this matters depends on the quality of the rest of the diet. A diet containing a high proportion of cakes, biscuits and confectionery will have a low nutrient density and it is important that some of these foods are replaced by others containing more essential nutrients (e.g. bread, fruit and dairy foods). However, it makes little sense to deprive a 90-year-old of the pleasure of sugar in their tea if their diet is otherwise adequate. In the elderly person who is ill, convalescent or has a poor appetite, sugar in the form of sweetened drinks and snacks may be an important way of ensuring that energy needs are met.

Salt

A high salt intake may increase blood pressure and hence the risks associated with hypertension, particularly stroke[3]. Many elderly people do add a lot of salt to their food, either out of habit or because of declining taste sensitivity. It is recommended that salt intake in this age group should be reduced but this must be done in a way which does not impair appetite (by making food too bland) or compromise nutrient intake (by eliminating important sources of other nutrients, e.g. cheese or Marmite).

Iron

Anaemia is a common feature in this age group. Iron deficiency from a low iron intake is likely to be exacerbated by poor iron absorption and blood loss resulting from gastrointestinal disorders or the use of certain drugs. Iron requirements will also be increased by chronic infection or inflammation. Haem iron (from red meat) is particularly valuable in this age group because of its high absorbability and the fact that relatively large amounts can be obtained from a relatively small quantity of food. Those who obtain most of their iron in the non-haem form (e.g. cereals and vegetables) need to consume plenty of vitamin C.

Zinc

Zinc plays an important part in wound healing and the possibility of a low zinc intake should be considered in those with leg ulcers and pressure sores. As with iron, the richest and most available source of zinc is red meat.

Calcium

Calcium is important to help maintain bone mass. Bone tissue starts to be lost after the age of 30 and the rate of loss accelerates sharply after the menopause. Whether this results in clinical osteoporosis depends on the level of peak bone mass achieved during early adulthood and whether preventative measures such as hormone replacement therapy are instituted at an appropriate time (see Chapter 36, *Osteoporosis*). A high calcium intake in later life will not in itself prevent osteoporosis or restore the tissue lost from bone; it may however slow down the rate of calcium loss. Inadequate calcium intakes will almost certainly increase the rate of loss. Calcium intake is likely to be below the recommended intake if consumption of milk and dairy products is low.

Other minerals and trace elements

Intake of nutrients such as magnesium, potassium and copper may be at risk in elderly people who consume an unvaried diet of low nutrient density.

Vitamin D

Vitamin D controls calcium absorption and its deficiency in this age group can leads to bone softening and distortion (osteomalacia, see Chapter 37). Many elderly people have little sunlight exposure so are less likely to meet their vitamin D requirements from this source. Vitamin D supplementation ($10\,\mu g$/day) is a sensible precaution during the winter months and in those who are housebound or living in institutions.

B group vitamins

Thiamin and riboflavin intakes may be inadequate in those with low energy intakes and diets of a low nutrient density. Folate and B_{12} are often poorly absorbed in this age group and marginal intakes may result in symptoms of deficiency such as megaloblastic anaemia.

Antioxidant nutrients

Vitamins C, E, beta-carotene and selenium are especially important because of their role in immune function and wound healing, both of which tend to become less efficient with increasing age. Antioxidants may also help protect against cancer and heart disease. Elderly people often avoid, or have a low intake of, the most important sources of these nutrients (fruit, vegetables and wholegrain cereals). Encouraging the consumption of these foods is an important aspect of health promotion.

DIETARY GUIDANCE

All elderly people should be encouraged to:

■ Enjoy and maintain an interest in food.
■ Eat a varied diet.
■ Eat a balanced diet.

Because of the diversity of this population group, specific dietary guidance must be applied with the following factors in mind:

■ Age, health and degree of activity.
■ Residential circumstances (living alone, with others, in sheltered accommodation or in residential care).
■ The presence of underweight.
■ The presence of overweight.
■ The presence of disability.
■ Factors such as illness or convalescence.

Food choice

General dietary guidelines which can be used both as a basis for giving advice and for assessing the likelihood of nutritional inadequacies are:

Bread, other cereals and potatoes group: 4 or more servings per day

These foods should form an important part of every meal. They are cheap, convenient and a valuable source of many nutrients, particularly B vitamins and minerals. Consumption of a breakfast cereal (fortified with vitamins and minerals) should be encouraged.

Wholegrain and wholemeal cereal foods are the best sources of insoluble fibre (and thus the most effective in treating or preventing constipation) but all types of foods in this group provide some fibre. A high fibre intake is inadvisable in those with poor appetites.

Fruit and vegetables group: 4 or more servings per day

Consumption of foods from this group usually needs to be encouraged. People who find it difficult to eat raw fruit may be able cope with softer canned or cooked fruit. Fruit juice is a useful source of vitamin C.

People who find the preparation of fresh vegetables difficult should be encouraged to use more frozen or canned vegetables instead (elderly people often mistakenly assume that these have no 'goodness' in them). Elderly people should be dissuaded from the common practices of overcooking green vegetables or adding bicarbonate of soda to the cooking water, both of which destroy vitamin content.

Milk and dairy foods group: 3 servings per day

These are valuable sources of protein and riboflavin and essential providers of calcium. Younger elderly people who are fit and active should be encouraged to consume reduced-fat milk and milk products. People who are ill, have small appetites or are underweight should use full-fat products because of their higher content of energy and vitamin A.

Meat, fish and alternatives group: 2 servings per day

Red meat is particularly useful because of its content of iron, protein and zinc. The quantity consumed does not have to be large; a small amount of lean meat provides a lot of nutrients. Nor need the most expensive cuts be chosen; casseroled cheaper cuts of meat and foods such as liver are just as nutritious and usually popular with this age group.

Regular consumption of oily fish, such as sardines, pilchards, herrings, mackerel and salmon, may help reduce the risk of thrombosis. Canned varieties are easy to use and usually good value for money.

To reduce the risk of salmonella, eggs should be well-cooked. The consumption of raw egg (e.g. a drink of raw egg and milk) should be strongly discouraged.

Fatty and sugary foods group

As in other age groups, consumption of these foods should not be at such a level that it prevents the consumption of more nutrient-rich foods. People who are overweight obviously need to watch their food intake from this group. But for most elderly people, the maxim 'a little of what you fancy . . .' is applicable.

OTHER DIETARY ASPECTS

Physical activity

Maintaining physical activity is also important, not only to avoid obesity but also to help minimise bone loss, maintain muscle mass and for cardiac health.

Store-cupboard advice

A list of store cupboard suggestions may be helpful for those who live alone, as a reserve for times when illness or bad weather make shopping difficult. Such items are:

Cartons of longlife milk
Cartons of longlife fruit juice

Canned or packet soups
Canned meat or fish (e.g. sardines, pilchards, tuna, corned beef)
Canned vegetables, packets of instant mashed potato
Canned fruit, dried fruit
Canned milk puddings and custards
Breakfast cereals
Crackers and biscuits
Marmalade, jam, peanut butter, Bovril, Marmite
Malted milk or hot chocolate drinks
Complan or Build-up

ASSESSING NUTRITIONAL ADEQUACY

Food intake

A 24-hour recall (or, if memory is poor, building up a picture of a typical day's food intake) cannot provide an accurate quantitative guide to nutrient intake but is nevertheless a valuable starting point for assessing dietary adequacy. Comparison of the representation of different food groups within a person's usual diet with those recommended for dietary balance (see above) will reveal any major dietary shortcomings. A low intake of foods from one of the four major groups (particularly milk or meat) or virtual absence of a food group (e.g. fruit and vegetables) increases the probability of dietary deficiency. A poor meal pattern (e.g. no breakfast or long periods without food) and a lack of variety in food choice (e.g. the tendency to eat the same foods every day) also increases the likelihood of nutritional inadequacies, particularly if intake is borderline.

Psychosocial factors

Individual circumstances should also be considered. The risk of an inadequate energy and nutrient intake is increased in people who:

- Live alone and with little family support.
- Are housebound.
- Find shopping and cooking difficult.
- Do not have at least one hot meal every day.
- Have a poor appetite.
- Have eating difficulties (e.g. poor dentition or swallowing disorders).
- Have a chronic illness, especially of gastrointestinal origin.
- Are in general poor health.
- Are depressed.
- Have suffered recent bereavement of a close friend or relative.
- Suffer from memory loss or dementia.
- Have a low income.

The more of these factors that are present, the greater the likelihood of nutritional inadequacy.

Body weight

Body weight is one of the most important indicators of nutritional status in elderly people. Low body weight often reflects poor nutritional status and is associated with an increased risk of infections, fractures, pressure sores or venous ulcers. A fall in body weight is suggestive of developing disease or dietary problems and requires investigation (see 'Underweight' in 'Diet-related problems' below).

Excess body weight also has important health risks in terms of morbidity and mortality. Obesity exacerbates joint disorders making mobility painful or difficult and also increases the risks from joint replacement surgery. It also increases the likelihood of hypertension and diabetes which in turn enhances the risk of stroke and coronary heart disease. The diagnosis and management of overweight and obesity in elderly people are discussed later in this chapter.

PEOPLE LIVING IN RESIDENTIAL CARE

Only a small proportion of elderly people live in residential homes but this still represents about three-quarters of a million people and the numbers are increasing[4]. The quality of nutritional care within residential homes is variable. Most institutions attempt to provide meals which meet the needs of elderly people as a group. Many are less successful at identifying or meeting the needs of particular individuals, particularly where there are financial constraints or staff shortages. It is the failure to consider individual need that usually leads to nutritional problems.

Factors which are most likely to result in a diet of low nutritional quality are listed below.

Inadequate food provision

- General lack of fresh foods.
- Heavy reliance on convenience foods of low nutrient quality (e.g. rissoles, fishcakes).
- Over-boiled vegetables of low vitamin content.
- Lack of fresh fruit (too time-consuming for staff to peel).
- Dull, bland, unappetising food.
- Lack of food choice at a meal.
- An over-repetitive menu offering little variety.

Lack of attention to individual need

- Portion sizes all the same irrespective of need.
- Inflexible timing of meals.
- Long periods without food (e.g. last food of the day provided at 5PM).
- Inadequate help given to those with feeding difficulties or behavioural disturbance.
- Inadequate time allowed to consume a meal before it is cleared away.
- Little monitoring of developing overweight or underweight.
- Little thought given to drug-nutrient interactions.
- Little attention paid to dental health or dentition.
- High prevalence of use of laxatives and suppositories.
- General imposition of fluid restriction to minimise incontinence.

DIET-RELATED PROBLEMS

Underweight

Energy requirements often increase during illness or following physiological stress such as a fracture or surgery. At the same time, appetite and food intake are likely to be reduced and there is a high likelihood of energy needs not being met. Fat stores and then muscle tissue will be used as an energy source resulting in body wasting. If energy intake remains inadequate, dietary protein will primarily be used for energy creation rather than for tissue maintenance or repair. Low energy intake is also likely to result in a low intake of micronutrients and this further compromises immune competence thus perpetuat-

ing the situation by prolonging illness or delaying healing.

Whether caused by increased requirements, inadequate intake or a combination of the two, the presence of underweight always indicates that energy intake is inadequate and increasing this is the first dietary priority. Boosting protein or vitamin and mineral intake should be seen as a useful adjunct to a good supply of energy but should not be a substitute for it. By themselves, these nutrients can exert little benefit while the energy deficit remains.

Practical ways of increasing energy and nutrient intake in people with small appetites or high requirements are discussed in Chapter 8, *Nutritional Support and Supplementation*. The use of sip feed energy supplements can be a valuable way of improving nutritional status in underweight elderly people.

If body weight is below 45 kg in women and 50 kg in men, referral to a dietitian is advisable.

Overweight and obesity

BMI (weight/height squared) is a less useful measurement of adiposity in elderly people than in other adults because the height component of the index is often difficult to measure accurately. Some elderly people are bed-bound or unable to stand upright; others may have lost height as a result of spinal bone loss or narrowed vertebral discs and this will reduce the validity of the calculated BMI. An alternative method of assessing body size in elderly people is the demispan which is the distance from the web between the fingers to the middle of the chest when the arm is outstretched. This can easily be measured from a person sitting, or even lying down. This measurement can then be used to calculate an similar index to the BMI, the 'Demiquet Index' (weight in kg divided by the squared demispan in metres). Alternatively, a simpler version the 'Mindex' (weight divided by the demispan) can be derived. Normal ranges for these indices, which can be used to identify people at both extremes of the range (i.e. either high or low adiposity), are given in the Department of Health report *Nutrition of Elderly People*, p. 19[1].

Obesity in elderly people is undesirable because it greatly increases the risk of diabetes and joint disorders. Prevention is always better than cure and an important aspect of health promotion in younger elderly people is the avoidance of weight increase with age, particularly if activity level declines.

For those who become overweight, strict dieting is not advisable as this reduces the intake of essential nutrients. Instead people should be encouraged to alter the balance of their diets, eating fewer foods from the fatty and sugary foods group and more from the bread, other cereals and potatoes, and fruit and vegetables groups. Increasing the amount of regular, gentle exercise undertaken will also help achieve slow, steady weight loss.

Constipation

Elderly people are particularly likely to suffer from constipation because:

- They often find it difficult to eat fibrous foods.
- They may take little exercise (exercise stimulates gastrointestinal motility).
- They may have a low fluid intake (due to fears of incontinence or having to get up at night).

Laxative use is high among elderly people and they are often given routinely to those in residential care. In the vast majority of cases this is totally unnecessary. Chronic laxative use tends to compound the problem and some types of laxatives, e.g. liquid paraffin, impair nutrient absorption.

Attempts should always be made to treat constipation by dietary means such as increasing consumption of fluid and fibre. This need not mean eating lots of wholemeal bread or coarse vegetables. Eating more cereal foods generally (white bread, breakfast cereals, etc.) and soft veg-etables (e.g. mashed potato; diced vegetables added to casseroles) will all increase fibre intake.

Bran should not be added to food; it reduces the absorption of many minerals and can, if consumed without sufficient fluid, cause intestinal obstruction.

Drug-nutrient interactions

Elderly people frequently take medication, often for prolonged periods of time. Many drugs have nutritional implications because they may:

- Decrease appetite (e.g. cytotoxic drugs).
- Cause nausea, vomiting or diarrhoea (e.g. antibiotics).
- Alter gut flora (e.g. warfarin).
- Reduce nutrient absorption (e.g. liquid paraffin).
- Interfere with nutrient metabolism (e.g. tricyclic antidepressants).
- Increase nutrient excretion (e.g. diuretics).

In people who are nutritionally depleted or on the borderline of nutritional adequacy, drug-nutrient interactions may be sufficient to precipitate an acute deficiency.

Swallowing difficulties
(see Chapter 29)

Physical disability (see Chapter 18)

REFERENCES

1   Department of Health (1992) *The Nutrition of Elderly People*. Report on Health and Social Subjects 43. HMSO, London.

2 Shipley, M.J. *et al.* (1991) Does plasma cholesterol concentration predict mortality from coronary heart disease in elderly people? 18 year follow-up in the Whitehall Study. *British Medical Journal* 303, 89–92.

3 Department of Health (1994) *Nutritional Aspects of Cardiovascular Disease.* Report of the COMA Cardiovascular Review Group. Report on Health and Social Subjects 46. HMSO, London.

4 Central Statistical Office (1993) *Social Trends 23.* HMSO, London.

Davies, L. (1993) *Easy Cooking in Retirement.* Penguin, London.

Help the Aged (1994) *Healthy Eating: A Help the Aged Advice Leaflet.* Produced in association with the Nutrition Advisory Group of the British Dietetic Association with support from Heinz. Available from: Help the Aged, St James's Walk, London EC1R 0BE, Tel: 0171 253 0253.

National Dairy Council (1992) *Nutrition and Elderly People.* Fact File 9. NDC, London.

National Dairy Council/Health Visitors' Association (1992) *Good Nutrition for Older People.* A practical interpretation of the Department of Health's report on *The Nutrition of Elderly People.* National Dairy Council, London.

FURTHER READING

Ageing Well (UK) (1994) *Health Promotion with Older People. Ideas for Primary Health Care Teams.* Available from: Age Concern England, Astral House, 1268 London Road, London SW16 4ER on receipt of A4 sae (at the 60 g+ rate).

Caroline Walker Trust (1995) *Eating Well for Older People.* Report of an Expert Working Group. Further details from: 'Older people', Broadcast Support Services, PO Box 7, London W3 6XJ.

USEFUL ADDRESSES

Age Concern England, Astral House, 1268 London Road, London SW16 4ER. Details of resource material for primary health care teams available on request. Mail order: Tel: 0181 679 8000.

Help the Aged, St James's Walk, London EC1R 0BE. Tel: 0171 253 0253. Details of resource material for elderly people available on request.

18

People with Physical or Learning Disabilities

People with disabilities have the same nutritional needs as everyone else but because the practical difficulties of meeting these needs are so much greater, their diets are more likely to be inadequate or inappropriate. This risk is not confined to people with severe difficulties such as those confined to wheelchairs. People who can do very little for themselves may have good support services; those with milder disabilities who have to fend for themselves often have a much poorer diet.

PHYSICAL DISABILITIES

Physical disability affects food procurement. People may find it difficult to:

Obtain food: Shopping and carrying heavy bags may be difficult.

Prepare food: Peeling vegetables or opening a tin may be impossible.

Cook food: Lifting pans of water on and off a cooker may be hazardous.

Eat food: They may not be able to hold a knife and fork.

Swallow food: Their disability may result in swallowing difficulties.

These problems may be compounded by factors such as low income, loneliness and isolation and depression.

All these factors affect the types of foods consumed and often result in a diet with a limited choice of foods, sometimes of a soft or liquidised texture, consisting of few fresh foods (especially fruit and vegetables) and a high proportion of convenience foods, cakes and biscuits. In nutritional terms, the diet can be low in vitamins, minerals and fibre but high in fat and sugars. Such a diet is likely to have an energy content which exceeds energy requirement (usually decreased as a consequence of the physical inactivity) thus leading to overweight and obesity.

Tackling these problems requires more than healthy eating guidance; the underlying difficulties causing the dietary problems also need to be addressed. These include:

- Ensuring that people know how to obtain all the benefits to which they are entitled.
- Making people aware of local facilities for providing help, e.g. good neighbour schemes, food delivery services, equipment loan and other support available from social services or local/national charities.
- Suggesting ways of making life easier. Sometimes a simple measure such as using an electric can opener, adapted cutlery or non-slip plate mats can make a great difference.
- Obtaining specialist dietetic help for people with severe nutritional problems such as swallowing difficulties, underweight or obesity.

LEARNING DISABILITIES

People with severe learning disabilities often have feeding problems which necessitate specialist care and support. Those living in an institutional setting are usually adequately fed but rarely ideally fed; problems such as lack of food choice and variety, foods of low nutrient density and scant attention paid to individual needs are still commonplace and similar to those of elderly people living in residential homes (see pp. 128–9).

People with milder learning difficulties who live in the community are a particularly vulnerable group in terms of nutrition, particularly those who have previously been in institutional care. Dietary problems are more likely to stem from inappropriate food choice rather than difficulties in obtaining food. Many people in this group:

- Find it difficult to understand what they should eat.
- Find it difficult to remember any guidance given.
- Find it difficult to decide what to eat.
- Find it difficult to manage money (they may forget to keep enough available for food).
- Find it difficult to read or understand food preparation instructions.
- May have poor cooking and food storage facilities.
- Are easily influenced by advertising or peer pressure.

In addition, many in this group are unemployed and consequently have a low income and little to do. The day may be filled by sitting in pubs, cafés or fast food restaurants; the money spent there may leave little for other food.

Many learning disadvantaged people living in the community are isolated and have little support. Health professionals may not be in a position to give direct support but they can help people obtain support from whatever facilities are available locally. In some areas there may be drop-in centres where people can meet, eat and find friends. Practically-orientated local health promotion initiatives, such as cookery classes or supermarket tours, can be very successful.

USEFUL ADDRESSES

The Disabled Living Foundation, 380/384 Harrow Road, London W9 2HU. Tel: 0171 289 6111. Provides an information service for disabled people and carers about gadgets and adaptations which can help make life easier.

MENCAP, 123 Golden Lane, London EC1Y 0RT. Tel: 0171 454 0454.

RADAR (Royal Association for Disability and Rehabilitation), 25 Mortimer Street, London W1N 8AB. Provides an information service about manufacturers and stockists of aids. Can advise on transport, wheelchairs and holidays.

SCOPE (formerly The Spastics Society), 12 Park Crescent, London W1N 4EQ. Tel: 0171 636 5020.

19

People on Low Incomes

There is wide health divide between the richer and poorer sections of society[1,2]. People in low income groups have a higher prevalence of obesity, hypertension, high serum cholesterol and anaemia and are more likely to suffer a premature death from coronary heart disease or cancer. Their children are more likely to have a low birthweight, birth abnormalities, poor growth, dental caries or to die in the perinatal period.

Many factors, such as smoking, poor housing, inactivity and stress, contribute to these differences but diet is also likely to be a major factor. Virtually every dietary survey shows the same pattern: that lower income groups consume a diet containing fewer essential nutrients but more fat and sugars than those in higher income groups[3,4,5]. As income declines, people eat fewer fresh foods and more low nutrient density convenience foods such as cheap meat products, chips, biscuits, cakes and sugary drinks. The difference in the consumption of fruit and vegetables (and hence the protective antioxidant nutrients which they provide) is particularly striking[3].

INCOME AND HEALTHY EATING

Most people can make beneficial changes to their diets without spending more on food (see p. 41). However, for those on low incomes it is much more difficult to do so, not simply because less money is available to spend on food but because of the many other factors which act as a constraint on food choice and availability. These may include:

- *Limited choice of food* Lack of transport may mean that people have to rely on small local shops which may not stock healthier food choices and where fresh foods may be of poor quality.
- *Higher cost of food* Food usually costs more in small local shops than in edge-of-town supermarkets. The price differential of staple items, such as bread, milk and fruit, can be considerable.
- *Lack of purchasing power* Even if people can get to supermarkets, they may not have the funds to make bulk purchases of food or take advantages of special offers.
- *Lack of storage facilities* People cannot buy food in advance if they don't have refrigeration or freezer facilities.
- *Poor cooking facilities* Poor housing usually also means poor cooking equipment. Fuel bills may be an added worry. Those living in bed and breakfast accommodation often have very limited access to cooking facilities.
- *Lack of cooking skills* Some people in disadvantaged circumstances have never learnt to cook, particularly men who live alone and people with learning disabilities.
- *Fear of wastage* People are reluctant to try new foods in case this turns out to be a costly mistake.
- *Psychological factors* Depression over living

conditions and continual worry over how to make ends meet can have a marked effect on food intake. People may not have the mental energy to think about healthy eating; the priority is simply to provide the family or themselves with enough food to stave off hunger.

- *Food expenditure is a high proportion of income* Low income families usually spend less money on food in total than those with higher incomes but this represents a much greater proportion of their income. In the population as a whole, food expenditure on food comprises about 12% of income; in low income groups, food expenditure often exceeds 30% of available income[5].

- *Other pressures on expenditure* People on low incomes are often well aware of healthy eating messages and are keen to eat the right foods. But practical constraints mean that food expenditure is way down the list of priorities; bills for rent, fuel, council tax, etc., are a more immediate concern. Expenditure on food is often determined by what is left after these have been paid.

DIETARY GUIDANCE

Identifying the dietary problems of people on low incomes is usually easy. Finding solutions to them is not. Dietary education alone is not the answer because lack of knowledge is not the sole problem. Healthy eating leaflets and static displays may heighten people's awareness that they have a problem but will not alter the circumstances which have lead to it.

Dietary education will only make a difference if it is applied in a way which is personally relevant to the situation in which people find themselves. Changes in eating habits are more likely to occur if some of the practical difficulties affecting food choice can be overcome. Healthy eating campaigns have to aim to make life easier for people, not more difficult.

The most successful health promotion programmes are those which:

- Focus on the needs and problems of a clearly identified group (e.g. single mothers, people living in bed and breakfast accommodation, particular ethnic groups).
- Have a clear attainable objective (e.g. improving the iron intake of toddlers).
- Don't try to achieve too much all at once (e.g. trying to persuade someone to eat a healthy diet and stop smoking, and reduce alcohol consumption, and take more exercise).
- Operate in a group setting, enabling people to make friends and meet others with similar problems thus reducing feelings of isolation.
- Are practically orientated giving people the opportunity to prepare, taste or obtain foods.
- Create an interactive partnership between clients and health workers so that each side can gain from and respond to the experience of the other.

Some of ways in which these may be achieved are:

- Healthy eating awareness days at a local community centre with foods to try and recipes to take away.
- Cook and eat sessions.
- Drop-in centres where a health worker or dietitian is available for informal one-to-one chats.
- Lunch clubs.
- Supermarket shopping tours highlighting good and poor value nutritional choices.
- Arranging transport facilities to out-of-town shopping facilities.
- Setting up local food co-operatives or shopping clubs to improve food availability.

The most effective strategies are often those which strengthen links within a community. Depression, apathy and low morale often stem from feelings of isolation. Getting to know other people with similar problems means that worries can be shared, difficulties discussed and mutual support given, and this can dramatically improve self-esteem and the ability to cope. It is at this point that knowledge concerning health is more likely to be translated into action.

REFERENCES

1 DHSS (1980) *Inequalities in Health.* Report of a research working group. HMSO, London.
2 Davey-Smith, G. *et al.* (1990) The Black Report on socioeconomic inequalities in health ten years on. *British Medical Journal* **301**, 373–7.
3 Gregory, J. *et al.* (1990) *The Dietary and Nutritional Survey of British Adults.* HMSO, London.
4 Department of Health (1989) *The Diets of British Schoolchildren.* COMA Report on Health and Social Subjects 36. HMSO, London.
5 MAFF (1993) *National Food Survey, 1992.* HMSO, London.

FURTHER READING

Brown, J. *et al.* (1992) Organising dietary education in a General Practice setting. *Health Visitor* **65**, 273–4.
James, J. *et al.* (1992) Improving the diet of under-fives in a deprived inner city practice. *Health Trends* **24**, 161–4.
MAFF (1992) *The Cost of Alternative Diets.* Food Science Division, Paper CP (92) 9/3. MAFF Consumer Panel Secretariat.

National Dairy Council (1993) *Nutrition and Low Income Families.* NDC, London.
Seymour, J. (1992) *Give us a chance: children, poverty and the Health of the Nation.* Child Poverty Action Group, Health Visitors Association, Save the Children.

RESOURCES

National Dairy Council (1993) *Nutrition and Low Income Families: A Pack for Primary Health Care and Community Workers.* Provides background information and material to help health educators develop nutrition education programmes with low income families. Includes the booklet *Nutrition and Low Income Families* (see Further reading above). Details available from: National Dairy Council, 5–7 John Princes Street, London W1M 0AP.
National Food Alliance (1995) *Healthy Eating on a Low Income.* A resource pack for health care professionals and others working with people on low incomes. Details available from: National Food Alliance, 3rd floor, 5–11 Worship Street, London EC2A 2BH. Tel: 0171 628 2442.

USEFUL ADDRESSES

Child Poverty Action Group, 4th Floor, 1–5 Bath Street, London EC1V 9PY. Tel: 0171 253 3406.

20

Minority Ethnic Groups

The 1991 census showed that over 3 million of the UK population (5.5% of the population) are of minority ethnic origin, almost half of whom were born in this country. The largest groups of people are those of Asian origin (2.7% of the population) and those of Afro-Caribbean origin (0.9% of the population).

People in minority ethnic groups generally have poorer health than the majority of the population and are at greater risk from premature mortality[1]. Some of these differences may be genetic in origin but most are associated with environmental factors such as poor housing, overcrowding and diet.

Asians have an increased risk of:

Diabetes
Coronary heart disease
Central obesity
Rickets and osteomalacia
Perinatal death (particularly in Pakistani infants)
Thalassaemia

Afro-Caribbeans have an increased risk of:

Hypertension
Stroke (twice the death rate of white people)
Mental illness
Diabetes (the risk is almost as high as in Asians)
Sickle cell disease
Lactose intolerance

ASIAN PEOPLE

Nutritional considerations

There is enormous diversity of nutritional intake among this group of people. Some of the younger members who have been born and brought up in this country consume a totally Westernised diet with its attendant disadvantages of being high in fat and sugar and low in nutrient density. Older people and those observing more traditional religious or cultural beliefs may have a very different type of diet and quite different dietary problems.

The traditional diets of different groups of Asian people vary according to their place of origin and its associated religious and cultural practices (see Table 20.1). Depending on the degree to which orthodoxy is observed, this may have the dietary influences shown in Table 20.2. As a broad guideline, East African Asians are least likely to follow religious customs while Pakistanis and Bangladeshis are most likely to observe orthodox practices.

In general terms, traditional Asian diets comprise:

Table 20.1 Sub-groups of Asian people living in the UK.

Place of origin	Religion
India:	
Gujerat	Usually Hindu; occasionally Muslim
Punjab	Usually Sikh; occasionally Hindu
Pakistan	Muslim
Bangladesh	Muslim
East African Asians	Variable. Religious beliefs less likely to affect diet

Table 20.2 Religious influences on diet.

Religion	Dietary restrictions
Hindus	Beef not eaten
	Vegetarianism common
	Some are vegan
	Fast days common
Sikhs	Beef and pork not eaten
	Some are vegetarian
Muslims	Pork not eaten
	All meat must be halal (killed by a method of ritual slaughter)
	Dawn-to-dusk fasting observed during Ramadan
	Alcohol not consumed

A staple cereal (usually chapattis and/or rice)
Pulses
Vegetables and fruit
Milk, yogurt and sometimes curd cheese
Cooking fat such as ghee (concentrated butter) or sometimes groundnut or mustard oil

If meat is eaten, it is usually in the form of chicken or mutton. In general, use of fish and eggs is low.

In many respects this type of diet can be considered a healthy one – it is generally high in carbohydrate and fibre and low in saturated fat. Problems usually arise when this balance becomes disturbed in some way, either as a result of tradi-tional foods not being available, lack of facilities preventing their preparation or Western influences resulting in foods such as fruit and vegetables being displaced by convenience foods, snacks and confectionery.

Common nutritional problems

Low nutrient density

In vegetarian diets, over-reliance on vegetables and insufficient use of pulses can result in a diet with low mineral and vitamin content. Lack of dietary variety and fresh foods may compound the problem. Vitamins may also be lost as a result of cooked dishes (such as a vegetable curry) being prepared in sufficient quantities to last several days. In the younger generation, the tendency to consume fast foods, confectionery and fizzy drinks outside the home adds little to nutritional quality or dietary balance. Obesity, particularly central obesity, is a major health problem among Asian people.

Lack of vitamin D

Asian people, particularly women, who observe traditional customs concerning clothing have little exposure to sunlight. Vitamin D synthesis there-fore tends to be low and dietary intake of this vita-min is also likely to be low in those who consume a vegetarian diet. In addition to this, there is some evidence that Asian people may have a lower ability to convert vitamin D to its active metabolite. All these factors greatly increase the risk of vitamin D inadequacy and the development of rickets or osteomalacia (see Chapter 37). Supplementary vi-tamin D is essential in children and pregnant or lactating women and may be advisable in elderly Asian women.

Iron and anaemia

The iron content of many Asian diets is low and anaemia is relatively common in women and chil-dren. Children are particularly vulnerable at the weaning stage when there may be over-reliance on cows' milk and very little intake of iron-containing foods. Commercial weaning foods are in theory useful but in practice the savoury varieties providing the most iron may be considered unsuitable because they are not vegetarian or halal, while sweetened desserts are acceptable but usually contain little iron. The use of an iron-fortified follow-on milk can be highly beneficial.

Infant feeding practices

There are considerable variations in infant feeding practices, not only between different Asian groups but also within them. They are affected by:

- *Traditional cultural influences* In general breast feeding is more common and more prolonged in those following orthodox traditions and who have only been in the UK for a short time. Breast feeding is more common among Pakistani Asians and less common among Bangladeshi Asians.

  In some cultural groups (especially Punjabi Indians) female infants may be less likely to be breast fed than male infants.
- *Western influences* Bottle feeding may be seen to have prestige value and a sign of Western affluence.
- *Social circumstances* Overcrowded living conditions may discourage breast feeding because of the lack of privacy.

  The necessity for a rapid return to work often deters breast feeding.

Weaning problems may include:

- Early weaning.
- Late weaning (common in Pakistani Asians observing traditional lifestyles).
- Early introduction of cows' milk, often with added sugar.
- Use of weaning foods of low nutrient density.
- Prolonged use of a bottle (up to and even beyond the age of 2 years).

Dietary guidance

Dietary guidance will be regarded as intrusive and unacceptable unless it takes account of individual dietary practices, cultural beliefs and the many factors influencing food choice within a particular family. Some of these factors may also inhibit dietary change; for example the views of older members of the family are usually greatly respected so a grandmother's opinion of how an infant should be fed may have more influence than that of a health visitor. Communication may also be a difficulty; someone who speaks English may still not find it easy to understand oral advice and may not be able to read written English at all. Older members of the community may not even be able to read material in their own language.

In general terms, dietary guidance for people in Asian communities may include:

- Encouraging the consumption of:
  Pulses (e.g. beans, peas and lentils, dhal)
  Milk and yogurt
  A variety of fruit and vegetables
  The staple cereal (rice and/or chapattis)
  Freshly prepared foods (rather than bulk quantities being cooked in advance).
- Decreasing the consumption of fat by:
  Using much less fat during cooking
  Using vegetable oils in preference to butter or ghee
  Not coating cooked chapattis with fat or adding it to dhal
  Using reduced-fat milk and dairy foods.
- Encouraging the use of iron-fortified milk, cereals and other products in the diets of young children.
- Ensuring that children and pregnant/lactating women take vitamin D supplements.

In most areas, resource material appropriate for the needs of the local community will be available for use as teaching aids and support material. The knowledge and skills within the Asian community itself should also be tapped. Practical initiatives such as healthy eating cookery classes led by an Asian person using traditional cooking practices are likely to have far more impact than a leaflet produced by someone with much less understanding of Asian culture.

AFRO-CARIBBEAN PEOPLE

Nutritional considerations

Afro-Caribbean diets are highly variable, some being totally European in character, others containing different degrees of influence from Caribbean, American, African and Chinese cookery.

Most Afro-Caribbeans are Christian so their diets are less likely to be constrained for religious reasons. A smaller sub-group are Rastafarians who observe dietary restrictions with varying degrees of strictness. This may entail:

- Vegetarianism, sometimes veganism.
- No processed foods (e.g. canned products) or anything containing additives.
- No alcohol.
- No added salt.

The traditional Afro-Caribbean diet comprises:

Cereals, principally rice, maize and wheat
Roots and tubers, e.g. yam, sweet potato, breadfruit, plantain
Other vegetables, e.g. aubergine, okra, spinach, callaloo
Fruits, e.g. mango, banana, lime, orange, guava
Pulses, e.g. black-eyed beans, split peas, lentils (often added to soups, stews or rice)
Chicken and fish, often salted
Fried foods
Sugared foods

Increasingly in the UK, fruit and vegetable consumption is being replaced by greater use of snack foods and confectionery. The common practices of frying foods and adding sweetened condensed milk to drinks and puddings also tend to increase the fat and sugar content of the diet. Many Afro-Caribbeans have 'a sweet tooth' so if sugar is added to foods or drinks it tends to be in large amounts. The taste of salt is also popular and the preference for salted meats and fish often results in high sodium intakes.

Dietary guidance

Healthy eating guidance in these groups therefore needs to focus on these aspects, particularly in an attempt to reduce the health risks from hypertension, stroke, obesity and diabetes:

- Consumption of cereal-based foods, fruits and vegetables should be encouraged.
- Consumption of fried foods should be reduced.
- Unsweetened, preferably fat-reduced milk should be used instead of condensed milk.
- The use of salted foods and added salt should be considerably curtailed.
- Heavy use of sugar in puddings and drinks should be avoided; if necessary artificial sweeteners can be used to achieve the desired level of sweetness.

REFERENCE

1 Balarajan, R. & Raleigh, V.S. (1993) *Ethnicity and Health – A Guide for the NHS*. Department of Health, London.

FURTHER READING

Clements, M.R. (1989) The problem of rickets in UK Asians. *Journal of Human Nutrition and Dietetics* **2**, 105–16.

Health Education Authority (1991) *Nutrition in Minority Ethnic Groups: Asians and Afro-Caribbeans in the United Kingdom.* Briefing Paper. HEA, London.

McKeigue, P., Marmot, M.G., Adelstein, A.M., Hunt, S.P., Shipley, M.J. & Butler, S.M. (1985) Diet and risk factors for coronary heart disease in Asians in north-west London. *Lancet* ii, 1086–90.

Tan, S.P. *et al.* (1985) *Immigrant foods. 2nd supplement to McCance and Widdowson's The Composition of Foods.* HMSO, London.

White, A. & Thompson, P. (1990) *The Caribbean Food and Nutrition Book.* Macmillan, London.

21

Vegetarians and Vegans

A well-planned vegetarian diet can be an extremely healthy way of eating. A poorly planned one can be a nutritional disaster area. It is important for health professionals to be able to distinguish between the two.

Vegetarianism has increased considerably in recent years, mainly for ethical reasons and concerns over animal welfare or because meat is believed to be unhealthy or unsafe. Surveys suggest about 4.5% of the population are vegetarians and about 12% no longer eat meat. As many as 25% of 16–24 year-olds may be non-meat eaters[1].

TYPES OF VEGETARIANISM

It is important to establish what people mean when they say they are vegetarian as there are many variations each with different nutritional implications. Vegetarianism may mean people:

- Avoid meat when possible but will eat it occasionally, e.g. out of politeness.
- Do not eat red meat (but will eat other types of meat such as poultry).
- Do not eat any meat (but do eat fish).
- Do not eat meat or fish.
- Do not eat meat, fish or eggs.
- Do not eat meat, fish, eggs, milk or milk products or anything derived from animals.

- Follow a cult diet such as a macrobiotic or fruitarian regime.

HEALTH BENEFITS OF VEGETARIANISM

Vegetarianism is often stated to have significant health benefits but these depend entirely on the way it is practised.

While it is true that vegetarian sub-groups of a population are less likely to suffer from diseases such as coronary heart disease and some cancers, this is not necessarily attributable to dietary factors *per se*[2]. Vegetarian people tend to be health-conscious in general and less likely to smoke, drink much alcohol or be overweight. Within a population, vegetarianism is often a marker of a healthy lifestyle and hence fewer health risks[3].

Many vegetarians do, however, consume a diet which is much closer to healthy eating targets than that consumed by most of the population. Avoidance of animal foods results in a low intake of saturated fats and a high consumption of fruit, vegetables and cereal foods results in a high intake of antioxidant nutrients and fibre. This will certainly be beneficial in terms of blood cholesterol, bowel function and protection against carcinogens.

Not all vegetarians consume a diet of this type. Some people avoid meat but give little thought as to what should take its place in nutritional terms. Heavy reliance on cheese as a main meal substitute may result in a diet rich in saturates and low in iron; vegetarian burgers, pies, pasties and pizzas have no nutritional advantage over the conventional variety and the only vegetables eaten by some teenage vegetarians are chips. Ironically some people who give up eating meat on 'health' grounds can end up eating a diet which is more unbalanced than it was before.

NUTRITIONAL CONSIDERATIONS

The effects of vegetarianism on food choice may be considerable. Strict vegetarians will avoid ordinary cheese (which is made using animal rennet) and many manufactured foods are also unsuitable because they contain ingredients derived from

Table 21.1 Nutritional risks of different types of vegetarianism.

Type of vegetarianism	Nutrients most likely to be deficient
Meat eaten rarely	Iron and zinc in vulnerable groups (e.g. children and young women)
No red meat/ any meat	Iron and zinc
No meat or fish	Iron, zinc and essential fatty acids from fish oils
No meat, fish or eggs	Iron, zinc, essential fatty acids and B_{12} Protein intake may be low in vulnerable groups
No meat, fish, eggs or milk	Iron, zinc, essential fatty acids, B_{12}, protein, essential amino acids, calcium, vitamin D, riboflavin, energy
Macrobiotic/ fruitarian diets	A wide range of deficiencies is almost inevitable

animals. Some brands of bread are unacceptable because they may contain emulsifiers derived from animal fats. Fortified breakfast cereals may be avoided if they contain animal-derived vitamin D. Any food containing lecithin may be avoided in case it has been extracted from eggs. Quorn, a mycoprotein sold as a meat substitute, may not be regarded as suitable because its production requires battery eggs and its safety evaluation involved animal testing. Some vegans will not consume medicine in gelatine-based capsules and may be reluctant to use any drug because of the animal-testing implications.

A well-constructed vegetarian diet is not deficient in any nutrient. Less well-balanced diets may have a low content of some nutrients. The more restricted the diet, the greater the risk of nutritional inadequacies, see Table 21.1.

Energy

Properly constructed vegetarian diets are high in fibre which means that they are bulky and of low energy density, i.e. have a relatively low calorie content for the volume of food consumed. In adults, this is usually beneficial, reducing the risk of overweight or obesity. In young children or people with small appetites it can be more of a problem because it may be difficult to consume sufficient food to meet energy and nutrient needs. Vegan children tend to be smaller and lighter than their peers[4]. Some energy dense foods such as vegetable oils may need to be included in the diet to help meet energy needs.

Protein

Many people think that lack of protein is the main risk of vegetarian diets. This is not the case; if foods such as milk, cheese and dairy products or eggs are eaten then protein intake is unlikely to be a problem.

Protein does become a significant consideration in vegans, i.e. those who eat no animal foods at all. This because animal protein contains all the essential amino acids required by the body whereas vegetable proteins are deficient in one or more of these amino acids. This problem can be overcome by eating mixtures of plant proteins because proteins of different botanical origin lack different amino acids. For example, pulses (i.e. peas, beans, lentils) are low in methionine but rich in lysine, while cereal foods contain little lysine but moderate amounts of methionine; a combination of the two therefore provides an appropriate amino acid mixture.

Fat

Total and saturated fat intake can be desirably low in vegetarians, although this is not always the case in those who consume a lot of cheese as a substitute for meat. In children total fat intake should not be too low or energy needs will not be met. Polyunsaturated fat intake often exceeds target levels and may even be near the recommended maximum although vitamin E intakes (necessary to metabolise polyunsaturated fat) are usually high too.

There are some concerns over the high ratio of n–6 to n–3 polyunsaturates in some vegan diets, particularly in the diets of children[5]. It has been suggested that this may impair the conversion of alpha-linolenic acid (an n–3 fatty acid) to docosahexaenoic acid (DHA) which is important in retinal and central nervous system development. DHA is virtually absent from many vegetarian diets as it is mainly present in animal foods (especially fish oils). Use of vegetable oils with a lower ratio of n–6 to n–3 fatty acids, i.e. soya bean or rapeseed oil, may be preferable to those with a higher ratio such as sunflower, safflower or corn oil.

Carbohydrate

Vegetarian diets can be beneficially high in complex carbohydrates and low in sugars. This is not always the case among teenagers who maintain their usual low fibre, high sugar diet by simply switching to brands of biscuits, cakes, doughnuts and confectionery, etc., which have 'suitable for vegetarians' on the food label.

Minerals and trace elements

Iron and zinc are always vulnerable in vegetarian diets because meat is such a concentrated source of these nutrients and it is present in a form which is particularly well-absorbed. It is not difficult to obtain sufficient amounts from other sources, i.e. by an increased intake of cereal foods and vegetables together with a good intake of vitamin C. The problem is that this is not always done.

Calcium intake only starts to be at risk when milk and dairy foods are excluded from the diet. Alternative sources of calcium such as soft-boned fish will usually be excluded too and calcium from vegetable sources can be poorly absorbed. A low calcium intake in children and young adults may have adverse effects on bone density in later life. Calcium supplements may be necessary if calcium intake remains poor.

A high fibre intake will reduce mineral absorption to some extent. This is not usually a problem because the foods providing the fibre are usually also rich sources of these nutrients as well. The effect may become significant in people whose mineral intake is of borderline adequacy, especially young children.

Vitamins

B group vitamins are most at risk in a vegetarian diet, the likelihood of deficiency increasing as the range of foods eaten decreases. Thiamin intakes may be low in those who exclude meat although this is unlikely to be a problem if wholegrain cereals and fortified breakfast cereals are consumed. The risk of riboflavin deficiency increases when people also exclude milk.

Vitamin B_{12} is only found in animal foods and will be deficient in vegan diets if a supplementary form is not consumed. In vegetarians consuming some animal foods, e.g. milk or eggs, B_{12} deficiency is much less likely.

DIETARY GUIDANCE

Whatever the degree of vegetarianism practised, it is important that a wide variety of foods is consumed. The more limited the consumption of foods, the higher the risk of nutritional deficiencies, especially in vulnerable groups such as children, teenagers and young women.

Vegetarians consuming some animal products

New vegetarians should experiment with a range of cereals, grains, pulses, nuts, soya products, fruit and vegetables rather than just trying to compensate by increasing their intake of milk, dairy products and cheese. Healthy eating guidance should be similar to that for non-vegetarians with people being encouraged to consume some foods from the four main groups.

Bread, other cereals and potatoes group

Plenty of these foods should be consumed. Some should be of a wholemeal or wholegrain type but exclusive use of such choices may not be appropriate in children or those with small appetites. If calcium intake is low (see below) white and brown bread (which in the UK is made with calcium fortified flour) may be better choices than wholemeal bread (made with unfortified flour).

Fruit and vegetables group

These foods are particularly important in non-meat eaters as a source of vitamin C to maximise the absorption of non-haem iron.

Milk and dairy foods group

If these are included in the diet, their use should be encouraged. If not, it is important that alternative sources of calcium are consumed such as:

Bread made with calcium fortified flour (white or brown)
Green vegetables
Pulses
Sesame seeds
Nuts (less suitable for young children)

Specialist dietetic advice should be sought for non-milk consuming children.

Alternatives to meat group

Foods which need to be encouraged as an alternative source of iron, zinc, protein and B group vitamins are:

Breakfast cereals
Bread
Dark green vegetables (e.g. spinach, broccoli, spring greens, watercress)
Peas (e.g. green, chick peas)
Beans (e.g. mung, kidney, soya, black eye, aduki)
Lentils
Dried fruit (e.g. apricots, raisins)
Nuts (and peanut butter)
Seeds (e.g. sesame seeds)

Fatty and sugary foods group

As in other people, consumption of these foods should not comprise a major part of the diet. Crisps, biscuits and confectionery and cola are just as likely to feature in the diet of vegetarian teenagers as in their non-vegetarian peers, and are just as undesirable.

Vegans

Many of the above considerations apply to vegans but because of the greater restriction of food choice, additional guidance is needed. The diet will need to include a range of foods from the following groups:

Cereals: Wheat, rice, oats, corn (e.g. bread, rice, pasta).

Fruit and vegetables: All types including potatoes. Avocado pears contain fat and are a useful source of energy in young children.

Pulses/beans: Peas, beans, lentils, soya products such as tofu.

Nuts/seeds: Nuts (e.g. almonds, hazelnuts, peanuts), sesame seeds, tahini.

Fats and oils: Vegetable oils and acceptable types of margarine.

Foods which are particularly useful for vegans (and vegetarians) are:

Bulgar wheat (burghul): derived from cracked wheat. Used as an alternative to rice or pasta.

Cous-cous: pasta-like granules made from semolina. Often used as the basis of a salad.

Miso: a product made from cooked fermented soya beans. Used for flavouring or as a stock substitute. Has a high salt content.

Tahini: a paste made from ground-up sesame seeds. Can be spread on toast or used as a constituent of salad dressing.

Tempeh: a meat substitute made from wheat flour.

Texturised vegetable protein (TVP): a meat replacement based on fungal/microbial protein available as dried chunks or granules. Strict vegans and vegetarians may not consume this because its development necessitated toxicity tests on animals.

Tofu: Soya bean curd with a soft rubbery texture like mozzarella cheese. Tofu provides protein, calcium, iron and folate.

Protein combining

In vegans, different types of vegetable proteins need to be combined together so that all essential amino acids are provided. Good combinations from a nutritional viewpoint are:

- Cereals + Pulses
  e.g.   Baked beans on toast
         Bean and lentil casserole with rice
- Nuts/seeds + Pulses
  e.g.   Nut and lentil loaf
         Hummus (chick peas and tahini)
- Cereals + Nuts/seeds
  e.g.   Tahini on toast
         Nuts and breadcrumb roast
- Vegetables + Pulses
  e.g.   Avocado with tofu
         Mashed potato and baked beans

This principle does not necessarily have to be applied too rigidly or even at every meal, but it is important that, over the course of a day, vegetable protein is obtained from cereals, pulses, nuts/seeds and vegetables.

A source of B_{12}

As this is only present in animal foods, vegans must either take B_{12} supplements or consume B_{12} fortified foods such as:

Yeast extracts
Fortified soya drinks
Fortified textured vegetable protein (TVP)
Fortified breakfast cereals

It is particularly important that adequate B_{12} (probably in supplementary form) is taken during pregnancy and lactation.

Vegan infants and children

This is a very vulnerable group in nutritional terms and specialist dietetic guidance is usually advisable to ensure that all nutrient needs are being met.

Infants who are not breast fed will require a soya-based infant formula milk. A specialist soya formula will also be necessary from the age of weaning as an alternative to cows' milk. Soya drinks available from health food shops are not suitable for young children because their content of vitamins, minerals and energy is too low to meet their requirements.

General weaning guidelines apply to vegan infants but particular care needs to be taken to encourage the consumption of a wide range of foods. In the initial stages, nuts and seeds must be ground to a paste to reduce the risk of choking. Foods such as tofu are a useful source of protein, calcium, iron and folate from the age of six months. If acceptable, commercial weaning foods fortified with iron and other micronutrients are helpful in ensuring nutritional adequacy.

As children grow and energy needs increase, it is important that energy dense foods, such as full-fat margarines, peanut butter, and avocado pears, form part of the diet. Vegetable oils derived from soya beans or rapeseed oils may be preferable in terms of their fatty acid composition to sunflower, safflower or corn oils.

Cult diets

Zen macrobiotic diets are progressively restricted diets from which foods of animal origin, and then fruit and vegetables are removed at various stages. At the final level only brown rice remains. The nutritional shortcomings of this are obvious. Another version of a currently fashionable macrobiotic diet consists of organically grown cereals, vegetables, pulses and small amounts of seaweeds, fermented foods, nuts and seeds.

A fruitarian diet is an extreme form of vegetarianism in which pulses and cereal foods are excluded as well as all foods of animal origin. Food consumption is mainly confined to raw and dried fruits, olive oil and nuts.

Children on these types of diet have been found to have multiple nutrient deficiencies, marked growth retardation and delayed development of motor and language skills[6].

REFERENCES

1   Realeat Survey Office (1995) *The Realeat Survey 1995*. The Realeat Survey Office, Howard Way, Newport Pagnell, Bucks MK16 9PY.
2   Thorogood, M. *et al.* (1994) Risk of death from cancer and ischaemic heart disease in meat and non-meat eaters. *British Medical Journal* **308**, 1667–71.
3   Dwyer, J.T. (1988) Health aspects of vegetarian diets. *American Journal of Clinical Nutrition* **48**, 712–38.
4   Sanders, T.A.B. (1988) Growth and development of British vegan children. *American Journal of Clinical Nutrition* **48**, 822–5.
5   Sanders, T. & Reddy, S. (1994) Vegetarian diets and children. *American Journal of Clinical Nutrition* **59** (supplement), 1176S–81S.
6   van Staveren, W.A. & Dagnelie, P.C. (1988) Food consumption, growth and development of Dutch children fed on alternative diets. *American Journal of Clinical Nutrition* **48**, 819–21.

FURTHER READING

British Nutrition Foundation (1988) *Vegetarian Diets*. Briefing paper no.13. BNF, London.

National Dairy Council (1990) *Nutrition and Vegetarianism*. Fact File 6. NDC, London.

Vandenbroucke, J.P. (1994) Should you eat meat, or are you confounded by methodological debate? *British Medical Journal* **308**, 1671.

USEFUL ADDRESSES

The Vegan Society, 7 Battle Road, St Leonard's-on-Sea, East Sussex TN37 7AA. Tel: 01424 427393.

The Vegetarian Society of the United Kingdom Ltd, Parkdale, Dunham Road, Altrincham, Cheshire WA14 4QG. Tel: 0161 928 0793.

PART 3

Diet and Disease

22

Coronary Heart Disease

Coronary heart disease (CHD) is currently the major cause of death in the UK, accounting for 30% of all male deaths and 23% of all female deaths[1]. The majority of these occur in people over the age of 65 years but a considerable proportion, almost one-fifth, occur before this age, many of them in men. CHD also results in considerable morbidity within the population.

CHD was relatively uncommon in the UK before 1925 and gradually increased until about 1980. Since then age-standardised mortality rates from CHD have declined although less rapidly than in other countries such as the USA and Australia. Within the UK, CHD death rates are highest in Scotland, Northern Ireland and northern areas of England.

CHD does not have a single cause but results from a complex interplay of various factors. For this reason no single dietary factor can be said to 'cause' CHD but a number of dietary components can increase or decrease the likelihood of its development.

Some of the factors which increase the risk of CHD, such as age, sex and genetic susceptibility, are unalterable. Prevention of CHD therefore focuses on reducing the risk from environmental or physiological factors which are subject to influence. The most important of these are believed to be:

- Smoking.
- Raised blood pressure.
- Raised blood cholesterol.
- Physical inactivity.

The prevalence of these risk factors within the population is high. The 1991 Health Survey for England[2] found that:

11%	had none of these risk factors
32%	had 1 risk factor
35%	had 2 risk factors
20%	had 3 risk factors
2%	had all 4 of these risk factors

Obesity, particularly central obesity, also enhances CHD risk via its influence on blood pressure, lipid metabolism and increasing the susceptibility to Type 2 diabetes which further increases the likelihood of CHD. In 1991, about 15% of women and 13% of men were found to be obese (BMI over 30)[2].

DIET AND THE DEVELOPMENT OF CORONARY HEART DISEASE

Dietary factors can directly affect two of the main stages leading to coronary occlusion and myocardial infarction:

- *Atherogenesis* The slow progressive build-up of fibrous plaque on the arterial wall following initial damage to the lining of vessel walls.
- *Thrombogenesis* The formation of a major

151

thrombus immediately prior to a coronary event.

Diet may also have direct or indirect effects on other factors which enhance risk, particularly hypertension and obesity.

Diet and atherogenesis

Dietary fat and blood cholesterol

The deposition of lipid material in atheromatous plaque is greatly influenced by the level of cholesterol in the blood. Most of this cholesterol in the blood is synthesised by the body (only a minute proportion is dietary cholesterol) and is carried around the body attached to lipoproteins. The total amount of cholesterol in the blood is the sum of the amount carried on different lipoproteins. The levels of these different lipoprotein fractions have different prognostic significance.

Most cholesterol in the blood is carried on low density lipoproteins (LDL). LDL cholesterol is the form in which cholesterol is taken to the tissues where it is required for many essential functions such as cell membrane and hormone synthesis. A smaller proportion is carried on high density lipoproteins (HDL) and HDL cholesterol largely reflects cholesterol being transported away from the tissues to the liver for excretion. A high LDL cholesterol level enhances atherosclerotic risk whereas a high HDL cholesterol is protective. The ratio between the two is a powerful indicator of risk because it reflects the balance between cholesterol synthesis and removal.

For practical purposes, total blood cholesterol (which is easier to measure than the separate lipoprotein fractions) is usually taken to be an indicator of atherogenic risk because LDL cholesterol comprises the major component of blood cholesterol. Total cholesterol is however a less sensitive indicator than the individual components; occasionally, a raised total cholesterol level will result from a beneficially high HDL cholesterol level.

The level of LDL cholesterol (and hence total cholesterol) is influenced by dietary fat content, particularly the level of saturated fat. A high fat intake increases the body's production of cholesterol and hence will raise LDL (and total) cholesterol. This is particularly likely to be the case if a high proportion of this fat is in the form of saturated fatty acids. Monounsaturated fatty acids (from olive oil) have a neutral or small lowering effect while n-6 polyunsaturated fatty acids (e.g. from sunflower or corn oils or polyunsaturated spreads) can significantly lower LDL cholesterol.

HDL is much less subject to dietary influences although can be increased by moderate amounts of alcohol and exercise and decreased by obesity and high intakes of n-6 polyunsaturated fatty acids. Dietary preventative measures therefore need to focus on lowering the level of LDL cholesterol.

There is a clear relationship between mean blood cholesterol levels and the prevalence of CHD. CHD is only common in countries where the average total blood cholesterol level exceeds 5.2 mmol/l (as in Britain). What has been harder to establish is the effect of reducing blood cholesterol level on subsequent CHD risk. Some studies have shown a reduction in CHD mortality but no overall reduction in mortality (i.e. death from some other cause rises). Some have shown a benefit only in high risk groups. Other studies have failed to show a reduction in either CHD or total mortality. However, a meta-analysis of evidence from 41 epidemiological studies[3,4] concluded that there is a causal relationship between blood cholesterol and CHD in both men and women throughout the age range. On a population basis, a long-term reduction in plasma cholesterol of 0.6 mmol/l (i.e. 10%) is associated with a 27% fall in overall CHD mortality. Experimental evidence suggests that lowering of blood cholesterol may not result in significant regression of atherosclerosis but does reduce its rate of progression. Plaques may also become more stable thus reducing the chance of a fissure and triggering thrombus formation.

Within a population, the risk of CHD increases progressively with blood cholesterol level:

Below 5.2mmol/l*	Low risk
5.2mmol/l–6.5mmol/l	Moderate risk
Above 6.5mmol/l	High risk

*On a population basis, cholesterol levels below 4.1mmol/l are associated with increased mortality from non-CHD causes, largely reflecting the presence of cancer.

The 1991 Health Survey for England suggested that about two-thirds of the UK population have a blood cholesterol level above 5.2mmol/l. It has been projected that if the *Health of the Nation* targets for dietary fat consumption were achieved, the resultant downward shift in mean cholesterol level could result in a 20% fall in CHD mortality[5].

This is a long-term population objective. Within an individual the immediate benefits from a reduction in a modestly raised cholesterol level may be small, particularly if few other major risk factors, such as smoking, hypertension or family history, are present. The greatest benefit will be to those with highest cholesterol levels particularly those with additional risk factors or those who have already had one coronary event.

It should also be borne in mind that dietary fat content is not the only dietary variable which may reduce CHD risk. Attention should not be focused on fat manipulation to the exclusion of other important dietary aspects.

Antioxidant nutrients

Recent understanding of the role of antioxidants and free radicals in the atherogenic process may explain some of the anomalies observed between diet, blood cholesterol and heart disease[6]. The main cholesterol-bearing lipoprotein LDL is subject to oxidative attack by free radicals (produced by phagocytic cells in the body or as a result of smoking) and the oxidation of LDL particles in the arterial intima is an initial step in the development of atheroma. Oxidised LDL is taken up by macrophages resulting in the production of cholesterol-laden foam cells. Foam cell death leads to deposition of a cholesterol rich mixture on the arterial wall, known as fatty streaks, and these rapidly expand into atherosclerotic plaque. The availability of antioxidants, such as beta-carotene, vitamins E

and C, and selenium, may therefore reduce the amount of oxidised LDL available for this process (and hence atheroma production). Conversely, a high level of free radical production (for example by cigarette smoking) will enhance LDL oxidation and atherogenesis.

This subject is still in its infancy and much remains to be learnt about the type and levels of antioxidant nutrients required to minimise lipid peroxidation and the extent to which they can retard or treat atherosclerosis. There is some evidence that vitamin E (a fat-soluble antioxidant which helps protect lipid molecules from oxidative attack) may be particularly important in this respect[7,8]. Other as yet little known antioxidants, such as flavonoids found in fruit, vegetables, tea and wine or other carotenoids, may also be significant. For this reason, increasing consumption of antioxidants by dietary means (e.g. increased consumption of fruit and vegetables) may offer greater benefit than supplementary antioxidants in tablet form.

It seems likely that the diet which offers greatest protection against atherogenesis is one which minimises both the production of LDL (i.e. is relatively low in fat) and also its oxidation (contains plenty of antioxidant nutrients).

Diet and thrombogenesis

Dietary factors can affect blood clotting mechanisms and hence thrombus formation. It has been known for a long time that societies which consume unusually large amounts of fatty fish (such as Eskimos) have a low prevalence of thrombotic diseases despite a high total fat intake. A number of prospective studies in Western populations have demonstrated that regular consumption of oily fish (2–3 portions/week) significantly reduces the incidence of primary and secondary coronary events[9,10]. This appears to be due to the content of long-chain n-3 polyunsaturated fatty acids such as docosahexaenoic acid (DHA) and eicosapentaenoic acid (EPA) in marine oils. EPA in particular has potent antithrombotic effects, possibly because it inhibits thromboxane production which causes platelet aggregation and vasoconstriction.

High plasma fibrinogen levels increase the risk of thrombosis and smoking significantly raises blood fibrinogen levels. A small reduction in fibrinogen levels may occur with consumption of fish oils and moderate amounts of alcohol.

A low fibrinolytic activity (a low ability to dissolve small blood clots as they form) may be a leading determinant of CHD in younger men (40–64). Fibrinolytic activity is inversely related to smoking and obesity, and positively associated with exercise.

tive to requirement either as a result of a high energy intake or a low level of physical activity or a combination of the two. Fat is the dietary component most likely to lead to an energy surplus because it is the most energy-dense nutrient, providing 9 kcal/g.

CHD risk increases considerably once BMI exceeds 30, partly as a result of its effect on blood pressure. Central obesity (a waist:hip ratio which approaches or exceeds 1.0) is particularly predictive of CHD because it is more likely to be accompanied by altered lipoprotein metabolism, insulin resistance and the development of Type 2 diabetes which itself increases CHD risk[11].

Diet and other cardiovascular risk factors

DIETARY GUIDANCE FOR THE PREVENTION OF CHD

Hypertension (see also Chapter 24)

Hypertension increases CHD risk because it increases the risk of damage to arterial walls and also increases the infiltration of blood components such as oxidised LDL into an area of damage.

There is evidence that a high sodium intake increases the risk of hypertension and that reducing salt intake may reduce that risk (see p. 160). However, such benefits probably take longer to be apparent in terms of CHD compared with stroke, possibly because its effects take longer to reverse or because initial damage has already begun to progress to atherosclerotic plaque.

An increased intake of potassium (found mainly in fruit and vegetables) may also be beneficial as it is a metabolic counterbalance to sodium so tends to offset its effects. Low serum potassium levels can result in cardiac arrhythmias.

High levels of alcohol consumption can increase hypertension, and obesity is also a major determinant of hypertension.

Obesity (see also Chapter 25)

No specific dietary component causes obesity. It always results from a surplus of energy intake rela-

Whether for primary or secondary prevention of CHD, it is important that dietary guidance aims to achieve overall dietary balance rather than focusing on one nutrient alone such as fat intake. However, the emphasis placed on particular types of dietary changes may differ according to individual circumstances. To some extent dietary prevention strategies for CHD should progress from the antiatherogenic to the antithrombogenic as people become older; fat reduction to prevent progression of atherogenesis may be more important in younger adults and consuming more fatty fish to help prevent thrombosis may be more important in elderly people.

Dietary advice should be based on healthy eating guidelines with particular aspects which may be relevant to CHD prevention being stressed. The guidance given will also need to take into account an individual's usual pattern of food consumption. For someone who already uses reduced-fat foods but eats little fruit and vegetables, encouraging consumption of the latter will be particularly important. The person whose daily food intake contains a high proportion of fatty and sugary foods will need to have their attention drawn to the four other important food groups.

Food choice

Bread, other cereals and potatoes group

Most people will need to eat considerably more of these foods. Increased consumption of these will help to displace fat-rich foods from the diet as well as providing high satiety value which may assist those who need to lose weight.

Oat-based breakfast cereals may offer a small benefit as a result of the hypocholesterolaemic effects of its soluble fibre (but any breakfast cereal is a better choice than either no breakfast or a fry-up).

Fruit and vegetables group

These provide important antioxidants and soluble fibre. At least 5 servings of these should be consumed every day, preferably from a variety of sources.

Milk and dairy foods group

Moderate amounts of these foods should be consumed because they are important providers of calcium, but it is important that low or reduced-fat products are chosen. Consumption of all types of full-fat cheeses (e.g. Cheddar, Stilton, Brie) should be kept to a minimum, preferably avoided altogether, because these are such concentrated sources of fat. Even those with a lower fat content (e.g. Edam, reduced-fat Cheddar) should be regarded with caution as they still contain significant amounts of fat.

Meat, fish and alternatives group

Moderate but not excessive amounts of these foods are an important part of a healthy diet.

Smaller quantities of leaner meat should replace larger amounts of fatty meats or fat-rich meat products. Poultry skin should never be consumed and surplus fat released on cooking should be drained off and discarded.

Ideally at least two servings of fish should be consumed every week, one of which should be an oily fish (e.g. mackerel, herring, salmon, pilchards, sardines) for its beneficial content of n–3 fatty acids. White fish contains few n–3 fatty acids but has a low total fat content so can be helpful in displacing higher fat main meal choices such as cheese, meat or poultry. Fish is also an important source of selenium (a dietary antioxidant).

The use of pulses, such as baked beans, kidney beans or lentils (valuable sources of soluble fibre), should be encouraged as a way of compensating for smaller portions of meat (e.g. in casseroles or other composite dishes).

Normally there is no necessity for people to avoid eggs despite the fact that egg yolk is a rich source of cholesterol. Dietary cholesterol has little effect on serum cholesterol at average levels of intake and has to be reduced to below 300 mg/day (which can only be achieved by means of a strict vegan diet) before endogenous cholesterol synthesis is reduced. However, people with familial hypercholesterolaemia (characterised by extremely high LDL cholesterol levels) may benefit from stricter control of dietary cholesterol intake which means limiting all types of animal foods including eggs.

Fatty and sugary foods group

Most people will need to curtail their intake of foods from this group and replace them with those from other groups, particularly bread/cereals and fruit/vegetables groups.

Fats and spreads: Full-fat products, such as butter and margarine, should be replaced by low-fat spreads derived from either monounsaturates (based on olive oil) or polyunsaturates (derived from corn oil, sunflower oil or soya oil). Although n–6 polyunsaturates have beneficial effects in terms of lowering blood cholesterol, excessive intakes may be counterproductive as they increase the susceptibility of LDL to lipid peroxidation. It is more important to choose a *low*-fat spread than one which contains polyunsaturates.

Cooking fats: Use of fat in cooking should be kept to a minimum and fried foods avoided as much as possible. If small amounts of cooking fat are essential, olive oil, rapeseed oil or soya oil may be the best choices.

Pies, ready meals, meat products (sausages, burgers, etc.): Although these composite foods contain components from other food groups, for the purpose of advice on heart disease they are probably best regarded as being in the 'fatty foods' group. These types of processed convenience foods need to be kept to a minimum for several reasons:

■ Most have a relatively high content of fat, especially saturated fat.
■ Many will be made using hydrogenated fats and thus contain *trans* fatty acids. Although the relevance of these to the development of CHD remains a matter of debate[12], someone who consumes a high proportion of processed convenience foods will almost certainly exceed the recommended maximum intake (2% of dietary energy).
■ Many will have a high content of sodium.
■ Heavy reliance on foods of this type often results in a diet containing very little fresh foods such as fruit and vegetables.

Sweetened pies, cakes, doughnuts, biscuits, chocolate, etc.: These also contain significant amounts of saturated and *trans* fatty acids and this, together with their sugar content, results in foods with a high energy content. Overconsumption of these foods increases the risk of energy surplus and hence obesity and also tends to displace more important foods from the diet. For these reasons, these foods should be discouraged.

OTHER DIETARY ASPECTS

Exercise

Exercise is vital for cardiovascular health, not only for the direct benefit on heart muscles as such but also for indirect benefits such as diminishing the risk of obesity and helping to alleviate stress.

Guidance issued by the Physical Activity Task Force in 1995 is that 30 minutes of moderate physical activity, such as a brisk walk, should be taken 5 times a week. (This replaced the previous advice of 20 minutes of vigorous exercise 3 times a week which most people found unrealistic). Those who are completely sedentary should be encouraged to be a little more active more often. It is important that people start gently and increase their activity level gradually. Sudden strenuous exercise in those unaccustomed to it can be hazardous.

Alcohol

The relationship between alcohol consumption and CHD is U-shaped, i.e. greatest mortality occurs at either very high or very low intakes. There may be several reasons for this. Moderate alcohol consumption tends to raise HDL concentration (which will be beneficial in terms of cholesterol removal) and alters haemostatic factors in a way which makes them less thrombogenic. Some alcoholic drinks, such as wine, are also rich sources of polyphenolic antioxidants which may be specifically protective. There is some evidence to suggest that wine consumption may partly explain the 'French paradox', i.e. why coronary mortality is so much lower in France and some southern European countries than would be expected from the prevalence of known risk factors. Moderate consumption of wine or other types of alcohol may therefore be of some benefit to cardiac health. However, high alcohol consumption can increase fibrinogen levels and hypertension and is obviously hazardous for other reasons.

Garlic

Garlic has been heavily promoted for its purported beneficial effects such as lowering cholesterol, enhancing fibrinolytic activity, inhibiting platelet aggregation and reducing blood pressure. Garlic has also been reported to have antioxidant properties. Experimentally there is some foundation for these assertions but whether they are of clinical significance has not yet been established[13].

REFERENCES

1 Department of Health (1994) *Nutritional Aspects of Cardiovascular Disease*. Report of the COMA Cardiovascular Review Group. Report on Health and Social Subjects 46. HMSO, London.

2 White, A. *et al.* (1993) *Health Survey for England 1991*. HMSO, London.

3 Law, M.R. *et al.* (1994) By how much and how quickly does reduction in serum cholesterol concentration lower risk of ischaemic heart disease? *British Medical Journal* 308, 367–72.

4 Law, M.R. *et al.* (1994) Systematic underestimation of association between serum cholesterol concentration and ischaemic heart disease in observational studies: data from the BUPA study. *British Medical Journal* 308, 363–6.

5 Bingham, S. (1991) Dietary aspects of a health strategy for England. *British Medical Journal* 303, 353–5.

6 Editorial (1993) Free radicals and vascular disease: how much do we know? *British Medical Journal* 307, 885.

7 Stampfer, M.J. *et al.* (1993) Vitamin E consumption and the risk of coronary heart disease in women. *New England Journal of Medicine* 328, 1444–9.

8 Rimm, E.B. *et al.* (1993) Vitamin E consumption and the risk of coronary heart disease in men. *New England Journal of Medicine* 328, 1450–56.

9 Kromhout, D. *et al.* (1985) The inverse relation between fish consumption and 20-year mortality from coronary heart disease. *New England Journal of Medicine* 312, 1205–1209.

10 Burr, M.L. *et al.* (1989) Effects of changes in fat, fish and fibre intakes on Death and Myocardial Reinfarction Trial (DART). *Lancet* ii, 757–761.

11 Larsson, B. *et al.* (1984) Abdominal adipose tissue distribution, obesity and risk of cardiovascular disease and death: 13 year follow up of the participants in the study of men born in 1913. *British Medical Journal* 288, 1401–1404.

12 British Nutrition Foundation (1995) *Trans Fatty Acids*. Report of a BNF Task Force. BNF, London.

13 Mansell, P. & Reckless, J.P.D. (1991) Garlic: effects on serum lipids, blood pressure, coagulation, platelet aggregation and vasodilation. *British Medical Journal* 303, 379–80.

FURTHER READING

Ashwell, M. (ed.) (1993) *Diet and Heart Disease. A Round Table of Factors*. British Nutrition Foundation, London.

Field, K. *et al.* (1995) Strategies for reducing coronary risk factors in primary care: which is the most cost-effective? *British Medical Journal* 310, 1109–112.

Imperial Cancer Research Fund OXCHECK Study Group (1995) Effectiveness of health checks conducted by nurses in primary care: final results of the OXCHECK Study. *British Medical Journal* 310, 1099–104.

National Heart Forum (1995) *Preventing coronary heart disease in primary care: The way forward*. HMSO, London.

USEFUL ADDRESSES

British Heart Foundation, 14 Fitzhardinge Street, London W1H 4DH. Tel: 0171 935 0185.

Coronary Prevention Group, 102 Gloucester Place, London W1H 3DA. Tel: 0171 935 2889.

23

Stroke

Stroke is the third biggest killer in the UK accounting for 9% of all male deaths and 15% of all female deaths, its incidence increasing sharply with age[1]. Every year about 100 000 people suffer a stroke and about one-third of them will die soon afterwards. A further 30 000 will die after a subsequent stroke. On the positive side, about half of those who have a stroke make a full recovery. Nevertheless, apart from the human suffering caused, the costs in terms of care and resources are considerable; at any one time there are about 350 000 stroke victims needing care within the community, many in nursing homes. Reducing the incidence of stroke is one of the *Health of the Nation* targets[2].

CAUSATION OF STROKE

Stroke can be broadly categorised into two types, ischaemic and haemorrhagic, the vast majority being ischaemic. As a result, many of the factors which are important for the prevention of atherogenesis associated with coronary heart disease (CHD) are also relevant to the prevention of stroke. There are, however, some differences in emphasis.

Hypertension is the most important risk factor for all types of stroke. Prospective studies have shown that adults with a diastolic blood pressure greater than 100 mmHg are 10–12 times more likely to have a stroke than those with a diastolic blood pressure of 80 mmHg[3]. It has been estimated that a fall in mean diastolic blood pressure of 7.5 mmHg could reduce stroke incidence by nearly half (46%)[3].

Treatment of hypertension has been found to have a much more rapid and greater effect on reducing the incidence of stroke than of CHD, probably because other risk factors are influencing the development of cardiovascular disease and the effects of prolonged elevated blood pressure on the cardiovascular system take longer to reverse[4].

Other factors such as obesity, smoking, heavy drinking, high salt intake and lack of physical activity are also strongly associated with the development of stroke although much of their influence may be exerted via their effects on blood pressure.

DIETARY GUIDANCE FOR THE PREVENTION OF STROKE

In general terms, dietary guidance to prevent a first occurrence or recurrence of stroke should be based on healthy eating principles along the lines of those given for the prevention of CHD (see Chapter 22). However, particular emphasis should be given to the following aspects:

■ *Reducing salt intake* particularly from processed manufactured foods.

- *Increasing potassium intake* via greater consumption of fruit and vegetables.
- *Preventing or correcting obesity.*
- *Increasing the level of physical activity* Moderate levels of physical activity have been shown to have significant benefits in terms of reducing the risk of stroke[5].

DIETARY GUIDANCE FOR THE TREATMENT OF STROKE

Stroke can have profound consequences on both the ability to eat and to obtain food. It may result in:

- *Swallowing difficulties (see also Chapter 29)* Acute stroke patients often have delayed swallow reflex necessitating either a semi-liquid or enterally-fed diet. Dysphagia usually improves with time but in some it may persist and measures are needed to ensure that food intake is of an appropriate consistency (liquidised food cannot be controlled and may cause choking) and adequate for nutritional needs.
- *Poor appetite (see also Chapter 8)* Depression is a common sequel to stroke and this often results in loss of appetite. Good nutritional intake may be important to the recovery process and people should be encouraged to eat small soft portions of appetising food. Supplements

in the form of sip feeds may be useful to help meet nutrient needs.

- *Disability (see also Chapter 18)* Stroke may result in permanent physical or mental disability and this may affect food intake if shopping or cooking become difficult, or if people forget to eat or eat inappropriate foods.

REFERENCES

1 Department of Health (1994) *Nutritional Aspects of Cardiovascular Disease.* Report of the COMA Cardiovascular Review Group. Report on Health and Social Subjects 46. HMSO, London.
2 Department of Health (1992) *The Health of the Nation: A Strategy for Health in England.* HMSO, London.
3 MacMahon, S. *et al.* (1990) Blood pressure, stroke and coronary heart disease. Part 1, prolonged differences in blood pressure: prospective observational studies corrected for the regression dilution bias. *Lancet* 335, 765–74.
4 Collins, R. *et al.* (1990) Blood pressure, stroke and coronary heart disease. Part 2, short-term reductions in blood pressure: overview of randomised drug trials in their epidemiological context. *Lancet* 335, 827–38.
5 Wannamethee, G. & Shaper, A.G. (1992) Physical activity and stroke in British middle-aged men. *British Medical Journal* 304, 597–601.

USEFUL ADDRESSES

The Stroke Association, CHSA House, Whitecross Street, London EC1Y 8JJ. Tel: 0171 490 7999. (This was formerly the Chest, Heart and Stroke Association.)

24

Hypertension

Raised blood pressure greatly increases the risk of coronary heart disease (CHD) and stroke. Within a population, a difference in diastolic pressure of 7.5 mmHg has been shown to be associated with a 29% difference in coronary heart disease risk and a 46% difference in stroke, irrespective of age, sex or ethnic group[1]. Reducing blood pressure has rapid and pronounced benefits, particularly in terms of stroke[2].

The 1991 Health Survey for England classified 16% of men (16–64 years) and 17% of women as hypertensive (systolic blood pressure above 160 mmHg and/or a diastolic above 95 mmHg)[3].

Hypertension is usually a primary disorder but can be secondary to renal or heart disease.

Factors which may contribute to primary hypertension are:

- *Genetic:* Some people are more susceptible to hypertensive factors than others.
- *Age:* Blood pressure tends to rise with age.
- *Sex:* Hypertension is less common in pre-menopausal women.
- *Stress:* Prolonged stress can exacerbate hypertension.
- *Diet/lifestyle:* High sodium intake
  Low potassium intake
  High alcohol intake
  Obesity
  Lack of physical activity.

DIET AND BLOOD PRESSURE

Sodium/salt

Sodium, because of its role in maintaining fluid balance, is essential for the maintenance of blood pressure. Whether excessive sodium intake causes raised blood pressure has been more difficult to establish for two reasons. First, blood pressure is regulated by a variety of mechanisms and influenced by many factors. Second, it is notoriously difficult to obtain an accurate assessment of habitual sodium intake from short-term dietary records such as those used in many epidemiological studies.

Recent comprehensive analysis evidence suggests that there is a relationship between the two. The Intersalt study[4], a large-scale multinational study, found positive associations between sodium excretion (a more reliable marker of sodium intake) and blood pressure and strong evidence that sodium intake accounts for much of the rise in blood pressure with age. Subsequent meta-analysis of 24 other major studies found that there was a quantifiable relationship between sodium restriction and fall in blood pressure[5]. The magnitude of the effect remains a matter of debate[6]. The effect of salt on blood pressure is probably smaller than that of obesity or alcohol, and salt restriction has more effect in older people and those with higher initial blood pressure. Nevertheless, it has been estimated that an average reduction of salt intake by 3 g/day (1.2 g or 50 mmol sodium/day) would result in an average reduction of systolic blood pressure of about 3.5 mmHg, and a larger effect could be expected in the long term as the rise in blood pressure with age was also reduced.

The *Health of the Nation* target is to reduce mean systolic blood pressure by 5 mmHg by the year 2005[7]. This will almost certainly necessitate the targets for obesity and alcohol to be achieved in addition to a reduction in salt intake.

A recent recommendation from the Department of Health is that average sodium intake should be reduced by one-third[8]. In the adult population, this means a fall from the current level of 9 g salt/day (3.6 g sodium/day) to 6 g salt/day (2.4 g sodium/day). The World Health Organization also recommends a maximum intake of 6 g salt/day.

A significant reduction in sodium intake can be achieved without drastic dietary alteration. About 15–20% of sodium intake is derived from salt added to foods at the table or during cooking. Much of the time this is done for reasons of habit rather than taste and many notice little difference if they use much less or leave it out altogether, particularly if they use more herbs or spices instead.

In most people's diets, the greatest proportion of sodium (about 60–70%) is derived from manufactured and processed foods. Heavy reliance on foods such as ready made pies and pasties, instant meals, canned soups and vegetables, savoury snacks, etc., inevitably results in a high sodium intake. Replacing some of these types of foods with more fresh foods, particularly fruit and vegetables, is likely to be beneficial in many dietary respects, not just in terms of sodium alone.

Potassium

Potassium counterbalances the effect of sodium. A high potassium intake may therefore be protective and a low one undesirable. The Intersalt study suggested that a 50% increase in potassium consumption would result in an average fall in systolic blood pressure of 1.6 mmHg[4]. Potassium intake can be increased by a greater consumption of fruit and vegetables.

Alcohol

Heavy drinking is associated with increased blood pressure. In one large population study, the difference in mean systolic blood pressure between non-drinkers and those consuming more than 30 units per week was 3.5 mmHg[5].

Obesity

Obesity is strongly associated with the level of blood pressure and weight reduction is an important part of the management of hypertension.

Physical activity

Increasing the level of physical activity helps to prevent or correct obesity but may also have independent hypotensive effects[8].

DIETARY GUIDANCE

People with hypertension should be strongly encouraged to consume a diet based on healthy eating guidelines in order to help minimise the risks from stroke and CHD. Particular emphasis should be given to:

- Reducing weight if necessary.
- Reducing salt intake by:
  - □ Avoiding adding salt directly to food.
  - □ Leaving salt out of recipes wherever possible; using more herbs and spices for flavouring.
  - □ Adding half the usual amount of salt to vegetable cooking water.
  - □ Using fewer manufactured processed foods or ready meals from packets, cartons or cans and using more fresh foods instead.
  - □ Avoiding highly salted foods (e.g. cheese, ham, salted fish).
- Increasing the consumption of fruit and vegetables.
- Keeping alcohol consumption within sensible limits.

Severe hypertension associated with renal or liver disease may require more drastic sodium restriction to 50 mmol/day (3 g salt/day) and possibly other dietary manipulations. Specialist dietetic advice is necessary in such cases.

REFERENCES

1 MacMahon, S. *et al.* (1990) Blood pressure, stroke and coronary heart disease. Part 1, prolonged differences in blood pressure: prospective observational studies corrected for the regression dilution bias. *Lancet* 335, 765–74.
2 Collins, R. *et al.* (1990) Blood pressure, stroke and coronary heart disease. Part 2, short-term reductions in blood pressure: overview of randomised drug trials in their epidemiological context. *Lancet* 335, 827–38.
3 White, A. *et al.* (1993) *Health Survey for England 1991.* HMSO, London.
4 Intersalt Co-operative Research Group (1988) Intersalt: an international study of electrolyte excretion and blood pressure. Results for 24 hour urinary sodium and potassium excretion. *British Medical Journal* 297, 319–28.
5 Law, M.R. *et al.* (1991) By how much does dietary salt reduction lower blood pressure? *British Medical Journal* 302, 811–19.
6 Swales, J.D. (1991) Dietary salt and blood pressure: the role of meta-analyses. *Journal of Hypertension* 9 (suppl. 6), S42–6.
7 Department of Health (1992) *The Health of the Nation: A Strategy for Health in England.* HMSO, London.
8 Department of Health (1994) *Nutritional Aspects of Cardiovascular Disease.* Report of the COMA Cardiovascular Review Group. Report on Health and Social Subjects 46. HMSO, London.

FURTHER READING

British Nutrition Foundation (1994) *Salt in the Diet.* Briefing Paper. BNF, London.

25

Obesity

Obesity is a serious public health problem because of its prevalence and associated health risks. The 1991 Health Survey for England showed that virtually half of the adult population (53% of men and 44% of women) could be considered to be 'overweight' (BMI >25) and that 13% of men and 15% of women were classified as 'obese' (BMI >30)[1]. The *Health of the Nation* target is to reduce this prevalence of obesity by about half (to 6% in men and 8% in women) by the year 2005 but more recent health surveys suggest that little progress is being made towards this target; if anything, the prevalence is continuing to rise[2].

THE HEALTH RISKS OF OBESITY

Obesity greatly increases the risk of mortality from heart disease, stroke, diabetes and some forms of cancers. It also results in greater morbidity from disorders such as gallstones and osteoarthritis and increases the risks from anaesthesia and surgery.

The health implications of overweight or obesity are usually evaluated by use of the BMI or Body Mass Index (weight in kg divided by height squared in metres) as this is a far better indicator of body fatness than consideration of body weight alone. A chart for measuring BMI in an individual is given in Appendix 4. Health risks are thought to increase once BMI exceeds 25, although to some extent this is an arbitrary cut-off point and a highly active person with a BMI of 28 may have lower health risks than an inactive person with a BMI of 25. However, there still seems little doubt that in adults, health risks accelerate sharply once BMI exceeds 30[3].

As well as the total amount of body fat, its distribution within the body may also have considerable prognostic value. People whose surplus fat is predominantly stored centrally, in the abdominal cavity, appear to have the greatest risk of metabolic complications such as heart disease, stroke, diabetes, gallstones and hormone-dependent neoplasms. Those whose fat is stored more peripherally, in hips and thighs, are less prone to metabolic diseases but more at risk from mechanical problems associated with carrying excessive weight, i.e. osteoarthritis, problems with load-bearing joints such as hips and knees, and varicose veins. These affect morbidity but are less serious in terms of mortality.

Fat distribution can be very simply assessed by the Waist-Hip Ratio (WHR) (waist circumference divided by hip circumference (see p. 55)). People with high WHR measurements have a predominantly central fat distribution (and have been colloquially termed 'apples'); those with a low WHR have a mainly peripheral fat distribution (and can be termed 'pears'). A ratio which exceeds 0.9 in men or 0.85 in women appears to be associated with increased risk of metabolic disease[3,4,5]. The UK population becomes increasingly apple-shaped with age and increasing BMI, and men tend to be more apple-shaped than women, a difference which may well explain much of the sex difference in prevalence of coronary heart disease (CHD)[6].

Since 'apples' are at greater health risk than 'pears' it has been suggested that obesity treatment is a far greater priority in this group. Those with central obesity are more likely to exhibit other risk factors, such as hypertension, high blood cholesterol levels and insulin resistance, which may be improved by weight loss. Furthermore, evidence suggests that intra-abdominal fat is more responsive to weight loss from diet or exercise than subcutaneous fat[7].

CAUSES OF OBESITY

The fundamental cause of obesity is simple and always the same – individual energy consumption has exceeded individual energy requirement. However, the factors which have led to this energy imbalance are complex and variable. To assume that obesity is always the result of gluttony is both wrong and unfair. Some of the most relevant factors are:

- *Genetic influences*   Obesity does tend to run in families although in some cases this may simply reflect the fact that the same inappropriate eating habits are adopted by successive generations. But undoubtedly there is variation between people in the way that energy-bearing nutrients are metabolised; those who are more efficient at producing and storing energy will need less of the fuel source (i.e. dietary fat, carbohydrate and protein) which provides it. Some people may also be more efficient at disposing of surplus energy than others.
- *Psychological influences*   Most people eat for reasons other than hunger, but in some people, comfort eating to combat loneliness or depression may result in a distorted eating pattern.
- *Physical activity level*   Lack of exercise will obviously help contribute to an energy surplus and once people become significantly over-

weight they often avoid exercise because they find the exertion difficult or because they are embarrassed by their appearance. Less obvious forms of physical activity may also account for some of the differences in energy requirements between people; restless, fidgety personalities will use up more energy during a day than those who are more placid.

- *Dietary composition*   Obesity is not caused by any specific nutrient, such as fat or sugar, only by a total energy intake which is higher than required. However, foods which contain a high proportion of fat are energy dense, i.e. provide a lot of energy relative to their bulk, and over-consumption of such foods can easily lead to a high energy intake. Sugar (i.e. sucrose) provides no more energy on a weight for weight basis than starch or protein; the problem is that sucrose tends to make foods highly palatable so it is easy to eat large quantities of them, and many of these foods also have a high fat and hence high energy content (e.g. cakes, biscuits and chocolates).

DIETARY MANAGEMENT OF OBESITY

In theory, treatment of obesity is simply a matter of correcting the energy imbalance by either reducing energy intake or increasing energy expenditure (or a mixture of the two). To say that is this is difficult in practice is a considerable understatement.

The statistics of dieting success are depressing with the vast majority of people who start to slim returning to their original weight. Repeated weight loss and gain, so-called 'yo-yo dieting', can even result in long-term weight increase as well as being associated with its own health problems such as osteoporosis. Following any type of diet is difficult (see Chapter 7, *Achieving Dietary Change*) but that required to achieve weight loss is probably most difficult of all because it tends to result in feelings of hunger and deprivation. Strict dieting makes people irritable and depressed and the trauma of keeping to the diet can seem far worse than the threatened health risks from not doing so.

Before a realistic strategy to achieve weight loss can be achieved, some of the physical and/or psychological factors which have led to the energy imbalance have to be identified. These will need to be addressed if any significant change in eating habits is likely to occur. Dietary assessment is the essential first step, although the objective of this is not to quantify usual calorie intake. In the primary care setting, attempting to do this is usually a waste of time because the type of dietary enquiry which can be made will not be capable of measuring this with any meaningful degree of accuracy (see Chapter 6, *Assessing Nutritional Adequacy*), particularly in a group of people who tend to under-report their food intake. What dietary assessment should aim to do is to build up a picture of typical dietary intake in order to identify:

- The typical meal pattern during the day.
- The degree of dietary balance between the four main food groups.
- The extent to which the fifth group, fatty and sugary foods, contributes to food intake.

These can be used as a basis to explore problems associated with what people eat, why they eat particular foods and when they eat them.

Several different types of eating patterns may emerge which have different implications in terms of management:

- *Heavy reliance on energy-dense convenience foods* People whose diet contains a high proportion of ready meals, take-aways and relatively few fresh foods, such as fruit and vegetables, are likely to be consuming a diet high in fat and energy content.
- *Inappropriate food choice* Some people avoid foods such as bread and potatoes in the belief that they are fattening and fill up with foods such as cheese or meat not realising that these are far more energy dense.
- *Over-indulgence* People whose lifestyle necessitates a lot of business or social entertaining or hotel life are often well aware that their weight

problems stem from too much rich food and alcohol.

- *Have a 'normal' food intake* Some obese people say that they eat very little and this is usually not true. However, if they say that they eat less, certainly no more, than other people who are much thinner this certainly can be true. In the thin person, 2000 kcal/day may not be enough to meet energy needs and may even cause weight loss; in the obese person, 2000 kcal/day may be too much and cause weight gain. Individuals differ both in terms of their energy needs and their ability to dispose of surplus energy intake. The person who needs least energy is, in a society where food is plentiful, most likely to exceed those needs and become obese. In many ways such people are the most difficult to treat because the unavoidable truth is that in order to remedy their obesity, they will have to consume an energy intake which is below the average for that of the population as a whole.
- *Behavioural eating problems* People whose eating pattern is significantly affected by psychological factors, such as anxiety, depression or low self-esteem, respond poorly to conventional dietary advice. In this group, counselling techniques and behavioural therapy are far more likely to be successful in effecting permanent change[8]. People with clear signs of bulimia nervosa or other eating disorders (see Chapter 26) should be referred for expert advice.

The way in which these different aspects are tackled will need to vary if treatment is to be successful in the long term, i.e. that it achieves a permanent change in eating habits so that weight loss can not only be achieved but maintained. Handing out a standard low calorie diet sheet to all-comers will be useless; obesity does not result from a standard set of dietary circumstances.

There are, though, common dietary objectives. All obese people need to consume less energy than their current level of intake – whatever that may be. This is likely to be less traumatic if the energy density of the food eaten is reduced rather than the total amount. In other words, the volume of the diet remains the same but the foods comprising it have a lower energy content. In general terms this means decreasing dietary fat content (the most energy-dense nutrient) and replacing it with carbohydrate and fibre-containing foods which provide more bulk but less energy. These measures are also healthy eating objectives which is why all overweight people should be encouraged to modify their existing diet along these lines.

Food choice

Bread, other cereals and potatoes group

Many overweight people regard these foods as 'fattening' and this misconception must be dispelled. These foods need to be a central part of the diet because of their satiety value, their nutritional value and because they will help to displace fat-rich energy-dense foods from the diet. Advice on the associated use of fat with these foods may be relevant; pasta should not be coated with butter, potatoes should not be fried, fat should not be liberally spread on bread.

Fruit and vegetables group

These are also vital components of the diet for many reasons but in those who are overweight are a particularly valuable way of decreasing dietary energy density. There is no need for people to live on a diet of salads as is often suggested. All types of vegetables and fruit, whether raw, fresh, frozen, canned or dried, can be liberally consumed. The only provisos are that they are not coated with fat (e.g. butter or cream) and that they are drained from any syrup.

Milk and dairy foods group

Reduced-fat sources of these should be encouraged for their content of calcium and other essential vitamins and minerals. Consumption of hard cheese should be watched; even types which contain less fat, such as Edam, are still a concentrated source of calories.

Meat, fish and alternatives group

These food choices should be of high nutrient density, e.g. lean meat rather than meat products, fish rather than breaded fish products. This need not incur greater cost; a smaller quantity of a higher quality product will meet nutritional needs and the difference in bulk can be rectified with greater use of vegetables, pulses or cereal foods.

Fatty and sugary foods group

Replacing many of these high energy, low nutrient foods with those from the other four major food groups is much more likely to produce a dietary balance leading to weight loss. These foods do not have to be excluded altogether – they do not have uniquely fattening properties. The problem is that their combination of high palatability and low satiety makes it easy for them to become undesirably dominant in the diet.

These guidelines need to be applied in the context of what someone usually eats and taking all the other factors which affect this (lifestyle, social and economic circumstances, self-esteem, readiness to change) into account. Change should not be expected overnight. Permanent change in eating habits – the ultimate objective – will be a gradual process and also one which is likely to require continued support and motivation (see Chapter 7, *Achieving Dietary Change*).

OTHER DIETARY ASPECTS

Exercise

Increasing the level of physical activity is a useful adjunct to a weight reducing diet. Not only does this improve physical fitness and general health, it also helps to distract attention from food, particularly in those who tend to eat out of habit or boredom. Beneficial exercise does not have to take the form of obvious sporting activities such as jogging or aerobics (although younger people may need only a little encouragement to try an activity of this type). But most people can find ways of gradually increasing their level of activity – using stairs rather than a lift, going for a walk every day, using the car less often. In some parts of the country, planned exercise programmes for slimmers or 'exercise prescriptions' are available as part of local health promotion initiatives.

Slimming clubs

Commercial or community-run slimming groups can be very helpful for some people because of the level of support they provide. A disadvantage is that people usually have to pay fees to attend them although this factor is probably part of the reason for their success; people are reluctant to waste their 'investment' by failure. Their effectiveness at achieving long-term weight loss is less certain but may well be better than many traditional forms of obesity advice.

Very Low Calorie Diets (VLCDs)

These are nutritionally complete high protein formula diets usually providing about 800 kcal/day and designed to act as a complete substitute for conventional meals. Sometimes they are used in conjunction with other products in the range such as snack bars or reconstituted meals provided in dried form. VLCDs can result in significant weight loss in the short term (in the initial stages most of it in the form of fluid rather than fat) but their long-term value is more questionable as they do little in terms of educating people how to adjust their normal diet so that they can attain and maintain permanent weight loss. They can occasionally be useful to convince the demoralised repeatedly-failed dieter that weight loss is possible and encourage them to achieve further weight loss by means of sensible eating habits.

'The latest diet'

The general public is very gullible when it comes to a new diet claiming to burn off fat or to be the definitive answer to quick and easy weight loss. Many such diets achieve initial rapid weight loss as a result of metabolic fluid loss which occurs with any form of energy restriction in the short term. If the long-term success rate matched the sales of some diet books, obesity would be a disappearing problem, not one which continues to increase.

Meal replacements

These are products, such as biscuits, snack bars or drinks usually containing added vitamins, mineral and cellulosic fibre, which are used as a replacement for one or more meals per day. These products are expensive and achieve little in terms of modification of eating habits.

Fibre supplements

These have been promoted as being an aid to weight loss. Some have been claimed to increase faecal energy excretion and although this may occur to a minor extent the significance in terms of overall energy balance is likely to be minimal. It is far preferable that people increase their consumption of fibre-rich foods.

Appetite suppressants

These should only be considered in people with severe eating disturbances.

PREVENTING OBESITY

The real answer to the treatment of obesity lies in its prevention, i.e.:

- Laying the foundations of good eating habits in children and ensuring that excessive weight is checked at any early stage.
- Encouraging teenagers and young adults not to be obsessed with slimming but rather to be an appropriate body weight for health.
- Persuading adults that middle-aged spread is not inevitable and to take steps to adjust their energy intake and activity level to match the fall in energy requirement with age, rather than waiting until they are two or three stone overweight.

REFERENCES

1 White, A. *et al.* (1993) *Health Survey for England 1991*. HMSO, London.
2 Bennett, N. *et al.* (1995) *Health Survey for England 1993*. HMSO, London.
3 Association for the Study of Obesity (1994) Consensus statement on obesity. *International Journal of Obesity* **18**, 189.
4 Larsson, B. *et al.* (1984) Abdominal adipose tissue distribution, obesity and risk of cardiovascular disease and death: 13 year follow-up of the participants in the study of men born in 1913. *British Medical Journal* **288**, 1401–4.
5 Lapidus, L. *et al.* (1984) Distribution of adipose tissue and risk of cardiovascular disease and death: 12 year follow up of participants in the population study of women in Gothenburg, Sweden. *British Medical Journal* **289**, 1257–61.
6 Ashwell, M. (1992) Apples and pears. *British Nutrition Foundation Bulletin* **17**, 13–14.
7 Krotkiewski, M. (1988) Can body fat patterning be changed? *Acta Medica Scandinavia* **723**, 213–23.
8 LeBow, M.D. (1981) *Weight Control: The Behavioural Strategies*. John Wiley, Chichester.

FURTHER READING

British Nutrition Foundation (1992) *The Nature and Risks of Obesity*. Briefing Paper 27. BNF, London.
Department of Health (1995) *Reversing the Increasing Problem of Obesity in England*. A report from the Nutrition and Physical Activity Task Forces. Available from: Department of Health, PO Box 410, Wetherby, LS23 7LN.
Garrow, J.S. (1988) *Obesity and Related Diseases*. Churchill Livingstone, London.
Health Education Authority (1991) *Obesity and Overweight*. A briefing paper. HEA, London.

26

Eating Disorders (Anorexia nervosa and Bulimia nervosa)

Eating disorders, of which anorexia nervosa and bulimia nervosa are the most common, are psychiatric disorders which manifest themselves in terms of food habits. The prevalence of each of these disorders has increased dramatically in recent years and is continuing to rise. Currently, about 125000 people in the UK suffer from bulimia nervosa and about 70000 from anorexia nervosa[1]. Many more cases are probably undiagnosed or unreported. In one study, fewer than a third of the people with bulimia had ever mentioned their eating disorder to their GP although many felt they needed medical help[1].

Treatment of eating disorders usually requires specialist psychiatric and dietetic care which is beyond the scope of the average general practice but it is important that those who work in the primary care setting are able to recognise developing signs of these disorders so that help can be sought at an early stage.

ANOREXIA NERVOSA

The seriousness of anorexia nervosa should not be underestimated since it carries a considerable risk of mortality; over 20% of sufferers die from the physical consequences of the disease and the risk of suicide is also high.

Typically anorexia nervosa occurs in young girls who have recently gone through puberty. The peak age of incidence is 18–19 years. Its most common features are:

- Pronounced self-imposed weight loss.
- Lack of concern over the weight loss.
- Distorted self-image, despite the emaciation the person still considers herself to be fat.
- Fear of weight gain.
- Obsessional interest in food despite little of it being eaten.
- Amenorrhoea

The physical effects of anorexia nervosa are those of severe starvation:

- Oestrogen deficiency.
- Bone loss (an anorexic patient can lose 10–15% of bone mass in one year).
- Bone marrow suppression and reduced red and white blood cell count.
- Muscle atrophy including that of the heart.
- Liver abnormalities.

Some of these may have lasting consequences such as impaired fertility, problems in sustaining a pregnancy, cardiac disorders and osteoporosis.

Body Mass Index (BMI), and the rate of fall of BMI, indicate the severity of the disorder. Those with a BMI above 13 can usually be treated on an out-patient basis. In-patient admission is needed if:

- BMI falls below 13.
- BMI is falling rapidly towards this level.
- The patient has marked electrolyte disturbances or myopathy.
- The patient is suicidal.

BULIMIA NERVOSA

Bulimia nervosa is much more common than anorexia nervosa. It shares some common features with anorexia nervosa but it is a quite distinct disorder. Bulimia is more difficult to treat than anorexia and 40% of cases remain chronically ill.

As with anorexia nervosa there is an overconcern with shape and weight and a rigid restriction of food intake, but there are also episodes of bingeing followed by self-induced vomiting or purging. Use of laxatives and excessive levels of exercise are common. Unlike the anorexic patient, the bulimic subject often does not look underweight, particularly facially. This is because the frequent presence of acid vomit in the mouth often results in benign enlargement of the parotid glands which gives a rounded appearance to the face making the patient look 'well'. Bulimia nervosa can therefore be missed because its presence only becomes apparent on questioning rather than from the patient's appearance.

Bulimics typically display obsessional symptoms. Some have signs of self-damaging behaviour (e.g. alcohol abuse, drug abuse, overdosing, cutting, burning, etc.); such patients are likely to be older (in their late twenties rather than late teens) and may have a history of sexual abuse or come from a home of alcohol abuse. Other clinical manifestations of bulimia nervosa are:

- Tooth enamel erosion resulting from the presence of acid vomit in the mouth.
- Electrolyte disturbances due to repeated vomiting (which results in potassium loss) and purging (causing loss of sodium and magnesium) may result in oedema, palpitations and tetany.
- Severe constipation and even rectal prolapse (caused by laxative abuse).

- Insomnia (can be caused by large quantities of caffeine-containing diet drinks).

DISTINGUISHING BETWEEN ANOREXIA NERVOSA AND BULIMIA NERVOSA

The principal difference between the two disorders is that anorexic patients look unwell but believe they are perfectly normal (and often fat); bulimics may look normal but are usually privately appalled by their eating behaviour and concerned at their inability to control it. The main contrasting features are shown in Table 26.1.

CAUSES AND RISK INDICATORS

The reason why these disorders manifest themselves is not really known other than that sufferers feel under pressure to be a certain size and form. Dieting greatly increases the risk, but many people diet and not all develop eating disorders.

For bulimia nervosa high risk factors appear to be:

- History of psychiatric disorder in family.
- Adverse experiences.
- Poor parenting.
- Obsessional personality.

Anorexia nervosa is more associated with:

- High IQ.
- Perfectionist personality.
- Response to stress.
- Response to pressure to lose weight.

Early intervention is important to minimise the physical damage which can result and to counter the psychological effects of the disorders which tend to perpetuate them and make them more refractory to treatment. Professional counselling and behavioural therapy is essential in most cases.

Table 26.1 Contrasting features of anorexia nervosa and bulimia nervosa.

Feature	Anorexia nervosa	Bulimia nervosa
Eating characteristics	Starvation	Starvation interspersed with bingeing/purging
Appearance	Emaciated	Often look well, especially facially
Patients' perception of the problem	Cannot see they have a a problem	Usually disgusted by their behaviour
Electrolyte disturbance	Usually only in later stages	Commonly occurs due to repeated vomiting

REFERENCE

1 Office of Health Economics (1994) *Eating Disorders: Anorexia Nervosa and Bulimia Nervosa*. Office of Health Economics, London.

FURTHER READING

Abraham, S. & Llewellyn-Jones, D. (1992) *Eating Disorders: The Facts*. Oxford University Press, Oxford.

Beumont, J.V., Russell, J.D. & Touyz, S.W. (1993) Treatment of anorexia nervosa. *Lancet* **341**, 1635.

Eating Disorders Association (1995) *Eating Disorders – A Guide to Commissioning and Purchasing Services*. Eating Disorders Association, Norwich.

Garner, D.M. (1993) Pathogenesis of anorexia nervosa. *Lancet* **341**, 1631.

Hogg, C. (1995) *Eating Disorders – A Guide to Primary Health Care*. Eating Disorders Association, Norwich.

USEFUL ADDRESSES

Eating Disorders Association, Sackville Place, 44–48 Magdalen Street, Norwich, Norfolk NR3 1JH. Tel: 01603 621414. Youth helpline (18 years and under): 01603 765050.

27

Diabetes Mellitus

The dietary management of diabetes has changed enormously in the last decade. Health professionals returning to this area of care after an absence of 10–20 years will probably find that some aspects of current dietary advice directly contradict those which they thought were correct. Long-established patients may also be puzzled at the apparent about-turn in guidance. There are very sound reasons for these changes and understanding what these are makes it easier to understand the new approach to dietary management.

Prior to the discovery of insulin in 1921, severe carbohydrate restriction represented the only hope of keeping the diabetic patient alive, and even this was not very successful. The availability of insulin dramatically changed the prospects of survival. In all the excitement, the role of diet was rather overlooked. It was assumed, although never scientifically shown, that carbohydrate was 'bad' for people with diabetes although it was accepted that a certain amount was necessary to counterbalance the hypoglycaemic effects of insulin. Consequently patients were given a diet low in carbohydrate, virtually devoid of sugar but rich in high fat, high protein foods such as cheese and meat. During the 1970s, doubts began to be expressed as to whether this was wise. It was becoming apparent that the threat to long-term diabetic survival was not so much from the diabetes itself (deaths from diabetic ketoacidosis are now rare) but from the vascular complications arising as a result of it, particularly the greatly increased risk of coronary heart disease. In this context, an atherogenic high fat, low carbohydrate diet seemed

unlikely to be beneficial. At the same time, epidemiological and experimental studies clearly showed that there was no necessity to restrict the carbohydrate intake of the treated diabetic patient. Although dietary carbohydrate has the greatest post-prandial effect on blood glucose levels, other factors such as total energy intake influence the baseline level of glycaemia. Diets containing a high proportion of their energy in the form of carbohydrate actually improve diabetic glucose handling as well as having many other advantages.

As a result of these deliberations, the dietary management of diabetes was re-evaluated and new recommendations were issued in the UK and other Western countries[1,2,3]. The primary objectives of diet in conjunction with other forms of therapy were to:

- *Help maintain near-normal glycaemia.* Keeping blood glucose levels as near to normal levels as possible has been shown to reduce the risk from peripheral vascular disease such as diabetic retinopathy (which can cause blindness), nephropathy (which can result in renal failure) and neuropathy (loss of nerve function).
- *Minimise the dietary factors which exacerbate atherogenesis* and so may increase the risk of cardiovascular disease.

The type of diet thought most likely to achieve this was one which:

- Contains an energy content which is appropriate to the individual's requirement.
- Contains a relatively high proportion of this energy in the form of carbohydrate.
- Contains a relatively low proportion of this energy in the form of fat, particularly saturated fat.
- Is not excessively high in protein or sodium.
- Contains most of its carbohydrate in a form which is not too rapidly absorbed, i.e. predominately starchy fibre-containing carbohydrate rather than sugar-rich foods.

NUTRITIONAL CONSIDERATIONS

Energy

Ensuring that the diet has an energy content which is appropriate for individual requirements is crucial. Preventing obesity (which will worsen glucose tolerance) is important but the chronic hyperglycaemic effects of continuous energy surplus will be seen long before overt obesity occurs. Conversely, in diabetic people who are obese, energy reduction (from any dietary source) will produce an immediate improvement in glycaemia long before weight reduction (which will further improve the situation) is achieved.

In diabetic children, dietary energy content is also an important consideration although ensuring energy sufficiency is usually the primary aim. The low carbohydrate diets of the past often resulted in severely restricted energy intakes with damaging consequences in terms of growth and development[4].

Tables of average energy requirements for sub-groups of the population are not a good guide to individual energy needs as the latter vary considerably. While it is possible to quantify individual energy requirements by means of formulae based on estimations of basal metabolic rate[5] this is rarely necessary in the primary care setting. A person's body weight is a good indicator of likely energy needs. If someone is overweight or even at the upper end of the normal range, or their weight is increasing, then they need to consume less energy than they do at present, irrespective of what that level is. A child whose growth rate is slow or slowing down almost certainly needs to consume more. Nor is it necessary to quantify usual energy consumption in terms of calorie intake. Simple assessment of the usual meal pattern and the proportion of food groups comprising the normal diet provides all the necessary information. If someone is of normal weight, their general level of food intake needs to stay more or less the same (although the types and times of consumption of some foods may need to change – see below). If overweight, they will need to eat less, and the proportions of foods from different food groups will reveal the types of adjustments which need to be made.

Carbohydrate

Most diabetic patients need to consume more energy in the form of carbohydrate (ideally at least 50% of dietary energy). This does not mean that people can eat as much carbohydrate as they like in addition to what they usually eat – that would simply result in energy overload. It is a proportional change in the context of an appropriate energy intake, i.e. of the total amount of energy consumed, more should be derived from carbohydrate and less from fat.

The type of carbohydrate consumed remains important. Most of it should come from starchy, fibre-containing foods such as bread, breakfast cereals, potatoes, rice and pasta. Large amounts of isolated sources of simple sugars, e.g. sugar-rich drinks or foods, should be avoided because of their rapid rate of absorption and influence on glycaemia. However, it is now generally acknowledged that there is no need to be obsessive about sucrose avoidance. Small amounts of sugar consumed with other foods or as part of a meal are not a problem.

LIVERPOOL
JOHN MOORES UNIVERSITY
AVRIL ROBARTS LRC
TEL. 0151 231 4022

In the past, carbohydrate intake has been strictly regulated by means of the carbohydrate exchange system. This specified the amount of a food providing 10g carbohydrate (e.g. an egg-sized potato, $\frac{3}{4}$ slice of bread, or a glass of milk) so that patients could exchange one food for another but still keep their carbohydrate intake constant. This system was seriously flawed. Equivalent amounts of carbohydrate do not have equivalent effects on blood glucose; the presence of other components in the food, particularly fibre, affect the rate of digestion and absorption, and other factors such as the composition of the rest of the meal or even the physical characteristics of the food (a whole apple has different effects from puréed apple) also confound the picture. Attempts have been made to derive a 'glycaemic index' which rates the effects of different carbohydrate foods on post-prandial glycaemia, but because people rarely eat particular foods in isolation (e.g. a potato on its own) but usually in conjunction with others (e.g. meat and vegetables which will alter the glycaemic effect of the potato) it has proved impossible to devise a glycaemic index based exchange system which is of any practical use. It is also being recognised that such a system is not really necessary. Ensuring that people eat regular amounts of carbohydrate foods of an appropriate type (i.e. mainly starch-based) is all that is necessary.

Fat

It is recommended that the fat intake of the diabetic population should be reduced to 35% of dietary energy – i.e. the same as that advocated for health for the general population. In practice this means that fat-reducing aspects of healthy eating guidelines are also appropriate for those with diabetes, i.e. using reduced-fat milk and dairy products, low-fat spreads, avoiding fried foods and unnecessary sources of fat and generally reducing the consumption of fatty foods (see p. 40). However, because people with diabetes have a much greater risk of developing coronary heart disease and other

vascular disorders than the rest of the population, it is much more important that this advice is followed.

Protein

There is some evidence that excessive consumption of protein increases microalbuminuria, an early sign of diabetic renal damage[2]. Patients should therefore be encourage to keep their consumption of meat, fish and alternatives to moderate levels, i.e. as recommended in current healthy eating guidelines.

Salt

Because of the greatly elevated risk of cardiovascular disease in the form of both coronary heart disease and stroke, any dietary measure which may reduce the risk of hypertension is obviously wise (see Chapter 24). Generally recommended measures such as a reduction in the use of added salt and processed manufactured foods are important for those with diabetes.

Fibre (non-starch polysaccharide)

Dietary fibre is as important for people with diabetes as it is for anyone else. Whether it is more important is debatable. Insoluble fibre present in starchy foods certainly plays a part in slowing the rate of glucose absorption but all cereal foods are beneficial in this respect and the additional advantage of wholemeal and wholegrain varieties over less fibre-rich types is probably not as great as has been suggested. Soluble fibre present in pulses such as beans may be more useful because it can lower both the rate of glucose absorption and the blood cholesterol level. However, the practical importance of this has to be kept in perspective; most people are not prepared to consume a diet containing large quantities of beans. Fibre-containing foods should be encouraged but need not be overemphasised.

Alcohol

People with diabetes should not exceed the levels of alcohol recommended for the rest of the population (see Chapter 4, *Sensible Drinking*). Insulin dependent patients also need to be aware that alcohol has a hypoglycaemic effect and so should never be consumed to excess or on an empty stomach. For this reason, those who do still use a carbohydrate exchange system should not count the carbohydrate content of any alcoholic drink (e.g. in beer) as part of their carbohydrate allowance.

Alcohol can react with sulphonylurea drugs and result in unpleasant side effects such as facial flushing in some people.

DIETARY GUIDANCE

General aspects of dietary management

The type of diet recommended for people with diabetes is actually very similar to the healthy diet advocated for the whole population, i.e. one which is relatively high in starchy carbohydrate and low in fat, sugars and salt and which avoids or corrects obesity. It is also one which is suitable for most of the family; the person with diabetes no longer has to consume a diet which is 'different' to that of everyone else, although the diabetic member of the family may have to be a little more careful about what and when they eat.

Standardised diets sheets have little place in dietary management. Instead the starting point for all dietary guidance is a person's usual dietary pattern – the types of foods they eat and when they eat them. Using this as a basis for dietary modification is more likely to result in a diet which is appropriate for an individual's energy needs and which is also acceptable and compatible with their lifestyle (and thus more likely to be followed).

Food choice

The proportion of food groups within a person's usual diet may need to be modified in line with those recommended for health.

Bread, other cereals, and potatoes group
These foods should be a major constituent of every meal and, particularly in insulin-dependent patients, may also be required as a between meal snack. The most important aspect is that these foods are eaten at regular intervals spaced throughout the day.

Fruit and vegetables group
At least 5 portions/day.

Milk and dairy foods group
Adequate amounts (2–3 portions/day), usually as reduced-fat products.

Meat, fish and alternatives group
Moderate (2 portions/day) but not excessive amounts of these should be consumed. Measures to minimise the amount of fat consumed (e.g. lean meat, avoidance of poultry skin, cooking methods) are important. Regular consumption (1–2 times/week) of oil-rich fish should be encouraged.

Fatty and sugary foods group

This group usually needs to receive close attention.

The consumption of cooking and spreading fats usually needs to be curtailed in order to reduce fat consumption. A low-fat spread should be used in preference to full-fat products such as butter or margarine. The use of cooking oil (and consumption of fried foods) should be kept to a minimum.

Large quantities of sugar-rich foods and drinks should be avoided as much as possible. Low sugar 'diet' drinks and products are an acceptable alternative. Intense sweeteners (e.g. aspartame, acesulfame-K or saccharine) can be used to sweeten drinks and some cooked desserts (see 'Sweeteners' in Chapter 10). These sweeteners cannot be used for baking (e.g. to make cakes) but a lower sugar alternative can be created by halving the amount of sugar in a recipe. The use of fructose and sorbitol or diabetic foods containing them is no longer recommended (see below). Small amounts of sugar-containing foods are acceptable.

INSULIN-DEPENDENT DIABETES (TYPE 1 DIABETES)

The general guidelines outlined above are also appropriate in this group but additional guidance is also needed as given below.

The need to balance insulin and carbohydrate

Achieving a balance between injected insulin and carbohydrate consumed is obviously important in order to avoid extremes of glycaemia. As mentioned above (under 'Carbohydrate') the traditional carbohydrate exchange system is gradually falling into disuse now that it is realised that it is not physiologically accurate. Nevertheless most insu-

lin-requiring patients (and the parents of newly diagnosed diabetic children) do require some initial guidance on an appropriate level of carbohydrate intake at each meal and this requires expert advice from a dietitian who is best placed to assess what is appropriate for that individual. In general people will probably need to eat about the same or possibly more starchy carbohydrate food than they normally do but it may need to be more evenly spaced throughout the day. Larger amounts may be required at some meals rather than others to match the peak activity of the injected insulin.

All insulin-dependent patients should be encouraged to make regular use of a home blood glucose monitor to ensure that glycaemic levels remain at moderate levels most of the time. Ideally, blood glucose should always be measured before each main meal and at bedtime. Occasionally it should also be measured 1–2 hours after a meal and this is particularly important in the early stages. Gradually, insulin-dependent patients will discover what they can (and cannot) eat in order to maintain acceptable blood glucose levels.

Hypoglycaemia

Inevitably people will not always get this balance right and hypoglycaemia (low blood glucose) will occur. This usually results from either a meal being missed or delayed, or from an unusually high level of physical activity (see below). All diabetic patients will be taught how to recognise the onset of this and the measures needed to deal with it but it is important that people closely associated with them (family members, school teachers, work colleagues, etc.) are also aware of its significance. Impending hypoglycaemia (e.g. sweating, shaking, feeling faint, sudden unexplained aggressive behaviour) needs to be treated promptly by the consumption of:

■ Firstly, about 10g of rapidly absorbed carbohydrate such as:

2–3 glucose tablets

or   2 teaspoons of sugar in water

or   a very small glass (about half a wine glass) of Lucozade

or   a small glass of any sugar-containing fizzy drink

or   2 teaspoons of jam or honey

or   4–5 soft sweets.

■ Secondly, this should be followed by about 10–20 g of slowly absorbed carbohydrate such as: a slice of bread or sandwich

or   a piece of fruit

or   a glass of milk and a biscuit

or   a meal if this is due.

It is very important that the second step follows the first one, otherwise the hypoglycaemia is likely to recur.

If the person becomes unconscious, a glucose containing gel such as Hypostop can be squirted on to the gums or glucagon can be given by injection.

Exercise

Exercise mimics the action of insulin and lowers blood glucose levels, so people taking insulin usually need an additional boost of carbohydrate prior to sporting or other forms of physical activity (e.g. a prolonged spell of gardening). Some of this carbohydrate can be in a rapidly absorbed (i.e. sugar-containing) form and this is a useful way of enabling diabetic children to consume ordinary sweets, normally unsuitable at other times. The amount and form of carbohydrate needed depends on the intensity and duration of the exercise about to be undertaken. For short bursts of activity (e.g. running about in the school playground at break-time) a small amount of rapidly absorbed carbohydrate in the form of chocolate or other source of sugar may be appropriate. If the activity will be more prolonged (e.g. a game of football) then a mixture of both rapidly and slowly absorbed carbohydrate

should be eaten, e.g. a couple of boiled sweets or glucose tablets plus some biscuits or a sandwich. A supply of glucose should be kept on hand during the exercise and further carbohydrate top-ups may be necessary.

It is particularly important that some slowly absorbed carbohydrate (e.g. biscuits or a sandwich) is also consumed at the end of a sustained period of exercise if a meal is not about to be consumed. The blood glucose level continues to fall during the recovery period and thus there is still a risk of hypoglycaemia for a few hours after the exercise has finished.

Illness

This can also easily upset the normal balance between diet and insulin. Illness, even if relatively mild, will cause a deterioration in diabetic control and if unchecked can lead to increasing levels of hyperglycaemia (high blood glucose) and other metabolic disturbances resulting in diabetic ketoacidosis and gradual loss of consciousness (diabetic coma). It is therefore vital that insulin continues to be taken, even if the appetite is severely diminished. But it is equally important that some carbohydrate is taken to counterbalance insulin activity and during illness this may need to be consumed in an easily assimilated form (see Table 27.1).

Blood glucose levels must be regularly monitored during illness.

NON-INSULIN DEPENDENT DIABETES (TYPE 2 DIABETES)

Non-insulin dependent diabetes is often considered to be a mild condition but its consequences in terms of diabetic complications are just as serious as in insulin-requiring patients.

Table 27.1 Alternatives to solid food.

The equivalent amount of carbohydrate to one potato or a small slice of bread (i.e. about 10g carbohydrate) can be derived from:

A very small glass (about $\frac{1}{2}$ wine glass)	Lucozade or grape juice
A small glass (about 1 wine glass)	Unsweetened fruit juice or ordinary cola
1 glass (tumbler size)	Milk, lemonade or other sugar-containing fizzy drink
1 cup	Thickened soup (canned or packet)
1 carton	Natural yogurt
$\frac{1}{2}$ carton	Flavoured yogurt
1 scoop	Ice cream
2 teaspoons	Drinking chocolate, Ovaltine, Horlicks or similar
2 teaspoons	Sugar, jam or honey

Unlike people with Type 1 diabetes, whose insulin production has virtually ceased altogether, people with Type 2 diabetes do still manufacture insulin but either in inadequate amounts or their tissues are resistant to its effects. Some of these patients will require oral hypoglycaemic drugs which either stimulate insulin production (sulphonylureas) or increase glucose uptake (biguanides). Others, particularly those who are overweight, can be managed by dietary measures alone, principally by regulation of energy intake.

General dietary aspects

The same general principles of dietary management apply to this group of patients as to insulin-dependent patients. Intake of starchy carbohydrate foods usually needs to be increased and evenly distributed throughout the day, while fat intake should be markedly curtailed. Foods supplying large amounts of simple sugars should be avoided.

In those who are overweight or obese, weight reduction will result in a dramatic improvement in blood glucose levels, usually as a result of the reduction in insulin resistance. Achieving a reduction in energy intake is thus the main priority. Contrary to belief, a diet does not have to be low in carbohy-

drate in order to achieve weight loss, either in diabetic people or in anyone else. A diet which is high in bulky starchy carbohydrate foods and fruit and vegetables, but greatly reduced in its content of fat-rich and sugar-rich foods, is far more likely to be successful and hence beneficial. The only difference which diabetes makes to the management of obesity is that food intake must be evenly spaced throughout the day, i.e. a person should not go without food for hours and then consume an enormous meal. This is especially important in those on oral hypoglycaemic drugs.

As with any person who has to achieve and sustain weight loss, supporting measures such as slimming groups, behavioural modification techniques, planned exercise programmes or exercise prescriptions may be additionally helpful. As long as such measures are based on sound science rather than gimmickry, they are not contraindicated for those with diabetes.

Patients on oral hypoglycaemic drugs

Whether or not the diet is restricted in energy content, it is particularly important that carbohydrate intake is distributed evenly throughout the day. For most people this means eating starchy carbohydrate foods at each of three meals per day; some will need intervening carbohydrate snacks.

Sulphonylurea drugs, such as glibenclamide or chlorpropamide, can cause hypos and these should be treated in the usual way with a mixture of short and slow acting carbohydrate (see above). Because sulphonylureas have a prolonged action, hypoglycaemic reactions can sometimes occur again a couple of hours later. If this problem persists, the drug dosage rather than the diet usually needs to be adjusted. Metformin (a biguanide) does not cause hypos.

Some patients on sulphonylureas may suffer side effects if they consume alcohol (see above).

Patients treated by diet alone

Timing of meals is less critical in this group than in diabetic patients on some form of hypoglycaemic therapy (either insulin or tablets). Nevertheless, meals should still be evenly spaced throughout the day.

For those who are overweight, dietary adjustment to reduce energy intake (particularly from fatty and sugary foods) is of paramount importance.

SORBITOL, FRUCTOSE AND DIABETIC FOODS

These are no longer recommended for diabetic patients in the UK[6]. Although sorbitol and fructose have less effect on post-prandial blood glucose levels than sucrose, in practical terms this benefit is minimal and outweighed by many other disadvantages. In large amounts these products cause osmotic diarrhoea, and children can be especially sensitive to this effect. In small amounts (e.g.

a teaspoon of diabetic marmalade on a slice of bread) the difference they make to blood glucose levels compared with the conventional alternative is negligible. Sorbitol, fructose and products containing them (e.g. cakes, biscuits and chocolate) have a high energy content so are not suitable for overweight people (the group which tends to use them most). These products are also expensive.

Now that carbohydrate restriction and total sucrose exclusion are no longer considered necessary, these products have outlived any use which they once had. Ordinary products found on the supermarket shelves which are 'low' or 'reduced' in sugar are much better alternatives (e.g. low calorie drinks, diet cola, reduced sugar jam). For baking purposes, non-overweight patients can use ordinary sugar to make cakes, etc., but using half the amount given in the recipe (the end-result is usually just as successful). Diabetic children should not be given diabetic sweets or chocolate but, if sweets are necessary, ordinary varieties should be used as carbohydrate top-ups prior to exercise (see above). Sugar-free chewing gum can be used freely at other times.

DIETARY MANAGEMENT OF DIABETES IN THE PRIMARY CARE SETTING

The trend towards the management of diabetes in the primary care setting means that dietary guidance is increasingly becoming the responsibility of the GP or practice nurse. In many ways it is entirely appropriate that routine dietary management becomes an integral part of diabetic care along with other aspects of treatment such as the use of insulin, oral hypoglycaemic drugs, glucose monitoring techniques or weight management. However, patients with continuing poor control which may be diet-related should be referred for expert dietetic assessment. It is also recommended that all patients with diabetes should receive their initial dietary guidance from a qualified dietitian and also be offered the opportunity of an annual dietetic review.

REFERENCES

1 British Diabetic Association Nutrition Sub-Committee (1982) Dietary recommendations for diabetics for the 1980s. *Human Nutrition: Applied Nutrition* **36A**, 378–94.

2 British Diabetic Association Nutrition Sub-Committee (1992) Dietary recommendations for people with diabetes: An update for the 1990s. *Diabetic Medicine* **9**, 189–202 (or available directly from the British Diabetic Association).

3 Nutrition Study Group, European Association for the Study of Diabetes (1988) Nutritional recommendations for individuals with diabetes mellitus. *Diabetes, Nutrition and Metabolism* **1**, 145–9.

4 British Diabetic Association Nutrition Sub-Committee (1989) Dietary recommendations for children and adolescents with diabetes. *Diabetic Medicine* **6**, 537–47 (or available directly from the British Diabetic Association).

5 Lean, M.E.J. & James, W.P.T. (1986) Prescription of diabetic diets in the 1980s. *Lancet* i, 723–5.

6 Thomas, B.J. & the Nutrition Sub-Committee of the British Diabetic Association (1992) Discussion paper on the role of 'Diabetic' foods. *Diabetic Medicine* **9**, 300–306 (or available directly from the British Diabetic Association).

FURTHER READING

British Diabetic Association (1994) *Balance for Beginners – Insulin Dependent Diabetes*. Available free from the British Diabetic Association (see 'Useful addresses' below).

British Diabetic Association (1994) *Balance for Beginners – Non-insulin Dependent Diabetes*. Available free from the British Diabetic Association (see 'Useful addresses' below).

Estridge, B. & Davis, J. (1992) *So Your Child has Diabetes*. Random Century, London.

Govindji, A. & Myers, J. (1992) *The Essential Diabetic Cookbook*. Thorsons, London.

Knopfler, A. (1989) *Diabetes and Pregnancy*. Optima Positive Health Guide. Macdonald & Co., London.

Mackinnon, M. (1993) *Providing Diabetes Care in General Practice – A Practical Guide for the Primary Care Team*. Class Publishing, London.

Sonksen, P., Fox, C. & Judd, S. (1994) *Diabetes at Your Fingertips*. 3rd edn. Class Publishing, London.

Wolever, T.M.S. & Brand-Miller, J. (1995) Sugars and blood glucose control. *American Journal of Clinical Nutrition* **Suppl 62**, 212s–27s.

USEFUL ADDRESSES

The British Diabetic Association, 10 Queen Anne Street, London W1M 0BD. Tel: 0171 323 1531. (This produces a wide range of information and offers many support services for both patients and health professionals.)

28

Dental Caries

The dental health of both adults and children has improved in recent decades. In 1968, 37% of adults in the UK had lost all their teeth; by 1988 this figure had fallen to 20% and by the year 2008 it is anticipated that it will be in the region of 10%.

The prevalence of tooth decay in children has also fallen over this period. In 1968, 40% of pre-school children had evidence of dental decay compared with 17% in 1995[1]. Between 1983 and 1993 the proportion of 15-year-olds free from dental caries rose from 7% to 37%[2]. Nevertheless, dental caries remains a significant health problem. Almost half of all 5-year-old children have some tooth decay, 60% of 9-year-old children have decayed, missing or filled primary teeth and the average 12-year-old has four diseased permanent teeth.

The prevalence of dental caries in children rises with age. While the average prevalence among pre-school children is 17%, within different age bands the figures are as shown in Table 28.1. Within all age groups there is also a greater prevalence of dental decay in the northern areas of the UK and in people from lower socio-economic groups.

CAUSATION

Dental caries results from the action of bacteria present in the mouth and tooth plaque (particularly *Streptococcus mutans*) on fermentable carbohydrate (sugars and starches in foods) resulting in the production of acid (mainly lactic and acetic acids). The acid produced attacks tooth enamel making it more porous and hence susceptible to further attack and tooth decay. Children's teeth are particularly vulnerable to this process.

Dental erosion causing progressive loss of enamel and dentine may also occur as a result of chemical action from acid present in some drinks rather than bacterial action. This is thought to be a significant contributor to dental damage in young children when tooth enamel is relatively soft and easily damaged.

FACTORS AFFECTING THE DEVELOPMENT OF DENTAL CARIES

Sugars and carbohydrates

All carbohydrates can cause dental caries but sugars (principally non-milk extrinsic sugars) cause the most damage because they are a readily available substrate for oral bacteria. Starchy carbohydrates are less likely to promote decay because they usually leave the mouth before being broken down to simple sugars.

Table 28.1 The prevalence of dental caries in pre-school children.

Age band	Caries prevalence
$1\frac{1}{2}$–$2\frac{1}{2}$ years	4%
$2\frac{1}{2}$–$3\frac{1}{2}$ years	14%
$3\frac{1}{2}$–$4\frac{1}{2}$ years	30%

The association between total intake of sugars and caries prevalence is not as strong as might be expected. There is much closer association with the *frequency* with which sugar-containing food is consumed. Small amounts of sugar consumed at frequent intervals (e.g. a packet of sweets) cause far more damage than the same or even a larger quantity of sugar consumed on a single occasion (e.g. in a drink). This is because acid conditions in the mouth tend to be neutralised a short time after a meal or snack by the buffering effect of saliva, inhibiting further acid attack and enabling small amounts of damage to tooth surfaces to be repaired. If, however, another sugary snack is consumed within a short interval, the conditions for acid attack will be recreated, damage repair will cease and the erosive process will continue.

The *texture* of a sugar-containing food is also relevant. Sticky chewable foods (e.g. toffee, muesli bars) will remain in the mouth longer and may leave small residues between the teeth where bacterial acid production can continue. Sugar in soft or liquid form (e.g. drinks or ice cream) will disappear from the mouth much more quickly.

Effective dental health promotion has to focus on these aspects rather than total sugar reduction alone. Most parents know that sugar is 'bad' for their children's teeth but many are unaware that it is far more important to watch frequency of consumption (especially the number of sugar-containing snacks between meals) than to worry about a few grams of sucrose present in a can of baked beans.

Acidity

The acid present in some foods or drinks can cause chemical erosion of tooth enamel, as distinct from erosion caused by bacterial action. Diet cola, which is highly acidic, may be just as damaging to teeth as ordinary cola, despite the absence of sugar. Fruit juice and fruit-flavoured drinks and sweets are also highly acidic, especially citrus varieties.

Foods such as milk and cheese contain phosphate and other components which help neutralise acid and may be protective when consumed at the end of a meal.

Saliva production

Saliva is important to help neutralise acid production in the mouth. Increased saliva production results in more bicarbonate being available as an acid buffer and also enhances the oral availability of minerals, such as calcium fluoride and phosphates, which are necessary for reversing the early stages of tooth decay. Chewing sugar-free gum after or between meals could be beneficial to teeth, particularly if this means that sugar-containing sweets are not consumed instead.

Oral hygiene

Poor oral hygiene results in build-up of plaque on the surface of teeth and enhances the conditions for acid attack. Regular brushing of teeth is a vital part of caries prevention.

Fluoride

Fluoride is incorporated into tooth enamel in the form of fluorapatite making it harder and more resistant to acid attack.

The introduction of fluoridised toothpaste is responsible for much of the decline in the prevalence of dental caries since the early 1970s[3]. The fluoride content of drinking water is also an important factor and caries prevalence is considerably lower in areas where water is naturally or artificially high in fluoride than in low fluoride areas. Water fluoridation is especially beneficial in deprived areas where take-up of other preventative measures is likely to be poor.

If local water fluoride content is less than 1 part per million, children will benefit from supplementary fluoride in the form of drops or tablets. Fluoride mouth rinses are useful for adults. Supplements are not advised in areas of high fluoride water content as excessive amounts can cause mottling of teeth. Large doses can be toxic. Local dental health officers can advise on the need for and appropriate levels of supplementation in a particular area.

GUIDANCE FOR PREVENTING DENTAL CARIES

General aspects to emphasise are:

- Use of a fluoride-containing toothpaste.
- Regular brushing and flossing of teeth using the correct technique.
- Regular visits to the dentist.
- Use of appropriate fluoride supplements in low water fluoride areas.

Dietary guidance should aim to:

- Reduce the frequency of consumption of sugar-containing foods, particularly those of a sticky or chewable nature.
- Avoid sugar-containing foods or drinks between meals.
- Encourage inveterate sweet-eaters to chew sugar-free gum instead.
- Keep consumption of acidic drinks, such as cola, to a minimum, and fruit juice to mealtimes only.
- End a meal with milk or cheese rather than fruit or fruit juice.
- Encourage the use of a feeding beaker for non-milk drinks and soya milks in infants over 6 months and discourage the use of a bottle altogether after the age of 1 year.

REFERENCES

1 Hinds, K. & Gregory, J.R. (1995) *National Diet and Nutrition Survey: Children aged $1\frac{1}{2}$ to $4\frac{1}{2}$ years. Volume 2: Report of the dental survey*. HMSO, London.
2 O'Brien, M. (1994) *Children's Dental Health in the United Kingdom 1993*. Office of Population Censuses and Surveys. Social Survey Division. HMSO, London.
3 Department of Health (1989) *Dietary Sugars and Human Disease*. Report of the COMA Panel on Dietary Sugars. Report on Health and Social Subjects 37. HMSO, London.

FURTHER READING

National Dairy Council (1995) *Diet and Dental Health*. Topical Update – 5. NDC, London.
Rugg-Gunn, A.J. (1993) *Nutrition and Dental Health*. Oxford Medical Publications, Oxford.

29

Dysphagia (Swallowing Disorders)

The process of swallowing is a complex manoeuvre requiring both voluntary and reflex actions. It can easily be disturbed by neurological damage or structural disorders and is a common consequence of strokes, motor neurone disease, multiple sclerosis, Parkinson's disease, head injury, cerebral palsy and surgery for cancer of the head or neck.

The effect of the lesion on the ability to swallow food depends on which of the phases involved in the swallowing manoeuvre are affected. This is usually assessed by a speech and language therapist who can also advise on the the correct texture and consistency of food for that particular patient.

FOOD CONSISTENCY

It is often assumed that dysphagic patients require a liquid diet but this is not the case (unless they are being tube fed). While dysphagic patients cannot cope with solid food which has to be chewed, they will also have difficulty in coping with runny liquids as these cannot be controlled. There is a high risk of aspiration with fluid and liquidised diets.

Instead, depending on the nature of the dysphagia, patients will usually be advised to consume foods in one of the following consistencies:

- *Thick fluids*   A consistency which can be sipped from a cup or through a straw.

- *Thin purée*   A consistency which can be sipped from a cup but not through a straw.
- *Thick purée*   A consistency which can be eaten with a spoon but does not hold its shape.
- *Soft food*   A consistency which can be eaten with a spoon or fork; holds its shape.

Alternatively patients may be recommended to consume foods which are either:

- *Slow moving drinks*   A straw placed in a cup of the liquid will fall slowly to one side.
- *Thick or semi-solid drinks*   A straw will stand up unsupported in the liquid on its own.

The correct consistency can be achieved by use of one of the commercial thickeners (prescribable for dysphagia) such as Thixo-D (Sutherland Health) or Vitaquik (Vitaflo). These are easy to use and do not impair the taste of the food or liquid.

For those who can swallow more solid material, suitable foods are those which are:

- *Soft but with some texture*   e.g. mashed potato. Anything which can be mashed with a fork is usually suitable. Foods such as soft bread tend to 'stick'.
- *Of an even texture*   i.e. no lumps such as in a casserole with pieces of meat or vegetables.
- *Of a single texture*   i.e. not mashed potato with gravy.
- *Moist but not runny*   i.e. no dry crumbly food or vegetables with tough skins.

Foods and liquids should be given at separate times; a bolus of food should not be washed down with a mouthful of liquid.

FEEDING TECHNIQUE

As well as providing food of the correct consistency, the correct feeding technique (e.g. positioning, amount, rate, suitable utensils, etc.) is also important and needs to be appropriate for each patient. Speech and language therapists will be able to provide expert guidance.

USEFUL ADDRESSES

Details of commercial thickeners may be obtained from:

Cow & Gate Nutricia Ltd, Newmarket Avenue, Whitehorse Business Park, Trowbridge, Wilts BA14 0XQ. Tel: 01225 768381. Brand name: Instant Carobel.

Fresenius Ltd, 6/8 Christleton Court, Manor Park, Runcorn WA7 1ST. Tel: 01928 579444. Brand name: Thick and Easy.

Nestlé Co Ltd, St George's House, Croydon CR9 1NR. Tel: 0181 686 3333. Brand name: Nestargel.

Sutherland Health Ltd, Unit 5, Rivermead, Pipers Way, Thatcham, Berkshire RG19 4EP. Tel: 01635 87488. Brand name: Thixo-D.

Vitaflo Ltd, West of Scotland Science Park, Unit 6.12, Kelvin Campus, Glasgow G20 0SP. Tel (freephone): 0800 515174. Brand name: Vitaquik.

30

Gastrointestinal Disorders

HEARTBURN (GASTRO-OESOPHAGEAL REFLUX)

Heartburn is a burning sensation felt at the base of the chest behind the breastbone, often spreading upwards from the stomach to the throat. Sometimes the pain extends into the arms mimicking angina. It typically starts about one hour after eating or at night and is caused by the reflux of acid from the stomach into the base of the oesophagus. Persistent reflux may lead to inflammation of the oesophageal lining (oesophagitis).

Reflux usually results from a weakened oesophageal sphincter in combination with either increased abdominal/intragastric pressure or lowered oesophageal pressure. Heartburn is sometimes accompanied by hiatus hernia which increases the likelihood of reflux.

Common precipitating factors are:

- Large meals (exert pressure on the oesophageal sphincter).
- Meals with a high fat content/fatty foods (take longer to leave the stomach).
- Excessive smoking, coffee and/or alcohol (may lower oesophageal pressure).
- Obesity (increases abdominal pressure).
- Pregnancy (increased abdominal pressure from the fetus; rising progesterone levels relax the oesophageal sphincter).
- Lying or bending down (loss of gravity on food movement).

Dietary guidance

- Eat smaller meals at regular intervals.
- Avoid food within 2–3 hours of bedtime.
- Avoid greasy or highly spiced foods or others which cause problems.
- Avoid excessive tea, coffee or alcohol.
- Avoid carbonated drinks and sparkling wines.
- Sleep on several pillows to keep the head above the chest.
- Lose weight if necessary.
- Stop smoking.

Antacids neutralise gastric acid secretion and can offer short-term relief but chronic use is inadvisable. Excessive use of bicarbonate preparation can cause rebound acid production and antacids containing magnesium or aluminium can impair absorption of minerals such as calcium, iron or zinc.

H_2-receptor antagonists, such as cimetidine, are very effective at suppressing gastric acid secretion.

GASTRITIS

This is generalised inflammation of the lining of the stomach which if severe and prolonged can lead to its breakdown and haemorrhage. The symptoms can include severe pain, typically at night. It is often associated with gastrointestinal reflux but can be caused by other irritants such as excessive smoking, alcohol or highly spicy foods (such as hot curries) or some drugs (especially aspirin). Infection with *Helicobacter pylori* may also be a factor in some cases.

Dietary guidance

- Adopt a sensible pattern of eating, i.e. not going for long periods without food and not eating enormous meals at any one time.
- Avoid irritants such as spicy foods, or others known to cause problems.
- Avoid excessive amounts of caffeine or alcohol.

General dietary measures which minimise reflux (see above) may also be helpful.

PEPTIC ULCER

A peptic ulcer is a localised area of erosion in the lining of the gastrointestinal tract in areas where there is contact with gastric juices, i.e. the lower end of the oesophagus, the stomach or the duodenum.

Treatment of peptic ulcers has been revolutionised by H_2-receptor antagonist drugs, such as cimetidine or ranitidine (which are powerful inhibitors of stomach acid and pepsin secretion), and antibiotic treatment for *Helicobacter pylori* infection. These measures relieve pain and promote healing within weeks.

Dietary guidance

Guidance on sensible diet and lifestyle is, however, often appropriate. Many ulcer patients have a lifestyle which is characterised by long periods without food interspersed with the occasional large meal, alcohol, coffee and cigarettes.

Some ulcer patients still believe that they should consume large quantities of milk (in the past the mainstay of peptic ulcer diets). This is not the case; the alkalinity of milk can have a rebound effect on gastric acid production and make the underlying situation worse.

While symptoms remain acute, dietary guidance as for gastritis (see above) may be helpful.

GASTRECTOMY

The body adapts well to removal of some or all of the stomach but some problems can remain:

- *Early satiety, sometimes with discomfort during or after a meal* This necessitates small, frequent meals. To reduce volume, fluids should be consumed separately from, not with, food.
- *Dumping syndrome* The loss of the stomach's function as a reservoir means that a large load of nutrients can be delivered much more rapidly than usual into the jejunum. This can cause tachycardia and hypotension making people feel nauseous, giddy and faint. Symptoms similar to those of hypoglycaemia can also occur about 2 hours after a meal due to of overproduction of insulin in response to the rapid absorption of large quantities of glucose.

  Dumping syndrome usually recedes with time but for those in whom it is a problem, smaller meals with a reduced content of readily absorbed carbohydrate (e.g. sugar-rich drinks and desserts) are advisable.

- *Low energy intake and weight loss* Early satiety often results in a low food intake and generalised low intake of nutrients and energy. Consumption of small regular meals of high nutrient density should be encouraged. Sip feed supplements may be helpful if food intake is particularly poor (see Chapter 8, *Nutritional Support and Supplementation*).
- *Iron deficiency* Iron deficiency anaemia is common because limited food choice may result in a low iron intake and gastrectomy also tends to reduce the absorbability of non-haem iron. Iron supplements may be needed.
- *B_{12} deficiency* Gastrectomy results in loss or reduced production of intrinsic factor secreted by the stomach which is essential for vitamin B_{12} absorption. Megaloblastic deficiency is inevitable in cases of total gastrectomy unless B_{12} is given by injection.

CROHN'S DISEASE

The inflammatory process underlying Crohn's disease is similar to that of ulcerative colitis and these two disorders are often grouped together under the heading Inflammatory Bowel Disease. The symptoms and effects are different.

Crohn's disease is a chronic auto-immune inflammatory disorder which can affect any part of the gastrointestinal tract but most commonly the terminal ileum. The inflammation causes thickening of the intestinal wall which can result in strictures, obstruction and fistulae. The symptoms of abdominal pain and diarrhoea are often accompanied by signs of malnutrition, particularly loss of weight and anaemia, resulting from a combination of poor appetite and malabsorption. Crohn's disease commonly starts in young adulthood and, like many inflammatory disorders, tends to be characterised by periods of active disease followed by partial remission.

The condition is difficult to treat. Steroids, 5-aminosalicylate compounds and other drugs can reduce inflammation and relieve symptoms but cannot cure it. Surgical resection may become essential if obstruction occurs but removal of the diseased part of the intestine rarely cures the disease; inflammation usually restarts nearby.

Dietary guidance

Dietary management of Crohn's disease always requires specialist dietetic care to minimise malabsorption and correct nutrient deficiencies. During the active phase of the disease, remission may be induced by complete bowel rest and the use of either parenteral feeding or elemental diets.

During periods of remission the main aims are to improve appetite, increase weight and correct nutritional deficiencies. There is no reason why most people should not follow a diet along healthy eating guidelines although the diet should not be too high in fibre because:

(1) It makes the diet too bulky (and too low in energy) for the likely level of appetite.
(2) It may increase the risk of obstruction.

Energy supplements may be beneficial and vitamin and mineral supplementation may be necessary. The malabsorptive state associated with Crohn's disease may result in poor tolerance to lactose, and some patients may benefit from a milk-free diet. Ileal resection may result in other dietary problems (see below).

There have been suggestions that food intolerance may trigger or exacerbate the inflammatory response underlying Crohn's disease. While food sensitivities can be identified in some patients, particularly to foods such as cereals, dairy products and yeast, there is little evidence that their exclusion significantly affects remission. Since food and nutrient intake is often poor in Crohn's patients, it is usually unwise to subject them to the rigours of diagnosis and treatment of food intolerance for what may be minimal, if any, gain.

ULCERATIVE COLITIS

Like Crohn's disease, ulcerative colitis is an auto-immune inflammatory disorder usually characterised by periods of active disease and remission. Unlike Crohn's disease, it only affects the colonic and rectal mucosa and can be completely cured by large bowel resection. Ulcerative colitis causes severe diarrhoea accompanied by the passage of blood and mucus, abdominal pain, low grade fever and general malaise. Apart from being an extremely debilitating condition, both physically and socially, it can lead to the life-threatening complications of toxic megacolon, bowel perforation, fistulae and haemorrhage. People with ulcerative colitis have a greatly increased risk of colo-rectal cancer if the disease has been present for more than 10 years.

There is no medical cure although corticosteroids and sulphasalazine can provide some relief. Corticosteroids seem to be most effective after initial attacks but less beneficial thereafter. Sulphasalazine is more effective in mild cases and seems to reduce the likelihood of flare-ups. Total colectomy will provide permanent relief although this necessitates an ileostomy or construction of a rectal pouch (see below).

Dietary guidance

Diet appears to have little influence on either the causation or the relief of symptoms of ulcerative colitis. Unlike Crohn's disease, elemental or peptide diets do not induce remission. During periods of remission, most patients can eat a normal healthy diet without any problem. Nevertheless patients do benefit from dietetic advice. Poor appetite and chronic diarrhoea and blood loss may leave patients severely nutritionally depleted, particularly in terms of iron. Many are also extremely anxious about eating for fear of triggering acute symptoms and consume a very limited diet. Patients should be discouraged from avoiding too many foods, only those which are known to exacerbate symptoms.

INTESTINAL RESECTION AND OSTOMIES

The effects of intestinal resection depend on both the location and the length of the part removed. Resection in the small intestine results in loss of surface area for digestion and absorption and there may be significant malabsorption of nutrients, reduced absorption of fluids and loss of bile salts. Resection in the large intestine results mainly in the loss of areas for storage and water absorption, and perhaps sphincters to release faeces. Problems are usually worst immediately post-surgery; in time some adaptation will occur.

Small intestine resection

The body usually adapts well to the loss of a segment of small intestine but if more than 70% is removed (i.e. if less than 100 cm remain) symptoms of malabsorption known as short bowel syndrome usually occur. This may result in severe diarrhoea with the passage of undigested food, and the malabsorption of many nutrients, particularly fat, lactose, fat-soluble vitamins, iron, folate and B_{12}. Excessive loss of bile salts may exacerbate the malabsorption. Initially, losses of nutrients and energy may be high (over 50% of the amount ingested) so in effect people need to consume twice as much as they did before. If these needs are not met, nutrient depletion and weight loss are inevitable. Electrolyte disturbances are also likely to occur.

Management of severe short bowel syndrome requires specialist dietetic help as the measures needed to provide symptom relief, correct multiple deficiencies and find forms of supplementary nutrients which can be tolerated by the patient are complex. Despite the fat malabsorption, fat restriction is not usually recommended as this severely reduces energy intake. If dietary fat restriction does become necessary, energy supplements in the form of carbohydrate will be essential (see Chapter 8, *Nutritional Support and Supplementation*). Some patients may require pancreatic supplements to offset pancreatic insufficiency caused by the malnutrition. A small proportion of cases will need long-term parenteral nutrition and fluids.

Large intestine resection

Removal of part of the colon is much less likely to result in nutritional depletion although if resection is extensive there may be some energy loss from the reduced bacterial fermentation of unabsorbed carbohydrate and, in the initial stages, faeces may be of a liquid consistency as a result of the reduced colonic absorption of fluid. Total colectomy will have nutritional implications arising from ileostomy (see below).

Ileostomy and colostomy

Resection of the rectum necessitates the creation of a stomal opening for the elimination of waste. If part of the colon remains, the end of the remaining segment is brought to the surface to form a colostomy. If the entire colon and rectum are removed, the terminal end of the ileum is brought to the surface to form an ileostomy. An ileostomy or colostomy may be temporary or permanent.

It takes time for people to adjust to the psychological and practical consequences of living with a stoma and most people benefit from advice and support from stoma care specialist nurses. Eating, particularly in the early stages, is a major worry to most people. They are terrified of leaks, odour and

subsequent embarrassment and are well aware that what they eat or drink may affect this. Most can be reassured that they will soon learn how to avoid problems and, perhaps with a few minor dietary precautions, be able to eat a normal diet.

The nutritional implications of ileostomies and colostomies are different:

Ileostomies:
- Result in the passage of a greater volume of much more liquid waste material.
- Waste material is passed frequently.
- Dehydration and electrolyte depletion are much more likely.
- Nutrient deficiencies can occur (especially B_{12} since its site of absorption may have been removed).
- Blockages are more likely because fibrous material in the diet may not be sufficiently broken down.
- The discharge fluid contains digestive enzymes which can cause inflammation of peristomal skin.
- Constipation does not occur.

Colostomies:
- The waste material is much more solid and like normal stools.
- Waste material is passed relatively infrequently.
- There is a low risk of electrolyte and fluid depletion.
- Nutrient deficiencies are less likely.
- Blockages are less likely because fibrous material is more likely to have been broken down.
- Digestive enzymes are not excreted so peristomal skin problems are less likely.
- Constipation can occur.

Dietary guidance for people with a stoma

General aspects
All stoma patients should be encouraged to consume a varied well-balanced diet. Some people

seem to be able to eat anything but others find that certain foods cause problems, particularly in the early stages. People will discover their own tolerances through trial and error.

Food should be well chewed, especially if it contains fibrous material. Certain high fibre foods may upset some people but fibre should not be avoided altogether as a certain amount is essential for stoma function.

Problems which may occur are:

- *Blockage* Fibrous foods passing rapidly through the gut will not be digested. Most of the time they will be expelled through the stoma without problem but occasionally blockage may occur. This is less likely to happen if fibrous food is well chewed before being swallowed. If chewing is difficult (e.g. in an elderly person with poor dentition) chopping food into small pieces or mincing it may avoid the problem. Foods which are most likely to cause blockage are:
    Celery, asparagus
    Nuts, especially peanuts consumed in large
      quantities
    Segments of orange or other citrus fruit
    Dried fruit, especially dried apricots
    Fruit and vegetable skins (particularly those
      from apple, tomato or potato)
    Cabbage
    Bean sprouts
    Peas or sweetcorn
    Coconut
- *Odour* Foods most likely to cause odour are:
    Onions, leeks, garlic
    Cabbage, Brussels sprouts
    Fish
    Eggs

Parsley and yogurt may help diminish odour production.
- *Diarrhoea* Some patients find that certain foods will produce an unpleasant liquid discharge. There are no foods which always produce these effects although common culprits are:
    Green beans
    Broccoli and spinach
    Raw fruit

    Beer
    Highly spiced foods

Stoma patients should be aware that diarrhoea can also result from infection, just as in anyone else, and that people with an ileostomy have an increased risk of contracting gastroenteritis. If this occurs it can result in rapid and extensive loss of fluid and electrolytes causing serious dehydration and electrolyte depletion. Oral rehydration therapy is essential in these circumstances and should be given until symptoms subside. Ileostomy patients should always have a supply of oral rehydration medication available.

Additional points for ileostomy patients

A good fluid intake is essential because more fluid is lost in stools, particularly in the initial few months after the ileostomy. People should be strongly discouraged from restricting fluid intake in an attempt to reduce stomal output because this is likely to lead to dehydration. Additional fluid will be needed in very hot weather.

While fluid loss remains high, some fluid should be taken as fruit juice (rich in potassium) and savoury drinks such as soups or Bovril (high in sodium) to replace lost electrolytes. Severe diarrhoea will require balanced oral rehydration therapy (see above).

Large amounts of high fibre foods are inadvisable but fibre should not be avoided altogether. Supplements of some minerals and vitamins (especially B_{12}) may be advisable if the diet seems restricted or inadequate.

To prevent unnecessary alarm, ileostomy patients should be warned that some highly coloured foods such as blackcurrant juice, beetroot or spinach can affect the colour of stools.

Additional points for colostomy patients

Plenty of fluid and an adequate fibre intake from cereal foods and vegetables are essential to help prevent constipation (hard stools passed infrequently). Bran should never be added to foods as it may cause blockage. Laxatives, particularly irritant ones such as senna, should be avoided.

Fermentation of food in the remaining part of

the colon may cause problems with flatus production. Foods which tend to cause most problems are:

Onions, leeks, garlic,
Cauliflower, cabbage, broccoli, Brussels sprouts,
Beans
Foods rich in resistant starch (e.g. reheated mashed potato)
Cucumber
Beer and other yeast-containing foods

Irregular meals and fizzy drinks may also exacerbate the problem.

IRRITABLE BOWEL SYNDROME

Irritable bowel syndrome (IBS) is a common disorder possibly affecting as many as 25% of the population to some degree and accounting for about half the referrals to gastroenterology clinics. It causes symptoms of abdominal pain and distention accompanied by either diarrhoea, constipation or an alternation between the two. In itself, IBS is a benign disorder (although it certainly makes life miserable for some people) but because its symptoms are also those of more serious diseases, the presence of these has to be excluded.

The cause of IBS is poorly understood but its effects may result from some abnormality in the enteric nervous system and consequent disordered bowel contraction or motility. It is commonly associated with stress or anxiety.

Attempts have been made to classify IBS sufferers into symptom-specific sub-groups such as those with predominantly either constipation or diarrhoea, since it seems likely that the cause and treatment of these two extremes may differ. However, this is not an infallible classification because:

■ Some IBS patients fluctuate between different sub-groups.
■ Not all patients with similar symptoms respond to the same treatment suggesting that differences in underlying aetiology remain.
■ Treatment sometimes improves one symptom but exacerbates another leaving the patient little better off.

Dietary guidance

The benefits of different types of dietary treatment on IBS are hard to evaluate because many studies show a marked placebo effect; the effect of someone taking a sympathetic interest in what can be a distressing condition can be as beneficial as dietary manipulation. It is also difficult to evaluate the effects of diet on IBS objectively because many of its symptoms (e.g. bloating, discomfort, pain) are vague and subjective.

For many years dietary treatment was to avoid 'irritating' foods, usually those with a high fibre content. More recently, high fibre diets, particularly those rich in cereal fibre, have been advocated although it is now clear that these are not helpful in all cases[1]. Given the heterogeneity of both IBS and of 'dietary fibre' this is not really surprising. More studies are needed to evaluate the effects of different types of fibre before its effects and benefits can be clearly established.

Results to date suggest that subjects who suffer from symptoms of constipation are more likely to benefit from treatment with fibre than if diarrhoea, distension, flatulence or abdominal pain are present[2,3]. If fibre is increased it should be done gradually to avoid adverse effects of flatulence and bloating. Bran supplements should be avoided as they can exacerbate existing symptoms.

Lifestyle changes and other measures which reduce or help people cope better with stress may be more helpful in other cases of IBS.

DIVERTICULOSIS AND DIVERTICULITIS

Diverticulosis is the symptomless presence of sacs or pouches (diverticuli) in the wall of the colon. Diverticulitis occurs when infection or inflammation occurs within these pouches.

Diverticuli are caused by pressure within the colon being exerted on weak points of the colon wall, usually the sigmoid colon where the contents are more solid. They are primarily a consequence of a low fibre diet because small, hard stools require more pressure to move them.

Dietary guidance for diverticulitis

Initial treatment for attacks of diverticulitis is rest and and a predominantly fluid diet. Once symptoms have receded, treatment is primarily that for constipation (see below).

CONSTIPATION

Many people assume constipation to be the absence of a daily bowel movement; this is not the case. There is great variability in the pattern of bowel movements among healthy people and a bowel movement every few days may be perfectly normal. Constipation occurs when the stools are not just infrequent but also hard, small and sometimes painful to pass.

As a result of this misconception, there is considerable overuse of laxatives among the general population. Genuine constipation should be avoided because of the risk of associated disorders such as haemorrhoids, diverticulitis and appendicitis. Occasionally, usually in children or elderly people, constipation can result in faecal impaction. Prolonged faecal transit time may also increase the risk of some colo-rectal cancers. However, regular laxative use is not the answer and overuse can make bowel function worse. Unless it results from organic disease, constipation is always a dietary problem.

Dietary guidance

This needs to focus on two dietary aspects:

■ Increasing the intake of fibre, particularly from cereal and vegetable foods.
■ Increasing the intake of fluid.

Regular moderate exercise also acts as a gentle stimulant to colonic function.

Dietary fibre

While most people are aware that 'fibre is good for constipation', fewer understand what this means in terms of foods.

Insoluble fibre, such as that found in cereal foods such as bread and breakfast cereals, is most effective at preventing or treating constipation because it absorbs water, swells up and increases faecal bulk. Wholemeal or wholegrain sources of cereals provide the greatest amounts and these food choices should be encouraged but a general increase in all types of bread and cereal foods will also improve dietary fibre content. Cereal fibre consumption should be increased gradually to avoid problems of distention and flatulence which may initially occur.

Consumption of vegetables and fruit should also be increased. Those which contain fibrous material will also increase faecal bulk and those containing mainly soluble fibre may have other protective effects against some bowel diseases.

In general adding raw bran to foods is not an appropriate way of increasing dietary fibre content. Although bran is a component of cereal fibre which will increase faecal bulk, its isolated use can be hazardous, especially in children or elderly people.

It swells considerably once it comes into contact with intestinal fluids and, if fluid intake is low, can cause obstruction. The high phytate content of bran also tends to impair the absorption of essential minerals such as iron, calcium and zinc.

Fibre supplements containing ispaghula husk, a natural plant product containing both soluble and insoluble fibre, can be effective at relieving constipation but should not be regarded as a long-term alternative to an increased intake of dietary fibre.

Fluid

The importance of fluid in preventing or alleviating constipation is often underestimated. The beneficial effects of fibre depend on there being sufficient fluid within the gut for it to swell. A low fluid intake will result in hard stools.

Many people do not consume sufficient fluid, particularly elderly people with restricted mobility who try to avoid having to make frequent trips to the lavatory. Those who are restricting fluid for this reason should be encouraged to consume at least one glass of water or soft drink with every meal or, if appetite is small, between every meal. This should not cause too many problems. The stronger diuretic effects of tea or coffee are more likely to result in frequency or urgency.

DIARRHOEA

Diarrhoea may result from:

- Bacterial, viral or protozoal infection.
- Disease of the gastrointestinal tract (e.g. carcinomal obstruction, ulcerative colitis).
- Malabsorption (due to lack of digestive enzymes, bile salts or reduced absorptive capacity).
- Food intolerance or osmotic overload (e.g. excessive quantities of sucrose or lactose).

Where diarrhoea is secondary to a chronic underlying disorder, treatment obviously depends on the management of the primary problem. Drugs which reduce gastrointestinal motility may be necessary in some circumstances.

Antidiarrhoeal drugs, many of which are available over the counter, are rarely an appropriate way of treating diarrhoea resulting from gastrointestinal infection (although they can be useful in awkward situations). Simple infective diarrhoea is best treated by allowing the body to eliminate the offending organisms and by replacing solid food with glucose-containing fluids until symptoms subside. Children and elderly people should be prescribed drinks specially formulated for oral rehydration, particularly if there is associated vomiting. These products can also be purchased directly from pharmacies. Alternatively an oral rehydration solution can be made at home using:

6–8 teaspoons of sugar $+\frac{1}{2}-1$ teaspoon salt dissolved in 1 litre ($1\frac{3}{4}$ pints) cooled boiled water.

REFERENCES

1 Rees, G.A., Trevan, M. & Davies, G.J. (1994) Dietary fibre modification and the symptoms of irritable bowel syndrome – a review. *Journal of Human Nutrition and Dietetics* 7: 179–89.
2 Lambert, J.P. *et al.* (1991) The value of prescribed high-fibre diets for the treatment of irritable bowel syndrome. *European Journal of Clinical Nutrition* 45, 601–609.
3 Muller-Lissner, S.A. (1993) Constipation and the Irritable Bowel Syndrome. *European Journal of Gastroenterology and Hepatology* 5, 587–92.

FURTHER READING

Ellis, P. & Cunningham, D. (1994) Management of carcinomas of the upper gastrointestinal tract. *British Medical Journal* 308, 834.
Farthing, M.J.G. (1995) Irritable bowel, irritable body or irritable brain? *British Medical Journal* 310, 171–5.
Forgacs, I. (1995) Clinical gastroenterology: recent advances. *British Medical Journal* 310, 113.
Kelly, M.P. (1992) *Colitis*. Routledge, London.
Thompson, W.G. (1993) Irritable bowel syndrome: pathogenesis and management. *Lancet* 341, 1561.

USEFUL ADDRESSES

British Colostomy Association 15 Station Road, Reading, Berks RG1 1LG. Tel: 01734 391537.

IA (The Ileostomy and Internal Pouch Support Group), PO Box 23, Mansfield, Notts NG18 4TT. Tel: 01623 280999. (Formerly the Ileostomy Association of Great Britain and Ireland.)

IBS Network, St John's House, Hither Green Hospital, Hither Green Lane, London SE13 6RU.

National Association for Colitis and Crohn's Disease (NACC), PO Box 205, St Albans, Herts AL1 1AB. Tel: 01727 844296.

31

Pancreatitis

Pancreatitis results from activated pancreatic enzymes attacking the pancreatic tissue itself resulting in inflammation and autodigestion. It is an extremely serious disorder with a high mortality rate. Acute pancreatitis requires hospital admission and specialised care.

Chronic pancreatitis may develop after repeated acute attacks, or as a result of underlying disease or prolonged alcohol abuse. Patients with chronic pancreatitis are nearly always underweight, partly as a result of malabsorption but also as a result of a poor food intake. The recurrent attacks of abdominal pain are often associated with eating so food aversion is common. Patients with alcoholism are often deficient in thiamin and other B vitamins.

DIETARY TREATMENT

Poor nutrition is bound to cause further deterioration in the patient's condition. Promoting weight gain – or preventing further weight loss – and correcting nutritional deficiencies are important. Steatorrhoea should not be treated with fat restriction (as is often the case) but by the provision of enteric-coated pancreatic enzymes to improve digestion. These should be taken with all meals and fat-containing snacks. The consumption of small, frequent meals and snacks comprised of nutrient-dense foods should be encouraged. If appetite, or compliance, is poor, nutrient dense fluid supplements are essential (see Chapter 8, *Nutritional Support and Supplementation*). Abstinence from alcohol should be strongly recommended for all patients.

About 20% of patients with chronic pancreatitis develop diabetes. This further exacerbates the weight loss and requires specialist dietetic management.

32

Cystic Fibrosis

Cystic fibrosis is a genetic disorder resulting in severe dysfunction of the exocrine glands, particularly the mucus-producing glands in the respiratory tract, the sweat glands and the pancreas.

Along with physiotherapy and control of bacterial infection, diet is a vital part of treatment because of the high risk of chronic malnutrition and, in children, poor growth and development. Energy requirements are greatly increased in cystic fibrosis mainly because of the greater effort involved in breathing, but the effects of the disease make it difficult to meet these high needs because of factors such as malabsorption from lack of digestive enzymes, excessive expectoration, frequent vomiting and generally poor appetite. Apart from the effect on growth and development, inadequate energy intake results in muscle wasting and further diminishes respiratory strength, increasing the risk of pulmonary infections. It is now recognised that there is a relationship between improved nutritional status and improved survival[1].

About 10–15% of cystic fibrosis patients have diabetes, a prevalence which is likely to rise as life expectancy increases.

DIETARY TREATMENT

Cystic fibrosis always requires expert dietetic management but since many of the primary care team will meet these patients as part of their routine care, it is important to understand what dietary measures are trying to achieve.

Dietary management of cystic fibrosis flouts all healthy eating principles. Prior to the 1980s, cystic fibrosis patients were given very low fat diets in an attempt to minimise the problems of malabsorption. This measure often resulted in severe growth failure and malnutrition. The development of enteric-coated replacement pancreatic enzymes made it possible for diets to be more liberal in terms of fat content and, now that the benefits of a high energy intake are well-established, people with cystic fibrosis are advised to consume a diet high in both fats and sugars. Parents of affected children are often understandably concerned at being encouraged to give their child what appear to be 'unhealthy' foods and need to be reassured that, for those with cystic fibrosis, such a diet is indeed 'healthy'.

Achieving a high energy intake

Foods high in fats and sugars must be encouraged, for example:

- Use of full-cream milk, full-fat cheeses, creamy yogurts.
- Adding extra butter or margarine to vegetables; spreading it thickly on bread.

- Adding extra milk or cream to soups, cereals, desserts, mashed potatoes.
- Eating plenty of meat, fish and eggs.
- Frying foods.
- Liberal (but not exclusive) use of sugar, sweets and chocolate (not surprisingly this aspect of the diet can cause problems with other siblings in the family).

Pancreatic enzyme replacement

These should be taken with every meal or snack. The newer enteric-coated microspheres or microtablets, e.g. Creon (Duphar), Nutrizym GR (Merck) or Pancrease (Cilag), result in much better absorption than the previous less acid-resistant forms of pancreatin. Enteric-coated preparations should be able to achieve 90% absorption of fat provided the dosage level is appropriate. This varies with the degree of pancreatic insufficiency and the size of the meal, and should be adjusted according to stool consistency and frequency, and abdominal discomfort. Higher dosage preparations of enteric-coated pancreatin, e.g. Creon 25000 (Duphar); Pancrease HL capsules (Cilag) and Nutrizym 22 (Merck), have recently been introduced.

Vitamin supplements

Deficiency of fat-soluble vitamins remains a risk due to fat malabsorption and increased requirements. The following supplements should be given:

Vitamin A	8000–10000iu (2400μg–3000μg) daily
Vitamin D	800iu (20μg) daily
Vitamin E	infants 50mg; children 100mg; teenagers/adults 200mg daily

Iron supplements may also be needed.

Energy supplements

If diet or weight gain remain poor, additional energy supplements are necessary (see p. 63). Many are ACBS prescribable for cystic fibrosis. Those which are particularly useful are:

- Standard/high energy sip feeds, e.g. Fresubin (Fresenius); Fortisip (Nutricia)
- Carbohydrate polymer supplements, e.g. Hycal (SmithKline Beecham)
- Fat and glucose polymer mixtures, e.g. Duocal (SHS)
- Fortified puddings, e.g. Formance (Ross)

Supplements or products with a high protein content are usually less suitable, particularly in younger age groups.

More intensive supplementary measures such as nocturnal nasogastric or gastrostomy/jejunostomy feeding may be necessary in some cases. Short-term total enteral or parenteral feeding is sometimes successful in stabilising lung function and improving nutritional status.

REFERENCE

1 Corey, M. & McLaughlin, F.J. (1988) A comparison of survival, growth and pulmonary function in patients with cystic fibrosis in Boston and Toronto. *Journal of Clinical Epidemiology* **41**, 583–91.

FURTHER READING

British Paediatric Association Working Party on Cystic Fibrosis (1988) *Cystic fibrosis in the United Kingdom 1977–1985: an improving picture.* British Medical Journal **297**, 1599–602.

Goodchild, M.C. & Dodge, J.A. (1985) *Cystic Fibrosis: Manual of Diagnosis and Management.* Baillière Tindall, London.

Royal College of Physicians (1990) *Cystic Fibrosis in Adults. Recommendations for Care of Patients in the UK.* RCP, London.

Webb, A.K. & David, T.J. (1994) Clinical management of children and adults with cystic fibrosis. *British Medical Journal* **308**, 459.

USEFUL ADDRESSES

The Cystic Fibrosis Trust, Alexandra House, 5 Blyth Road, Bromley, Kent BR1 3RS. Tel: 0181 464 7211.

33

Gallstones

Gallstones are clumps of solid material which form in the gall bladder. Most gallstones are comprised of cholesterol together with small amounts of calcium salts. Occasionally pigment stones derived from bile pigments, such as bilirubin, may form. Stones vary in size and can be as large as an egg. Smaller ones cause the most problems because they can move into the bile ducts, blocking the flow of bile and causing pain and jaundice.

DIETARY TREATMENT

Surprisingly, there is little evidence that a low-fat diet is necessary for most gallstone sufferers, although this is commonly recommended. It is probably only appropriate for the minority of people with steatorrhoea. However, some people do find that certain fatty foods upset them in which case these should be avoided. Many female gallstone sufferers are also overweight and reducing fat intake as part of general weight reducing measures is advisable. In general though, fat consumption need not be any more restrictive than that recommended for healthy eating.

In severe cases, removal of the gall bladder will resolve the problem completely. This does not seem to affect the digestive processes.

34

Hyperuricaemia and Gout

Uric acid is the end product of purine metabolism. Purines are components of every cell in the body because they are a constituent of DNA. Cell turn-over results in the release of purines which are then broken down into uric acid and transported via the blood to the kidneys for excretion. Dietary purines (derived from cell nuclei present in food) are also broken down to uric acid and about two-thirds of this is absorbed into the blood prior to renal excretion, the remainder being excreted via the gut. There is no dietary requirement for purines as they are synthesised by the body as required for DNA manufacture.

Uric acid circulates in the blood in the form of urate. If urate concentration exceeds a certain level some will precipitate as crystals of uric acid which may then be deposited in joints. These can cause inflammation and result in the painful symptoms of gout. Uric acid may also be deposited in soft tissues or as stones in the kidney.

There is a strong genetic tendency to gout and the condition is much more common in men than women. Diet is rarely the sole cause of gout but it can be a triggering factor. Normally any rise in plasma urate from dietary purines is accompanied by increased renal excretion, but in people with low plasma urate clearance and perhaps high endogenous purine synthesis, a high dietary purine intake may exacerbate the formation of uric acid crystals. Obesity and hypertension also reduce renal urate clearance and hence increase the risk of gout.

DIETARY TREATMENT

Diet no longer plays a major part in the treatment of gout. Acute attacks are usually effectively treated by non-steroidal anti-inflammatory drugs or colchicine. Once symptoms have subsided, longer-term treatment with drugs which either reduce uric acid formation (e.g. allopurinol) or increase its excretion (e.g. probenecid) help prevent uric acid deposition.

In mild cases of gout, particularly if accompanied by obesity or over-indulgence, dietary measures which result in weight loss and healthier eating can avoid the need for long-term medication. Avoidance of large quantities of purine-rich foods (typically those rich in cell nuclei) may also be helpful:

Foods rich in yeast (e.g. beer), yeast extracts and yeast tablets
Offal
Meat
Shellfish
Fish roes
Myco-protein (i.e. meat-substitutes such as Quorn).

35

Renal Stones

Kidney stones can vary in composition but the vast majority are comprised of calcium salts, principally calcium oxalate.

DIETARY TREATMENT

All types of stones

The one dietary factor which is of most relevance to the formation of all types of stones is fluid intake. A low fluid intake significantly enhances stone risk and all patients with stones should have a fluid intake which produces at least 2.5 litres of urine per day. It is particularly important that some fluid is consumed before going to bed (urine flow is at its lowest during the night) and that extra fluid is consumed in hot weather and when abroad in hot climates.

Calcium stones

Calcium intake
The relationship between calcium intake and stone formation remains unclear. Between 20–40%

patients with recurrent stones have raised blood calcium levels and elevated urinary calcium excretion, and dietary calcium restriction is often recommended. This advice is now being questioned. No prospective study has yet shown that lowering calcium intake decreases the risk of stone formation but there is evidence that it may be detrimental in terms of bone mass (and hence increases the risk of osteoporosis)[1].

Oxalate intake
The more important dietary influence on stone formation may be oxalate (the other major component of calcium stones). While most oxalate within the body is endogenously produced, there is evidence to suggest that high dietary intakes of oxalate, or a low intake of minerals (including calcium) which bind it in the gut and inhibit its absorption, may affect stone formation. This may explain the recent finding from one large-scale prospective study that high dietary calcium intakes were protective in terms of stone formation[2]. The main sources of dietary oxalate are tea (which is the major contributor in the average diet), rhubarb, spinach, beetroot, chocolate and nuts.

Mega-doses of vitamin C (in excess of 1 g/day) produce hyperoxaluria and an increased risk of kidney stones because oxalate is the main end product of ascorbic acid metabolism.

Malabsorption and ileal resection also cause hyperoxaluria because more free fatty acids are present in the gut which preferentially bind calcium thus leaving more free oxalate available for absorption. The presence of unabsorbed bile salts in the colon also increases colonic permeability to oxalate.

Uric acid stones

These are a consequence of hyperuricaemia which may also cause gout (see Chapter 34). There is some evidence that a high dietary intake of purines may be more likely to trigger uric acid stone formation than other symptoms of gout. Those prone to stone formation may be well-advised to avoid rich sources of purines (see p. 201).

Cystine stones

These are very rare and a consequence of cystinuria, an inborn error of metabolism requiring specialised dietary management.

REFERENCES

1   Lemann, J. (1993) Composition of the diet and kidney stones. *New England Journal of Medicine* 328(12), 880–81.
2   Curhan, G.C. *et al.* (1993) A prospective study of dietary calcium and other nutrients and the risk of symptomatic kidney stones. *New England Journal of Medicine* 328(12), 833–8.

36

Osteoporosis

Osteoporosis literally means 'porous bone' and results from loss of bone tissue. A certain amount of bone loss is an inevitable consequence of ageing but osteoporosis is said to be present when bone tissue has been lost to such an extent that the bone loses strength and becomes abnormally susceptible to fracture.

Osteoporosis is not a new disorder – adult skeletons from ancient civilisations show signs of osteoporosis – but its prevalence has greatly increased in recent decades and, without preventative measures, is likely to continue to rise as the population becomes increasingly aged in composition. Currently, almost 1 in 4 women over the age of 50 have been shown to have a level of bone density which predisposes to osteoporotic fracture, particularly of the hip, vertebra or wrist. By the age of 70, nearly half of all women will have experienced one of these fractures. In men, low bone density is less common but about 1 in 20 men over the age of 70 can be considered to be at risk of osteoporotic fracture[1].

Osteoporosis has enormous costs in terms of morbidity, mortality and NHS resources. Hip fractures alone account for over 50 000 hospital admissions per annum and about one-quarter of these cases die soon afterwards and about half lose their independence or have subsequently impaired quality of life. Osteoporosis may also account for 50 000 wrist fractures each year. Vertebral or spinal fractures are less common but can cause considerable pain, distortion, loss of height and many secondary problems. Osteoporosis is often not diagnosed until fracture or noticeable height loss occurs.

The causes and prevention of osteoporosis and the role of the primary care team in diagnosing and managing the disease are discussed in a recent report from the Department of Health's Advisory Group on Osteoporosis[1].

CAUSATION

Bone is not a static structure but is constantly being remodelled; old bone is continuously being removed and new bone created. The adult skeleton is entirely replaced every 7–10 years. During childhood, more bone is created than lost, hence enabling growth to take place. By late adolescence, bones reach their maximum size but continue to increase in density for a further decade or so until *peak bone mass* is reached at about the age of 30–35. After this there is a slow net loss of bone tissue with age.

Factors which influence bone loss are:

- *Age* The longer people live, the more bone tissue will be lost. On average there is a net loss of about 0.5% bone tissue every year after the age of 35. Trabecular bone (the interior bone meshwork) tends to disappear first; cortical bone (denser outer bone) starts to be lost between the ages of 40–50. Other factors also compound the risk of osteoporosis with age; elderly people are less efficient at absorbing dietary calcium and tend to be less active (or even immobile). Unsteadiness, the use of sleeping or analgesic drugs, or poor eyesight also increase the likelihood of falls.

■ *Sex* Women are much more at risk of osteoporosis than men for a number of reasons.

  □ *Hormonal* Oestrogen has a protective effect on bone. Loss of oestrogen production at the menopause (or as a result of surgical removal of the ovaries) results in a greatly accelerated rate of bone loss (3–5% bone mass per annum) for a period of about 5 years. Women who have an early menopause have an increased risk of osteoporosis (unless hormone replacement therapy is given). Amenorrhoea due to anorexia nervosa or strenuous exercise (such as that which can occur in female athletes or ballet dancers) also greatly increases the risk of osteoporosis.

  □ *Bone density* Women have bones which are smaller and less dense than those of men. Women therefore have less bone to lose before the 'fracture threshold' is reached.

  □ *Longevity* Women tend to live longer than men and so more are affected by age-related bone loss.

■ *Genetics* Heredity accounts for some of the variation in bone density and hence osteoporosis is more common in some families. Peak bone mass is thought to be 80% determined by genetic factors and 20% by environmental factors.

■ *Ethnic group* Afro-Caribbeans have much greater peak bone mass than Caucasians. Osteoporosis is therefore less common among this group of people.

■ *Body frame size and weight* People with smaller bones have fewer reserves to withstand age-related bone loss. Overweight women also produce more protective oestrogen than thin people. People who have had anorexia nervosa have a greatly increased risk of osteoporosis.

■ *Smoking* Women who smoke tend to be thinner, have lower oestrogen levels and to have an earlier menopause, all of which increase the osteoporotic risk.

■ *Exercise* Load-bearing exercise has an important effect on bone. The movement of muscles applies pressure to bones which respond by becoming stronger (e.g. professional tennis players have denser bones in their serving arm than on their non-serving side). Conversely, immobility or paralysis results in rapid loss of calcium from bone and reduction in bone mass. Some of the increased prevalence of osteoporosis almost certainly reflects the increasingly sedentary lifestyle in Western societies.

■ *Diet*

  □ *Calcium* An adequate calcium intake during childhood, adolescence and early adulthood is essential for maximum peak bone mass to be achieved. Intakes below 500 mg/day may reduce peak bone mass and increase osteoporotic risk in later life. Once the point of peak bone mass has been passed, it is unclear to what extent calcium intake influences bone loss. Most studies have failed to show a relationship between post-menopausal bone loss and habitual calcium intake[2,3]. Current evidence suggests that a habitually high calcium intake at this stage of life does not by itself prevent osteoporosis although it does seem likely that very low calcium intakes will exacerbate calcium loss and so make matters worse. The value of calcium supplementation remains debatable; high calcium intakes may retard the rate of bone loss but cannot alone restore calcium to bone[4]. However, calcium supplements may be helpful in conjunction with other forms of therapy.

Other dietary factors which may have an indirect effect because of their adverse effects on calcium balance are:

  □ *Inadequate vitamin D* Vitamin D is essential for the absorption of calcium. Low intakes of vitamin D usually result in incorrect formation of bone (i.e. rickets/osteomalacia) rather than loss of bone tissue (i.e. osteoporosis). However, inadequate vitamin D may impair the body's ability to adapt to either a low calcium in-

LIVERPOOL
JOHN MOORES UNIVERSITY
AVRIL ROBARTS LRC

take or high requirement by increasing the amount of calcium absorbed from the gastrointestinal tract. Combined supplements of vitamin D (20 μg/day) and calcium (1.2 g/day) have been shown to reduce the risk of osteoporotic fracture in elderly women[5].

☐ *Excessive protein intake* High protein intakes increase calcium excretion although to some extent this is offset by the high phosphate content of many sources of protein.

☐ *Excessive salt intake* A high intake of sodium increases calcium excretion.

☐ *Excessive fibre intake* Cereal fibre contains phytates which bind calcium making it less available for absorption. Some vegetables contain oxalates which reduce calcium absorption.

☐ *Excessive alcohol intake* This increases the rate of bone loss.

☐ *Excessive caffeine intake* This increases calcium excretion.

☐ *Low fluoride intake* Fluoride is incorporated into bone and, in the same way that it makes teeth more resistant to caries, can strengthen bone and make it less liable to fracture.

Secondary Osteoporosis

Osteoporosis may also be secondary to an underlying disorder (such as rheumatoid arthritis, hyperthyroidism, chronic liver disease or alcoholism) or prolonged use of certain drugs (such as corticosteroids).

PREVENTION OF OSTEOPOROSIS

Women of menopausal age

Those who are at greatest risk of osteoporosis:

- Have a family history of osteoporosis.
- Have an early menopause.
- Smoke.
- Are thin.
- Are white.
- Are sedentary.
- Have a history of anorexia nervosa or exercise-induced amenorrhoea.
- Had a low intake of milk and milk products in childhood.

Bone density can be measured by dual x-ray absorptiometry (DEXA) and DEXA screening of menopausal women is being increasingly recommended as a way of identifying those who would most benefit from protective measures such as:

- *Hormone replacement therapy (HRT)* This significantly retards bone loss. Bone loss is most rapid in the five years following the menopause; HRT therefore needs to commence at an early stage to have the maximum benefit.
- *Exercise* Encouraging people to maintain regular exercise may be a vital preventative measure.
- *Diet* While it is important that people over the age of 50 consume sufficient calcium, there is little evidence to suggest that high calcium intakes in the form of supplements are by themselves protective. For many people, this measure is simply too late. At this stage of life, the aim should be to guard against low calcium intake which could exacerbate bone loss. People should be encouraged to consume a diet providing plenty of calcium in the form of milk

and dairy products and which also follows healthy eating guidelines and so is not excessive in terms of salt, alcohol and caffeine.

Elderly people

The risk of osteoporotic fracture is increased in those who:

- Are confined to bed or a wheelchair.
- Are housebound.
- Are unsteady on their feet due to arthritis, drug treatment, transient ischaemic attacks.
- Have a generally poor diet.

The most important preventative measures are:

- *Home safety* In this age group, home safety is an important aspect of minimising the risk of falls and osteoporotic fracture. Checking the home for obvious hazards, such as poor lighting, loose rugs and trailing flexes, and installing handrails are simple but important aspects of prevention.
- *Encouraging mobility* Mobility should be encouraged in those where this is still possible. Among younger, still fully mobile elderly people, gentle regular exercise should be strongly advocated.
- *Healthy eating* A well-balanced healthy diet which maintains a good calcium intake in the form of milk and dairy products should be encouraged. Housebound people may need vitamin D supplements to ensure adequate calcium absorption.

Childhood and adolescence

Although osteoporosis does not, in normal circumstances, *occur* in this age group, preventative meas-

ures, particularly a good calcium intake, to decrease the risk in later life need to start at this age, i.e.:

- Adequate calcium intake to achieve peak bone mass.
- Regular exercise.

Children who dislike or consume little milk or dairy products should be given expert dietetic advice to ensure that calcium intake is adequate. Calcium supplements should only be used under medical/dietetic supervision.

Young adulthood

This age group is unlikely to spend much time worrying about the prospect of crippling bone disease in later life but they should be made aware that diet and lifestyle at this age undoubtedly affect the level of peak bone mass achieved at the age of 30–35 and hence the risk of future osteoporosis. The following are particularly important:

- Good calcium intake (i.e. plenty of milk and dairy products in the diet).
- General healthy diet.
- Avoidance of risk factors such as smoking and heavy drinking.
- Maintenance of regular exercise.

TREATMENT OF OSTEOPOROSIS

Drug treatment

- *Calcitonin* This is the hormone which blocks the breakdown of bone and hence can both prevent and treat osteoporosis. It is, however, expensive and only available in specialist centres.

- *Disphosphonates* These inhibit bone resorption and also increase bone density. Drugs derived from this group probably offer a treatment for the future. Etidronate used in the treatment of Paget's disease is now prescribable for spinal osteoporosis.
- *Anabolic steroids* have a limited use because of their undesirable side effects. Nandralone decanoate can relieve pain in the elderly who have suffered vertebral fracture.
- *Sodium fluoride* has been used to reduce the risk of spinal fracture but there is some evidence it may increase the risk of fracture at other sites. Since there is a narrow margin between benefit and toxicity, specialists tend to be wary of using it.

Dietary treatment

Calcium supplements given in isolation are unlikely to be of any benefit. They may, however, be useful in conjunction with the above drugs.

REFERENCES

1 Department of Health (1994) *Report from the Advisory Group on Osteoporosis*. Department of Health, London.
2 Riggs, B.L. *et al.* (1987) Dietary calcium intake and the rate of bone loss in women. *Journal of Clinical Investigation* 80, 979–82.
3 Stevenson, J.L. *et al.* (1988) Dietary intake of calcium and postmenopausal bone loss. *British Medical Journal* 297, 15–17.
4 Dawson-Hughes, B. (1991) Calcium supplementation and bone loss: a review of controlled trials. *American Journal of Clinical Nutrition* 54, 274S–80S.
5 Chapuy, M. *et al.* (1994) Effect of calcium and cholecalciferol treatment for three years on hip fractures in elderly women. *British Medical Journal* 308, 1081–2.

FURTHER READING

National Dairy Council (1992) *Calcium and Health*. Fact File 1 (Revised edition). NDC, London.
National Osteoporosis Society (1994) *Priorities for Prevention. Guidance Document*. National Osteoporosis Society, Bath.
Peel, N. & Eastell, R. (1995) Osteoporosis. *British Medical Journal* 310, 989–92.

USEFUL ADDRESSES

The National Osteoporosis Society, PO Box 10, Barton Meade House, Radstock, Bath BA3 3YB. Tel: 01761 471771.

37

Rickets and Osteomalacia

Rickets and osteomalacia result from vitamin D deficiency. Vitamin D controls the absorption of calcium from the diet and its incorporation into bone. In conditions of vitamin D deficiency, bone development is abnormal and bones lack structural strength. Those which support body weight can become curved or deformed. These effects are most apparent in growing children in whom the condition is called rickets. However, since bone remodelling continues throughout life, vitamin D deficiency can also affect adults; this is called osteomalacia.

In most of the population, vitamin D requirements can be met by the action of sunlight on skin. Some sub-sections of the population are more reliant on a dietary source of vitamin D to meet their vitamin D needs. These are:

- People with little exposure to sunlight
  - Housebound elderly or disabled people.
  - People who keep most of their skin covered for religious/cultural reasons.
- People with high vitamin D requirements
  - Infants.
  - Children below the age of 5 years.
  - Pregnant and lactating women.

Those in at risk groups should ensure an adequate dietary intake of vitamin D from foods such as fortified margarines and breakfast cereals. Supplements may be necessary if consumption of these foods is low. All children should be given supplementary vitamin D (as A,D,C drops) from the age of one year and until the age of three, or until the age of 5 in those thought to be still at risk. Breast fed infants should be given A,D,C drops from the age of 6 months.

Rickets remains a public health problem among Asian children and the reasons for this remain unclear. Factors such as low skin exposure to sunlight, low vitamin D intake and a high fibre content which may impair calcium absorption explain some, but not all of the increased risk. Metabolic differences in the rate of conversion of vitamin D to its active metabolites may be partly responsible. Vitamin D supplementation is particularly important for Asian children.

FURTHER READING

Clements, M.R. (1989) The problem of rickets in UK Asians. *Journal of Human Nutrition and Dietetics* 2, 105–16.
DHSS (1980) Rickets and Osteomalacia. Report of the working party on fortification of food with vitamin D. Report on Health and Social Subjects 19. HMSO, London.

38

Arthritis and Rheumatism

Rheumatism is a general term for pain emanating from the joints or structures around them. Arthritis literally means 'inflammation' and is commonly used for any type of joint disease. The two major types of arthritis are osteoarthritis and rheumatoid arthritis.

Osteoarthritis (OA) is the most common type of arthritis affecting about 1 in 10 of the UK population. It is primarily a degenerative process associated with ageing and the result of general wear and tear on joints. Joint cartilage becomes worn away, particularly in the load-bearing joints such as the hips and knees, causing pain, joint deformity and disability. The joints may become acutely inflamed but this is not common. Osteoarthritis is the major cause of disability in the UK.

Rheumatoid arthritis (RA) is less common but more serious because it can ultimately affect other organs such as the heart and lungs as well as joints. It is an inflammatory condition where acute inflammation of joints is followed by destruction and deformity. RA is a chronic progressive disorder but characterised by periods of relapse and remission. The cause is unknown but it is thought to be an auto-immune disorder, i.e. an attack on the body's tissues by its own immune system. It usually occurs at a younger age than osteoarthritis and is more common in women. Unlike OA, smaller peripheral joints, such as those of the hands, wrists, feet and ankles, are often affected.

There is no cure for arthritis but the use of pain relieving and anti-inflammatory drugs and physiotherapy can help alleviate symptoms. Surgical replacement of joints such as the hip or knee can dramatically improve the quality of life for some people.

DIET AND ARTHRITIS

Diet is an important aspect of arthritis but not in the way that many people imagine; many of the dietary remedies and 'cures' currently advocated are little more than quackery. As with any condition characterised by remissions and relapses, people tend to try a particular remedy when symptoms are bad and any subsequent improvement is automatically assumed to be causal rather than coincidental.

GENERAL DIETARY IMPLICATIONS

The effects of disability (see also Chapter 18)

Difficulties with shopping, preparing and cooking food may mean that some people disabled by arthritis may have a limited diet comprised of a few easy to eat foods (such as biscuits or cakes) and generally poor nutritional status. Low intake of micronutrients, such as vitamin C and zinc, may impair immune competence which may be of particular relevance to those with rheumatoid arthritis. The combination of an imbalanced diet and lack of mobility increases the risk of obesity which makes moving around even more difficult and painful.

The effects of drug therapy

Many of the drugs used to treat arthritis have nutritional implications. Non-steroidal anti-inflammatory drugs (NSAIDS) can cause indigestion, gastric irritation and lead to gastric ulcers. This is less likely if they are given in combination with H_2-receptor antagonists such as cimetidine. Steroids, such as prednisolone, may be used in the treatment of rheumatoid arthritis. These can have a number of long-term effects such as weight gain, diabetes and ulcers.

SPECIFIC DIETARY CONSIDERATIONS

Osteoarthritis

The primary aim of diet should be to correct or prevent overweight and obesity. Excessive weight increases the strain on load-bearing joints, such as hips or knees, and weight reduction can be enormously beneficial in reducing pain and improving mobility. Weight loss may also be advisable prior to joint replacement surgery, both to reduce the risks from the surgery itself and to make it easier to regain mobility afterwards.

Dietary advice should focus on the need to eat a healthy diet containing plenty of foods from the bread/cereals and fruit/vegetable food groups and fewer from the fatty/sugary foods group. This is particularly important advice in those with reduced mobility who are at particular risk of becoming overweight.

No other dietary measures or supplements have been shown to have any beneficial effect on non-inflammatory forms of osteoarthritis.

Rheumatoid arthritis

In addition to the importance of a varied well-balanced diet, there are a number of other dietary considerations in people with RA.

Poor appetite
Loss of appetite is common in RA patients as a result of pain, depression or drug therapy. Their diets may therefore be nutritionally inadequate, particularly in terms of micronutrient content, and this may impair immune competence.

Iron
Anaemia is a common feature of RA and may result from the disease process inhibiting the formation of haemoglobin, or gastric bleeding caused by anti-inflammatory drugs or poor iron absorption (vitamin C intake, which improves the absorption of non-haem iron, is often low in RA patients). All RA sufferers should be encouraged to have a good intake of iron, ideally as haem iron from meat, and vitamin C. Iron supplements may be necessary in some cases.

Fish oils
Omega-3 fatty acids, such as eicosapentaenoic acid (EPA) and docosahexaenoic acid (DHA), found in fish oils may have a beneficial effect on inflammatory symptoms of arthritis. Controlled trials of fish oils in those with RA have been shown to reduce the symptoms of swollen and tender joints, morning stiffness and pain, possibly as a result of their

effect on suppressing production of leukotriene B_4 (known for its powerful inflammatory properties) and interleukin-1 (involved in the breakdown of cartilage)[1].

Intake of EPA and DHA can be increased by consuming marine oil supplements or more oily fish such as:

Mackerel
Salmon
Herring
Sardines
Pilchards

Fish oils supplements are unlikely to be beneficial to people with osteoarthritis unless acute joint inflammation is present.

Evening primrose oil

Evening primrose oil may also help relieve the pain and stiffness of rheumatoid arthritis[2]. This oil is a rich source of gamma-linolenic acid (GLA) which is necessary for the production of an anti-inflammatory prostaglandin PGE_1. Increased intake of GLA may stimulate production of this prostaglandin.

Combined supplements of both marine fish oils and evening primrose oil (e.g. Efamol Marine) are available although it should be emphasised that there is as yet no clear proof of their clinical benefit to RA sufferers. However, if patients wish to take these supplements, they are unlikely to be harmful and may be helpful.

Food intolerance

Food intolerance has been suggested to be a cause of RA and many populist self-help books advocate the use of exclusion diets, some of which are extremely restrictive. There is little scientific evidence to suggest that these measures are generally beneficial and some of these self-imposed restrictions are far more likely to create dietary deficiencies and unnecessary stress than symptom relief. As with other inflammatory disorders, it is possible that food intolerance may exacerbate symptoms in a small number of cases but if genuine food intolerance is suspected, patients should be referred to a dietitian.

ALTERNATIVE DIETARY REMEDIES

Dietary remedies which claim to alter 'acid/alkali balance', provide 'enzymes' or 'remove toxins' should be regarded with caution. Many such products rely on unsound science, are of unproven benefit, are expensive and may result in a diet which compromises the intake of important nutrients. People of course have the freedom to choose any remedy which they feel may be beneficial but health professionals should ensure that people do so on the basis of informed choice, not ignorance, and that dietary harm does not result.

REFERENCES

1 Kremer, J.M. *et al.* (1985) Effects of manipulation of dietary fatty acids on clinical manifestations of rheumatoid arthritis. *Lancet* i, 184–7.
2 Belch, J.J.F. *et al.* (1988) The effects of altering dietary essential fatty acids as requirements for non-steroidal anti-inflammatory drugs in patients with rheumatoid arthritis: double blind placebo controlled study. *Annals of the Rheumatic Diseases* 47, 96–104.

USEFUL ADDRESSES

Arthritis and Rheumatism Council, Copeman House, St Mary's Court, St Mary's Gate, Chesterfield, Derbyshire S41 7TD.
Arthritis Care, 18 Stephenson Way, London NW1 2HD. Tel: 0171 916 1500. (Information/counselling service for arthritis and rheumatism sufferers. Also a Helpline Freephone: 0800 289170.)

39

Multiple Sclerosis

Multiple sclerosis (MS) is a degenerative disease of the nervous system characterised by progressive demyelination of nerve sheaths and consequent impairment in the conduction of nervous impulses. It occurs more frequently in women and peak incidence is in early adult life. The symptoms, severity and course of the disease vary greatly between individuals. In most people, it is characterised by periods of relapse followed by remissions which can last months or years. In some people the symptoms gradually progress without remission and in a few cases there is rapid deterioration of motor function. But not everyone with MS becomes severely disabled; only one in five MS sufferers ever needs a wheelchair.

DIET AND MULTIPLE SCLEROSIS

The role of diet in the progression or remission of MS is unclear.

The myelin sheath is largely comprised of lipid material and there has been speculation that dietary fat content may influence its composition. MS is very rare in parts of the world where saturated fat intake is low. Long-term follow up of MS patients consuming a diet restricted in total fat (to 30% of dietary energy) and with a very low content of saturated fatty acids, but relatively high levels of omega-6 polyunsaturated fatty acids (principally linoleic acid), did show some evidence of benefit in terms of the severity of relapse and duration of remission, particularly in those with early disease[1]. But these effects were not seen in everyone and the dietary measures required to achieve these intakes were stringent.

A double-blind trial supplementing a diet already high in omega-6 polyunsaturates with omega-3 fatty acids from fish oils also showed some evidence of benefit in terms of the frequency, severity and duration of relapses[2]. As a result of these and other findings, supplements of evening primrose oil (a rich source of omega-6 fatty acids) and fish oils (providing omega-3 fatty acids) are sometimes taken by people with MS. As long as the rest of the diet is adequate, these supplements are unlikely to do any harm and may possibly do some good but there is as yet insufficient evidence to suggest that all MS patients should be encouraged to use them. The effects of these and other dietary fat manipulations undoubtedly merit further study but for the time being their benefits remain speculative rather than proven[3].

Nevertheless it is clear that current healthy eating objectives (which include eating less saturated fat and increasing consumption of marine oils) are compatible with any such benefits. A diet with good nutrient density will also meet other important needs of those with MS, namely to maintain good immune function and normal weight.

There is no scientific evidence that gluten-free diets have beneficial properties in terms of MS.

DIETARY GUIDANCE

It should be emphasised to people with MS that consuming a well-balanced healthy diet is an important way of making a positive contribution to the management of the disease.

Foods which should be particularly encouraged are:

- *Bread and cereal foods* to help keep the saturated fat content of the diet to a low level and as a source of insoluble fibre which will help prevent or alleviate constipation.
- *Fruit and vegetables* for vitamin C and other antioxidant nutrients important in immune function.
- *Fish* particularly oily fish for their omega-3 fatty acids.
- *Milk and dairy products* are a valuable source of nutrients but reduced-fat varieties should be chosen.

Foods which may need to be discouraged are:

- *Fatty foods* Sources of saturated fat, such as butter, lard, suet, hard cheese and cream, should be kept to a minimum. Vegetable oils and spreads should be used in preference.
- *Sugary foods* Consumption of these should be curtailed if body weight is increasing or too high.

People should also be encouraged to remain as active as possible within the constraints imposed by the disease in order to help prevent weight gain and for general physical health and well-being.

COMMON DIETARY PROBLEMS

- *Psychological effects on eating* Depression (perhaps at having MS) or anxiety (at the thought of its implications) can affect food intake and result in either anorexia or comfort eating, or even fluctuations between the two. People should be encouraged to think of eating well as something constructive they can do to assist their future health.
- *Fatigue* Many MS patients suffer phases of debilitating fatigue when tasks such shopping, cooking, even eating seem too much of an effort. Family, friends and neighbours may be able to offer support at these times and if necessary, sip feed type nutritional supplements may be helpful as a way of maintaining good nutritional intake.
- *Overweight* Being overweight is not helpful with a disease characterised by muscle weakness and fatigue. It can also make life more difficult for carers if people need to be lifted. However, rapid or drastic weight loss is not appropriate as this will only increase the risk of depression and fatigue.
- *Disability* (see Chapter 18) Progressive disability may result in poor food intake.
- *Swallowing disorders (see Chapter 29)* These are common in later stages of MS and may require expert dietetic assistance.

ALTERNATIVE DIETS

People who have a relentless progressive disease want to do as much as they can to halt its advance. Multiple sclerosis patients are very vulnerable to suggestions that certain diets or supplements may induce remission. While people should be free to try a course of action which gives them hope, it is important that they are discouraged from following a highly restricted diet which may jeopardise the intake of important nutrients (such as antioxidant nutrients) or that the cost of special preparations does not impose such a strain on the budget that people cut down on food.

REFERENCES

1 Swank, R.L. & Dugan, B.B. (1990) Effect of a low saturated fat diet in early and late cases of multiple sclerosis. *Lancet* ii, 37–9.

2 Bates, D. *et al.* (1989) A double-blind controlled trial of long-chain omega-3 polyunsaturated fatty acids in the treatment of multiple sclerosis. *Journal of Neurology, Neurosurgery and Psychiatry* **52**, 18–22.

3 Editorial (1990) Lipids and multiple sclerosis. *Lancet* **ii**, 25–6.

FURTHER READING

Povey, R., Dowie, R. & Prett, G. (1992) *Learning to Live with Multiple Sclerosis*. Sheldon Press, London. (Originally pub-lished by the Multiple Sclerosis Society of Great Britain and Northern Ireland.)

USEFUL ADDRESSES

The Multiple Sclerosis Society of Great Britain and Northern Ireland, 25 Effie Road, Fulham, London SW6 1EE. Tel: 0171 736 6267.

40

Food Allergy and Intolerance

'Allergy' has been a fashionable diagnosis in recent years and many people believe they are 'allergic' to one or more foods. Most will be mistaken since genuine food allergy is quite rare, although some may have some other form of food intolerance. Food allergy is only one of a number of types of adverse reactions to food.

Food allergy is most likely to occur during infancy or childhood because immaturities in the gastrointestinal tract mean that potential allergens are more likely to be absorbed and the immature immune system is more likely to react to their presence, particularly milk or egg protein. About 40% of children grow out of their sensitivity by the age of 5 years.

FOOD ALLERGY

Genuine food allergy results in the production of specific antibodies (IgE) to that food. Each time the food is eaten, an allergic response is provoked causing the release of chemical mediators such as histamine which then produce the symptoms of allergy such as swelling of oral tissues, vomiting, diarrhoea, skin rashes or respiratory distress. Only a minute amount of the allergen is needed to trigger the reaction and the reaction may be so severe that it causes anaphylactic shock and even death.

The most common causes of genuine allergy are:

Peanuts and other nuts (and the oils made from them)
Milk protein
Eggs
Fish
Shellfish
Soya beans (and oils made from them)

FOOD INTOLERANCE

Food intolerance is often mistaken for food allergy but is fundamentally different from it. Food intolerance reaction does not involve allergic sensitisation and therefore no production of IgE antibodies within the bloodstream. There are several possible causes of food intolerance:

- *Pseudoallergy* This most closely resembles food allergy because the symptoms are caused by histamine release from mast cells resulting in generalised gastrointestinal, skin and respiratory responses. However, no immunological mechanisms are involved in the histamine release, chemical factors in the food itself appear to be the trigger. Unlike genuine allergy, small amounts of the food often do not cause a response; usually relatively large amounts are required. Pseudoallergy does not cause anaphylaxis although its consequences can be acutely debilitating.

Common triggers of this type of food intolerance are:

Wheat
Orange and other citrus fruits
Strawberries
Fish and shellfish

- *Enzyme deficiency* Lack or deficiency of digestive enzymes (e.g. lactase) will result in an intolerance to certain food components (e.g. lactose). Rare metabolic enzyme defects may result in severe food intolerant disorders such as phenylketonuria or galactosaemia.
- *Pharmacological effects* People may react to pharmacologically active substances present in food such as:
  - □ *Caffeine* Caffeine, present in tea, coffee, cola drinks and some analgesics, is a stimulant and in large amounts causes palpitations, sweating, shaking and symptoms of anxiety. Some people are more sensitive to these effects than others.
  - □ *Vasoactive amines* These are powerful vasoconstrictors and in large amounts can cause unpleasant symptoms, particularly headache, nausea and giddiness. They may also trigger migraine in some, though not all, sufferers. The most common culprits are:

Histamine   Fermented foods such as
            cheese, sauerkraut, salami
            sausage
            Badly stored fish, especially
            mackerel
Tyramine   Cheese
            Yeast extract
            Chocolate
            Red wine
            Pickled fish
            Some fruit especially bananas,
            avocados and citrus fruits

Vasoactive amines are normally deactivated in the body by the enzyme monoamine oxidase (MAO). People taking MAO-inhibitor antidepressive drugs which suppress the activity of this enzyme must avoid foods rich in vasoactive amines.

- □ *Monosodium glutamate (MSG)* Large amounts of MSG can cause headache, palpitations, and even chest and arm pain mimicking heart attack. This has been nicknamed 'Chinese restaurant syndrome' as Chinese food often contains large amounts of MSG.
- *Irritants* Strong spices can directly irritate the gut mucosal lining. Sulphite, either present naturally or as an additive, can sometimes trigger asthma attacks (particularly if inhaled as sulphur dioxide gas given off by fizzy or acidic drinks).
- *Toxins* There are many natural toxins present in foods, e.g. in many types of fungi, undercooked kidney beans or solanine in green potatoes. Food contamination can also result in the presence of bacterial toxins (e.g. in shellfish) or fungal toxins (e.g. in mouldy bread) which may have gastrointestinal effects.
- *Food aversion* This form of food intolerance is of psychological rather than physical origin. People are convinced, often for quite irrational reasons, that a particular food or group of foods, or even all foods, cause harm or physical effects.

PREVALENCE OF FOOD ALLERGY AND INTOLERANCE

Many people believe they are 'allergic' to something they eat, a diagnosis which they have often made themselves. Food additives are often believed to be responsible[1]. A recent study in the UK showed that about 20% of a large population sample believed themselves to have a food intolerance but detailed investigation revealed the true prevalence to be in the region of 1.5%[2]. Other studies have reached a similar conclusion[3]. About 15% of the population appear to have a genuine sensitivity to some environmental factor such as dust, pollen, pet hair or feathers. Only about 2% of the population have some degree of adverse reactions to foods or food ingredients (and women are more likely to be affected than men) Thus:

- 2 in 10 people believe themselves to be intolerant to food.
- Only about 2 in 100 people actually are intolerant to food.
- Only about 1 in 10000 people is intolerant to food additives.

Nevertheless, although the numbers of true sufferers may be small, food allergy and intolerance must not be dismissed as being of no importance; for those with a genuine sensitivity, the consequences in terms of ill-health may be considerable and in a few cases, life-threatening.

DIAGNOSIS

Many cases of 'allergy' are self-diagnosed or are pronouncements by unqualified allergy 'specialists', sometimes after an expensive series of tests of dubious value[4].

There are in fact few reliable tests for food intolerance. Skin tests and the radio-allergen absorbent test can sometimes detect true allergy but even these can be unreliable giving both false-positive and false-negative results. These tests cannot be used at all for food intolerance since this does not provoke an immune response. Techniques such as hair analysis are useless.

Some specific types of food intolerance can be diagnosed by their characteristic effects, e.g. gluten intolerance causes flattening of intestinal villi so can be diagnosed by jejunal biopsy. However, in most instances, diagnosis of food intolerance necessitates dietary detective work, preferably by someone experienced in the following techniques.

Diet/symptom records

For people with symptoms suggestive of food intolerance but with no obvious cause, keeping a record of everything consumed over a period of time together with a record of symptoms and their severity is a first step. Sometimes this can be revealing, for example migraine attacks only occurring on days when a particular tyramine-rich food was consumed. More often the relationship between diet and symptoms is more diffuse, particularly if the intolerance is to a food component such as milk protein or wheat which may be present in many foods, sometimes quite unlikely ones (e.g. bread may contain milk protein, beefburgers may contain wheat). Dietetic expertise is usually necessary to spot any but the most obvious associations.

Exclusion diets

Simple exclusion diets
If the patient or a diet/symptom record suspects that a single food or food component is causing intolerance, excluding the item from the diet to see whether the symptoms disappear is an obvious step. Although simple in theory, this is not always simple in practice because there are so many hidden sources of food components in manufactured foods. Again, dietetic help is usually necessary in order to ensure that exclusion is total; if it is not, a diagnosis of genuine intolerance may be missed. Dietitians have access to the National Food Intolerance Databank which contains details of the components of manufactured foods and hence can advise on brands of foods which are free from certain ingredients. Patients may also need to be taught how to use food labels and recognise that for example 'lactoglobulin' means 'milk'.

Multiple exclusion diets
These are more complex and exclude a broad range of foods in an attempt to induce symptom relief. They are used where a diet/symptom record has produced no obvious links between the two but intolerance is still suspected. In some cases, an offending food may be such a ubiquitous part of the diet that there is no obvious pattern between consumption and symptoms; in others there may be a

reaction to more than one food. There are two main types of multiple exclusion diet:

(1) Foods are progressively removed in small groups (3–5 foods) at a time until symptoms disappear. Each excluded food is then reintroduced singly in order to identify the offending culprit(s).

(2) The patient may be placed on a diet which only contains two or three foods (such as lamb, rice, and pears which rarely cause any reaction) or even an elemental diet containing no food at all. Other foods are then added one at a time to the diet until reaction occurs.

Multiple exclusion diets always require dietetic supervision. The likelihood of a clear diagnosis depends on meticulous planning and close guidance and supervision of the patient. Because these diets are so restricted, the risk of nutritional deficiency is high and their use in children must always be under close medical and dietetic care. Patients have to be highly motivated in order to comply with the demands of a highly restricted diet for long periods of time, and also to cope with the possibility that their symptoms may turn out to be non-food related. Half-hearted attempts at multiple exclusion diets are a waste of time for all concerned. Nevertheless for some who have suffered for years from chronic gastrointestinal or other symptoms, identification of genuine food triggers and their subsequent avoidance can result in a dramatic improvement in the quality of life.

Confirmation of diagnosis

Ideally food intolerance (but not food allergy) should be confirmed by blind food challenge. This means administering the suspected food or foods in a disguised form to see if symptoms are reproduced. As this is a time-consuming and difficult procedure, it is rarely carried out but is advisable if there is any doubt as to the diagnosis or if it means the patient has to exclude an important food (such as milk). Food challenge is inappropriate in many cases of allergy because of the risk of anaphylaxis.

FOOD AVOIDANCE

Eliminating a reaction-provoking food or food component from the diet is sometimes straightforward (e.g. avoiding shellfish or strawberries) but more usually it is not. If genuine sensitivity exists then exclusion of the offending item must be total if any benefit is to result and, in some cases of allergy, to prevent the risk of anaphylaxis. In practice, achieving this can be difficult. Manufactured foods are a minefield of hidden components, some of which may be detectable from a food's ingredients list (if people know what terms to look for) but others will not, because they may be present as part of compound ingredients (which will not be itemised separately) or in an unspecified form (e.g. 'vegetable oil' may be derived from soya, groundnut or neither of these). Since manufactured foods also change in formulation quite frequently, any lists of suitable or unsuitable brands have to be updated regularly.

The nutritional implications of eliminating a food or group of foods from the diet also have to be considered. Removal of a food such as milk requires careful thought as to how the resulting loss of this major source of calcium is to be replaced, particularly in infants and children.

General guidance on dietary measures necessary in some of the most common causes of food allergy and intolerance are given below. In most cases, qualified dietetic assistance will also be essential if food avoidance is to be both effective and without harm.

Peanut avoidance

Peanut allergy is one of the most serious forms of food intolerance because the degree of sensitivity to it can be so high and the consequences so serious. The prevalence of peanut allergy has increased considerably in recent years, partly because nuts have become a more common ingredient of manufactured foods, such as biscuits, cakes and desserts, but mainly because of the extensive use of peanut or groundnut oil in many foods.

Because it is present in a disguised form in so many foods, and because of the high risk from exposure, anyone diagnosed with peanut allergy must be referred to a dietitian for expert advice.

Egg avoidance

Intolerance to egg is quite common but is usually quite easy to diagnose because symptoms usually appear fairly rapidly after consumption and the sufferer connects the two events.

As well as avoidance of eggs themselves, sufferers need to avoid foods which usually contain egg such as:

    Cakes
    Meringues
    Mayonnaise
    Egg pasta
    Quiche-type flans

Many other manufactured foods, particularly biscuits and sauces, will also contain egg. Sometimes this is readily obvious from the list of food ingredients on the food label (e.g. fresh egg, dried egg, powdered egg, egg white, egg yolk, egg lecithin) but other egg-derived ingredients are not (e.g. albumen, ovomucin, ovomucoid, ovoglobulin, ovovitellin, livetin, vitellin). In addition the food additive lecithin (E322) can be derived from egg although it is more usually extracted from soya.

Synthetic egg replacers suitable for use in baking are available.

Milk avoidance

Milk intolerance results from:

- Allergy or intolerance to cows' milk protein.
- Intolerance to lactose.

Cows' milk protein allergy/intolerance

This most commonly occurs in infancy and childhood but often disappears by the age of 5 years. As milk is such an important food for young children, dietetic guidance on suitable alternative sources of nutrients will be necessary. Formula fed infants will require an alternative to a cows' milk infant formula. In some cases a soya-based formula can be used instead but this is not suitable in all cases since some infants react to soya as well. A protein-hydrolysate formula may be necessary.

Exclusion of cows' milk protein from the diets of older children and adults requires avoidance of many foods as well as obvious sources of milk, such as cheese and yogurt, as many manufactured foods contain milk as an ingredient under various descriptions such as casein, caseinates, lactoglobulin or whey. Total exclusion usually requires dietetic help.

Lactose intolerance

This may result from a deficiency of the enzyme lactase, either as a result of genetic deficiency (common in many people of African, Asian or Mediterranean origin) or as a secondary consequence of disease or damage to the gastrointestinal tract.

Although milk is the primary source of both milk protein and lactose, dietary exclusions are not quite the same:

- All types of milk (cows', goats', sheep) contain lactose so all are unsuitable for lactose intolerance. (Goats' or sheep milk may be suitable for people sensitive to cows' milk protein.)
- Some milk products, such as butter and hard cheese, contain milk protein but very little lactose so need not be avoided.
- Low lactose milks available in longlife cartons are useful for lactose intolerance but are not suitable for cows' milk protein avoidance.
- Some medicinal products contain lactose as a filler; these are not contraindicated in cases of cows' milk protein intolerance.

In many cases of lactose intolerance, particularly that of genetic origin, a certain amount of lactose can be tolerated and complete exclusion of milk is unnecessary; this can be discovered by a process of trial and error. Secondary lactase deficiency as part of a malabsorption state will result in much lower tolerance to lactose and in such cases dietetic help will be needed to ensure lactose exclusion. As with those intolerant to cows' milk protein, all lactose intolerant children should be referred to a dietitian to ensure that milk exclusion does not jeopardise their nutritional intake.

Soya avoidance

Soya is present in many manufactured foods because 'vegetable oil' used as an ingredient is often derived from soya. Other sources of soya in foods are:

- Lecithin used as an emulsifier (E322) – this is derived either from soya or egg.
- Some types of hydrolysed vegetable protein.
- Soya flavouring.
- Soya protein products

Ascertaining whether a particular food contains soya usually requires recourse to the manufacturer or the National Food Databank.

Wheat avoidance

This necessitates avoidance of both wheat protein and wheat starch. Some of these food sources are obvious, e.g. bread, pasta, many breakfast cereals and any product containing flour (such as cakes, biscuits, pastry). However, wheat also creeps into many foods in the guise of rusk, cereal, edible starch, gluten, modified starch, thickener, binder and other variants so its exclusion is by no means straightforward. Other constituents such as hydrolysed vegetable protein may or may not be of wheat origin. Some people with a wheat intolerance also react to other grains, such as oats, rye, corn and barley, which makes dietary exclusion even more difficult.

Although gluten is a wheat protein, proprietary gluten-free foods are not necessarily wheat-free because some products contain wheat starch. Only those products which state that they are also 'wheat-free' will be suitable.

Many people believe themselves to be intolerant or even allergic to wheat. Because wheat avoidance results in the exclusion of so many important foods from the diet, it is important to establish that this is a necessary measure. Those with genuine intolerance should be given expert dietetic help.

Gluten intolerance (coeliac disease)

Intolerance to gluten, a protein found in many cereals but particularly wheat, results in coeliac disease. This results in a characteristic loss and flattening of the villi in the intestine causing malabsorption. Gluten intolerance can also present as the skin disease dermatitis herpetiformis. In the UK, the prevalence is about 1 in 2000, a figure which appears to be increasing. It is often thought of as a paediatric condition but it can appear at any age, most commonly in middle-age but sometimes in elderly people too.

The intolerance is permanent, and complete and life-long exclusion of gluten from the diet is important. This not only relieves symptoms by restoring normal intestinal function but also reduces the risk of gastrointestinal malignancy, particularly small bowel lymphoma.

A gluten-free diet is a major undertaking and always requires expert dietetic advice. It necessitates complete avoidance of wheat, barley, rye, usually oats, and all food products containing them. In practice this means exclusion of a vast number of manufactured foods, not just obvious sources of cereals, such as bread, breakfast cereals, pasta and anything containing flour, but also many types or particular brands of foods as diverse as beefburgers, fish fingers, baked beans, canned soups, gravy mixes, ice cream and vending machine coffee. Essentially anything which comes out of a can, packet or jar or which has been coated or modified in some way has to be suspected of containing gluten. Information on whether it does or does not contain gluten is also liable to change with time owing to product reformulation. The Coeliac Society of the United Kingdom maintains a constantly updated list of gluten-free manufactured foods and this is available to their members and dietitians.

A wide range of commercially produced gluten-free foods is now available, many of them ACBS prescribable for gluten intolerance, and it is essential that coeliac patients are offered and encouraged to use these products, otherwise their diets will either be very limited or not free from gluten. A broad guide to the types of prescribable products available is given in Table 40.1. Non-prescribable gluten-free foods (which patients may like to buy as an occasional treat) are listed in Table 40.2. Further details can be found in *MIMS*, the *British National Formulary* or obtained from

Table 40.1 Prescribable gluten-free foods.

Bread	Vacuum-packed	White bread sliced/ unsliced Wholemeal sliced/ unsliced Par-baked bread White rolls Wholemeal rolls
	Bread mixes Flour and pastry mixes	
Biscuits	Digestives Tea biscuits Crackers Crispbread	
Pasta	Spaghetti Spirals Tagliatelle Macaroni Vermicelli Lasagne	

Table 40.2 Non-prescribable gluten-free foods.

Breakfast cereals	Muesli breakfast cereal Hot breakfast cereal
Biscuits	Wafers Pretzels
Cakes	Madeira cake Ginger cake Fruit cake Mince pies Christmas pudding Rich fruit cake
Confectionery	Chocolate bars

dietitians or the manufacturers listed at the end of this chapter.

AVOIDANCE OF FOOD ADDITIVES

Genuine intolerance to food additives is very rare but when it does occur the effects can be profound. Those which are most likely to provoke serious reactions are as follows.

Sulphur dioxide and sulphites

Sulphur dioxide and sulphites are important and commonly used preservatives but they can have gastrointestinal or respiratory irritant effects. Sulphur dioxide gas released from food either from the sulphur dioxide itself or from the breakdown of sulphites can trigger asthma attacks. The presence of these substances in foods may be indicated as:

Sulphur dioxide	E220
Sodium sulphite	E221
Sodium bisulphite	E222
(or sodium hydrogen sulphite)	
Sodium metabisulphite	E223

Potassium metabisulphite	E224
Calcium sulphite	E226
Calcium bisulphite	E227
(or calcium hydrogen sulphite)	

Azo dyes

Azo dyes are synthetic dyes which colour foods yellow, orange or red but their use is being increasingly replaced with more natural alternatives such as beta-carotene or annatto. Azo dyes which have been known to cause reactions are:

Tartrazine	E102
Quinoline Yellow	E104
Yellow 2G	E107
Sunset Yellow	E110

BHA and BHT

These are antioxidants and are used in many manufactured foods to prevent rancidity. Their presence in foods may be indicated by either their full name or E number

| BHA (butylated hydroxyanisole) | E320 |
| BHT (butylated hydroxytoluene) | E321 |

OTHER DISORDERS ASSOCIATED WITH FOOD ALLERGY/ INTOLERANCE

Atopy (eczema and asthma)

The three associated problems eczema (atopic dermatitis), asthma and hay fever (collectively known as 'atopy') are very common affecting about 10% of the population.

It is recommended that infants with a family history of atopy should be exclusively breast fed for the first 6 months of life and that weaning should be delayed until at least 6 months[5]. This will not be totally protective because there will still be exposure to non-food triggers, but current evidence suggests it may prevent some cases or delay the appearance and severity of others[6]. When weaning does commence, potentially allergenic foods such as cows' milk, eggs and fish should be introduced with care, one at a time and the child closely monitored for any reaction.

There is little evidence that soya infant formulas have a protective effect against the development of atopic disease, nor are these products always suitable for infants allergic to cows' milk because sensitivity to cows' milk protein and soya protein often co-exist.

There is no evidence that the avoidance of cows' milk or other potentially allergenic foods by pregnant or breast-feeding women decreases the risk of atopy in their child.

Eczema

Older children with atopic eczema may sometimes benefit from withdrawal of cows' milk protein but this is a drastic step to take and should only be contemplated if the severity of the symptoms justify it.

Asthma

The reasons for the marked increase in asthma in recent years (now thought to affect 1 in 10 children and 1 in 12 adults) remain a matter of debate but it does seem likely that greater air pollution (particularly from vehicle exhaust gases) and the tendency to live in warm but poorly ventilated buildings are partly responsible.

Asthma attacks may result from exposure to an allergic trigger (such as house dust mites, pollens or animal fur) or non-allergic triggers (such as viral infections, air pollutants, exercise, stress or change in temperature) or a combination of both.

Diet is probably not an important trigger in most asthmatic people. Occasionally, asthma can be triggered by inhalation of sulphur dioxide present as a food additive or derived from sulphite preservatives (see above under 'Avoidance of food additives').

Some people with asthma can be shown to have food sensitivities although this tends to be in those with other symptoms of allergy such as eczema or hay fever and who are constantly reacting to other triggers such as pollen or house dust mites. In these circumstances, even if food is a contributory factor, its removal from the diet may in practice make little difference.

Migraine

Many factors trigger migraine and usually a combination of circumstances is necessary before an attack occurs. In a small number of cases, foods rich in vasoactive amines (e.g. cheese, wine and some types of fish, see p. 217) may have pharmacological effects which trigger an attack. In others, diet can indirectly cause migraine if it results in a low blood sugar, e.g. going for long periods without food or not eating after prolonged exercise. In many people, there are no links between diet and migraine.

Hyperactivity

In the past hyperactivity in children has often been attributed to food allergy, particularly to food addi-

tives such as azo dye food colours (see above). While genuine sensitivity to some additives can exist and can result in behavioural disturbance, this is extremely rare and certainly not the widespread problem many believe it to be. Genuine hyperactivity usually has a psychiatric or neurological basis. Some cases of hyperactivity diagnosed by parents are simply badly behaved children.

REFERENCES

1 Young, E. *et al.* (1987) The prevalence of reactions to food additives in a survey population. *Journal of the Royal College of Physicians* 21, 241–7.
2 Young, E. *et al.* (1994) A population study of food intolerance. *Lancet* 343, 1127–30.
3 Niestjil Jansen, J.J. *et al.* (1994) Prevalence of food allergy and intolerance in the Dutch population. *Journal of Allergy and Clincal Immunology* 93, 446–56.
4 Sethi, T.J. *et al.* (1987) How reliable are commercial allergy tests? *Lancet* i, 92–4.
5 Department of Health (1994) *Weaning and the Weaning Diet.* COMA Report on Health and Social Subjects 45. HMSO, London.
6 Burr, M.L. *et al.* (1993) Infant feeding, wheezing and allergy: a prospective study. *Archives of Diseases in Childhood* 68, 724–8.

FURTHER READING

Gray, J. (1986) *Food Intolerance: Fact and Fiction.* Based on the report of the Royal College of Physicians and the British Nutrition Foundation. Grafton Books, London.
MAFF (1991) *Food Allergy and Other Unpleasant Reactions to Food.* A Foodsense guide from the Food Safety Directorate. Reference no. PB1696. Available free (See Appendix 1).
MAFF Food Safety Directorate (1994) *Food Intolerance.* Fact Sheet 12. MAFF, London.
National Dairy Council (1994) *Adverse Reactions to Food.* Topical Update – 2. NDC, London.
Royal College of Physicians (1995) *Good Allergy Practice: Standards of care for providers and purchasers of allergy services within the NHS.* Details from: The Royal College of Physicians, 11 St Andrew's Place, London NW1 4LE.

USEFUL ADDRESSES

The Anaphylaxis Campaign, PO Box 149, Fleet, Hampshire GU13 9XU.

British Allergy Foundation, St Bartholomew's Hospital, West Smithfield, London EC1A 7BE. Tel: 0171 600 6127.

The Coeliac Society of the United Kingdom, PO Box 220, High Wycombe, Bucks HP11 2HY. Tel: 01494 437278.

The Migraine Trust, 45 Great Ormond Street, London WC1N 3HZ. Tel: 0171 278 2676.

Details of gluten-free food can be obtained from the following:

Cantassium Company, Larkhall Laboratories, 225 Putney Bridge Road, London SW15 2PY. Tel: 0181 874 1130. Brand name: Trufree Flours.

General Dietary Ltd, PO Box 38, Kingston upon Thames, Surrey KT2 7YP. Tel: 0181 336 2323. Brand names: Ener-G, Valpiform.

Gluten Free Foods Ltd, PO Box 178, Stanmore, Middlesex HA7 4XN. Tel: 0181 954 7348. Brand names: Barkat, Glutano.

Nutricia Dietary Products Ltd, Newmarket Avenue, Whitehorse Business Park, Trowbridge, Wilts BA14 0XQ. Tel: 01225 771801 or 768381. Brand names: Glutafin, Rite-Diet.

Scientific Hospital Supplies, 100 Wavertree Boulevard, Wavertree Technology Park, Liverpool L7 9PT. Tel: 0151 228 1992. Band Name: Juvela.

Ultrapharm, PO Box 18, Henley-on-Thames, Oxon RG9 2AW. Tel: 01491 578016. Brand names: Ultra, Aproten.

41

Cancer

In the UK, cancer affects over 200000 people each year and is the second leading cause of mortality (accounting for 25% of all deaths). Many of these cases of cancer are preventable. Smoking is thought to cause about one-third of cancer deaths and diet may be responsible for an additional third, particularly cancers of the digestive tract[1].

Diet appears to have both causative and protective effects; it may also enhance or diminish the effects of other carcinogenic agents such as tobacco, ultra-violet light, ionising radiation or environmental hazards[2].

The development of cancer is thought to involve several stages, typically:

- *Initiation* Exposure to carcinogens and damage to cellular DNA which may or may not progress.
- *Promotion* External factors trigger the expression of altered DNA.
- *Progression* Rapid replication of abnormal cells.

Diet is not thought to play a major part in the initiation process despite the fact that food contains numerous carcinogens. Most of these are of natural rather than man-made origin and are either normal components of plant or animal tissues, or created by heating and cooking (e.g. benzpyrines and pyrido-indoles) or present as a result of contamination (e.g. fungal aflatoxin produced by moulds). The body has sophisticated protective mechanisms, such as detoxifying enzymes, so that it can withstand the constant exposure to low levels of these substances. It is possible that excessive amounts of carcinogens from an unusually high intake of certain foods or a high level of contamination could swamp the body's ability to deal with them but in normal circumstances this seems unlikely to occur.

Diet probably has most influence at the stage of cancer promotion by either increasing or reducing the response to the effect of carcinogens. Dietary factors which may increase cancer promotion are:

- High fat intake.
- High energy intake.
- High alcohol intake.

Dietary factors which retard promotion are:

- High intake of antioxidant nutrients, particularly from fruit and vegetables. The protective effect of fruit and vegetables appears to be much greater than the promoting or protective effects of any other dietary component.
- High intake of fibre (non-starch polysaccharide).

The third step, cancer progression, may be influenced by nutritional effects on immune function.

DIET AND CANCER PROMOTION

Cancer enhancing factors

Dietary fat

In animals, a high fat intake enhances the development of breast cancer, although to some extent this effect is linked with that of total energy intake[3]. The type of fat consumed is also relevant. Linoleic acid (an essential fatty acid) appears to be particularly important for tumour development in mammals, although once the amount needed for tumour growth has been reached (about 4% of dietary energy), further linoleic acid probably has the same effect on cancer promotion as other types of fat[4]. The relevance of this to human breast cancer is less certain. Most epidemiological studies fail to show a significant relationship between the breast cancer and either the amount or type of fat consumed[5]. Current consensus is that if a high fat intake does enhance the risk of human breast cancer it is probably as a result of its contribution to energy intake and obesity[6] (see below).

There is some evidence that high fat diets may promote colorectal cancer although results from experimental and epidemiological studies are equivocal and may also be reflecting the effects of a high energy intake (see below). Additionally, a high fat intake is often associated with a low intake of complex carbohydrates and hence dietary fibre and it may be this latter factor which is the more significant.

Dietary energy

There is a positive association between energy intake and many types of cancers, particularly colorectal cancers[7]. Obesity, particularly central obesity, increases the risk of development of endometrial, cervical, ovarian and gall bladder cancers in women and prostate cancers in men[8], possibly as a result of its effects on steroid hormone or insulin production or altered metabolism. Reduced physical activity may also enhance cancer production.

Alcohol

High alcohol consumption increases the risk of cancers of the mouth, upper respiratory tract, oesophagus and liver. This risk is greatly enhanced if there is associated use of tobacco[9].

Other dietary components

There is little evidence that there is an independent effect of dietary protein or meat intake on cancer promotion. Although epidemiological studies show that vegetarians have a much lower cancer risk than non-vegetarians, this may well be due to factors such as their higher consumption of fruit and vegetables, lower energy intake and less use of alcohol and tobacco rather than to the dietary absence of meat *per se*[10].

Protective factors

Dietary fibre (non-starch polysaccharide)

There is little doubt that a high fibre intake is associated with a reduced risk of cancer, particularly that of the large bowel[11]. However, the nature of this association is difficult to unravel. Whether it is due to fibre *per se* is hard to determine owing to the confounding effects of other dietary variables (particularly dietary energy and antioxidants). 'Fibre' (or more correctly non-starch polysaccharide) is also not a uniform substance but a group of diverse compounds and consumption of different types of fibre may well have different protective effects.

Nevertheless it is plausible that some or all components of dietary fibre may be protective in cancer development. A high fibre intake, particularly of cereal fibre origin, increases stool bulk and speeds up intestinal transit time and therefore tends to reduce the exposure of the bowel mucosa to carcinogens and promoters. There is also evidence that some fibre components which are fermentable by colonic bacteria yield substances with protective effects[11].

More studies are needed to resolve these questions.

Antioxidant nutrients

There is growing evidence that dietary antioxidants have an important protective role in the development of cancer[12]. In most studies of diet and cancer there is a striking relationship between low consumption of fruit and vegetables and increased cancer risk[13]. The reasons and possible mechanisms for this association are complex but it seems increasingly likely that it reflects the protective antioxidant content of these foods. Oxidative damage and the generation of free radicals appears to be part of the mechanism involved in the initiation and promotion of cancer at the cellular level[14]. Dietary factors which help counteract the oxidative process are therefore likely to be protective.

Much remains to be learnt about dietary antioxidants and their differing effects. Early work suggested that vitamin A helped protect against some cancers, especially lung cancer. It now seems more likely that it is beta-carotene, the precursor of vitamin A, and probably other carotenoids present in fruit and vegetables which have most influence on cancer prevention[15]. Vitamin C may have particularly strong protective properties in terms of oral, oesophageal, gastric and pancreatic cancers, possibly because it may reduce the production of endogenous carcinogens (e.g. the formation of nitrosamines from nitric oxide released by cells as a bactericide). Vitamin C is also a powerful scavenger of free radical molecules, increases the activity of detoxifying enzyme systems and has an important influence on immune function[14]. The role of vitamin E in cancer prevention is more equivocal although its protective effect against lipid peroxidation and its close interaction with vitamin C make it likely that it is of some importance.

The trace element selenium may also have strong protective effects[16], partly from its role as an antioxidant and in detoxifying enzyme systems but possibly also because of its direct toxicity to proliferating cancer cells.

Other trace elements or as yet unidentified biologically active substances found in plants may also have anticarcinogenic effects. For this reason, pharmacological supplements of antioxidant vitamins may not necessarily be as protective as those consumed in the form of a mixture of fruit and vegetables.

DIETARY GUIDANCE TO REDUCE CANCER RISK

The European Prospective Investigation into Cancer (EPIC), which commenced in 1991 involving 415000 people in seven countries, may provide some definitive answers regarding the role of diet in the causation of cancer and help clarify which foods or food components promote cancer and which offer protection. However, it is likely to be some years before any significant conclusions emerge.

Meanwhile there is general agreement that fruit and vegetables are, whatever the reasons, protective against many types of cancers, particularly those of the oesophagus, stomach, colon, rectum and respiratory tract. Increased consumption of fresh fruit and vegetables is one of the recommendations listed in the European Code against Cancer, part of the 'Europe against Cancer' programme. The World Health Organization recommends that everyone eats 5–6 portions of fruit/vegetables a day (and this has been adopted in some healthy eating guidance as the '5-a-day' or 'Take 5' slogans).

This advice may be particularly pertinent for smokers. Smoking generates the production of free radicals and so greatly increases the risk of oxidative damage. The requirement for protective antioxidant nutrients is thus likely to be greatly increased but in practice many smokers have lower than average intakes of these nutrients, particularly vitamin C and beta-carotene[17]. This can only exacerbate the risk.

In practical terms, dietary guidelines for healthy eating are highly compatible with those currently thought to reduce cancer risk. An increased intake of foods such as fruit, vegetables and fibre-containing cereals may be specifically protective. Avoiding a high energy intake, particularly from foods rich in fat or which results in obesity, may reduce the likelihood of cancer development or progression.

Dietary guidelines for cancer prevention:

- Eat more fruit and vegetables (aim for 5 portions a day).
- Eat more fibre-containing cereal foods.
- Eat fewer fatty foods.
- Avoid or correct obesity.
- Keep alcohol intake within sensible drinking limits.
- Avoid excessive intakes of potential carcinogens from barbecued, smoked or salted foods.

DIETARY TREATMENT OF PATIENTS WITH CANCER

Dietary management of patients with cancer depends on the nature, site and management of the disease. Surgical procedures such as intestinal resection may have nutritional implications (see 'Intestinal resection' in Chapter 30). Radiotherapy may also have profound, although usually short-term effects on food intake as a result of nausea, vomiting, diarrhoea, reduced appetite or a sore mouth. General guidance for such problems can be found in Chapter 8 (*Nutritional Support and Supplementation*). Dietetic help should be sought if the symptoms are severe or persistent.

In people who are expected to make a good recovery, the importance of a healthy diet should be stressed. An increased consumption of fruit and vegetables should be particularly encouraged because of their protective effects on both antioxidant and immune function.

For those in whom the prognosis is poor, eating should be made as pleasurable as possible and dietary restrictions confined to those essential for symptom relief. Nutritional adequacy should be maintained for as long as possible, if necessary with the help of sip feed supplements if appetite is poor. People with severe eating difficulties, dysphagia, or malabsorption should receive expert dietetic assistance.

REFERENCES

1 Doll, R. & Peto, R. The causes of cancer: quantitative estimates of avoidable risks of cancer in the United States today. *Journal of the National Cancer Institute* 66, 1192–308.

2 Doll, R. (1990) An overview of the epidemiological evidence linking diet and cancer. *Proceedings of the Nutrition Society* 49, 119–31.

3 Freedman, L.S. *et al.* (1990) Analysis of dietary fat, calories, body weight and the development of mammary tumors in rats and mice: a review. *Cancer Research* 50, 5710–9.

4 Ip, C. (1987) Fat and essential fatty acids in mammary carcinogenesis. *American Journal of Clinical Nutrition* 45, Supplement 1, 218–24.

5 UK Nutritional Epidemiology Group (1993) *Diet and Cancer. A review of the epidemiological evidence.* Nutrition Society, London.

6 Williams, C.M. (1993) Food: its role in the aetiology of cancer. In: Waldron, K.W. *et al.* (eds) *Food and Cancer Prevention: Chemical and Biological Aspects*, pp. 3–11. Royal Society of Chemistry, London.

7 Albanes, D. (1992) Energy intake and cancer. In: Micozzi, M.S. & Moon, T.E. (eds) *Macronutrients: Investigating their Role in Cancer*, pp. 205–29. Marcel Dekker, New York.

8 Garfinkel, L. (1985) Overweight and cancer. *Annals of Internal Medicine* 103, 1034–6.

9 International Agency for Research on Cancer (1988) *Monographs on the Evaluation of Carcinogenic Risks to Humans: Alcohol Drinking.* Volume 44. IARC, Lyons.

10 Thorogood, M. *et al.* (1994) Risk of death from cancer and ischaemic heart disease in meat and non-meat eaters. *British Medical Journal* 308, 1667–71.

11 Bingham, S.A. (1993) Plant cell wall material and cancer protection. In: Waldron, K.W. *et al.* (eds) *Food and Cancer Prevention: Chemical and Biological Aspects.* pp. 339–47. Royal Society of Chemistry, Cambridge.

12 Waldron, K.W. *et al.* (1993) *Food and Cancer Prevention: Chemical and Biological Aspects.* Royal Society of Chemistry, Cambridge.

13 Block, G. *et al.* (1992) Fruit, vegetables and cancer prevention: a review of the epidemiological evidence. *Nutrition and Cancer* 18, 1–29.

14 Thurnham, D.I. (1993) Chemical aspects and biological mechanisms of anticancer nutrients in plant foods. In: Waldron, K.W. *et al.* (eds) *Food and Cancer Prevention: Chemical and Biological Aspects.* pp. 339–47. Royal Society of Chemistry, Cambridge.

15 van Poppel, G. *et al.* (1993) Carotenoids and cancer: an update with emphasis on human intervention studies. *European Journal of Cancer* 29A, 1335–44.

16 Diplock, A.T. (1991) Antioxidant vitamins and disease prevention: an overview. *American Journal of Clinical Nutrition* 53, 189S–93S.

17 Margetts, B. & Jackson, A. (1993) Interactions between people's diet and their smoking habits: the dietary and nutritional survey of British adults. *British Medical Journal* 307, 1381–4.

FURTHER READING

Austoker, J. (1994) Diet and cancer. *British Medical Journal* 308, 1610.

Health Education Authority (1990) *Diet and Cancer*. Briefing paper. HEA, London.

National Dairy Council (1995) *Nutrition and Cancer*. Fact File 12. NDC, London.

USEFUL ADDRESSES

BACUP (British Association for Cancer United Patients and their families and friends), 121–123 Charterhouse Street, London EC1M 2AA. Tel: 0171 608 1661.

Cancer Relief Macmillan Fund, Anchor House, 15–19 Britten Street, London SW3 3TZ. Tel: 0171 351 7811.

Cancer Research Campaign, 10 Cambridge Terrace, London NW1 4JL. Tel: 0171 224 1333.

42

HIV Infection and AIDS

By mid 1995, 11 184 cases of AIDS had been reported in the UK of whom 7640 had died; 24 000 people were recorded as having the HIV virus[1]. Even if, as predicted, the incidence of new cases will level off by the late 1990s and then begin to decline, HIV infection will remain a significant health problem for many years to come.

The role of diet in the management of HIV infection, particularly in its later stages, is an area of active investigation and the benefits of different types and degrees of nutritional interventions are currently being evaluated. What is already clear is that diet is an important aspect of care at all stages of HIV infection.

DIETARY ADVICE IN ASYMPTOMATIC HIV PATIENTS

The inevitable reaction to the diagnosis of being HIV positive is one of depression, even despair. People may think there is 'not much point' concerning themselves with healthy eating as they won't live long enough to benefit from it. They are almost certainly wrong. The relationship between nutrition and immune function is well-established and a diet which maintains immunocompetence may well delay the progression of the disease[2].

In order to maintain immune competence the diet must contain:

- *Sufficient energy to maintain body weight* If energy intake is too low, dietary protein will be used for energy needs rather than to maintain muscle mass and the immune system.
- *Sufficient intake of protein, vitamins and minerals* Dietary energy should predominately come from foods of high nutrient density rather than those providing mainly energy alone. In practice this means encouraging consumption of foods from all four major food groups, particularly fruit and vegetables.

As is typical with many incurable diseases, people with HIV infection are very tempted to try alternative or complementary nutritional therapies in the hope that these may be beneficial. Such hopes should be not be dashed but if such measures result in a diet which is clearly distorted or inadequate and so likely to do more harm than good, health professionals should suggest more rational alternatives. The use of megadoses of vitamins and minerals is very common but may not be advisable as some may be immunosuppressive[3]. If people are concerned about vitamins and minerals, or their intake appears to be lower than desirable, supplements providing Reference Nutrient Intake levels of intake can be recommended.

HIV patients in disadvantaged circumstances, perhaps sleeping rough and with a history of drug or alcohol abuse, often have a very poor nutritional intake and multiple nutrient deficiencies. Improved nutrition is an important objective but one which is difficult to achieve without the support of local agencies and outreach projects.

SYMPTOMATIC HIV INFECTION AND AIDS

Maintaining a nutritional intake adequate to maintain immune competence remains important at all stages of HIV infection. But as the infection becomes more active, additional dietary measures also become necessary.

Maintenance of body weight

Weight loss is a prominent feature of active HIV infection. It used to be thought that this was an unavoidable consequence of the disease itself as a result of hypermetabolism, but recent evidence suggests that this is not the case and that it simply reflects an inadequate energy intake[4]. Correcting weight loss is important as it may affect both morbidity and mortality. Body wasting results in weakness, fatigue and lethargy and so markedly impairs the quality of life. It may also decrease resistance to opportunistic infections. Weight loss is also associated with decreased survival time in those with AIDS[5].

Weight loss takes two forms:

- *Acute weight loss* This can be rapid and severe and typically accompanies opportunistic infections such as cryptosporidium-induced diarrhoea or *Pneumocystis carinii* pneumonia. It is possible to correct this in the post-infective period when there is considerable anabolic potential, provided that energy and nutrient intake is sufficiently high. This usually necessitates some form of nutritional support or supplementation (see Chapter 8).
- *Chronic weight loss* This is usually associated

with gastrointestinal disease and malabsorption. Early intervention to correct or minimise weight loss is important. This is likely to require the use of nutritional supplementation, preferably with dietetic assistance so that this is appropriate for the type of gastrointestinal problems present.

Food hygiene

People with advancing HIV become increasingly susceptible to infection. Food and water-borne infections which may be of little consequence in a healthy person can cause debilitating effects in the person with HIV. Those with HIV infection should be reminded of the important aspects of food safety recommended for the general population (see Chapter 11).

Factors affecting appetite and food intake

Some of the manifestations of advanced HIV disease have profound effects on food intake, particularly if their treatment necessitates drug or radiotherapy treatment. Common problems are:

- Anorexia.
- Nausea and vomiting.
- Diarrhoea.
- Dry or sore mouth.
- Changes in taste perception.
- Swallowing difficulties.
- Dehydration and electrolyte disturbances caused by night sweats.

Although general measures for dealing with these types of problems are covered elsewhere in this book (e.g. see cancer, Chapter 41; swallowing disorders, Chapter 29; small appetite,

Chapter 8), expert dietetic guidance should be sought when these problems are HIV-related because there are so many other nutritional implications.

In the later stages of HIV infection, palliative nutritional support, possibly in the form of home enteral or parenteral nutrition, may be appropriate for some patients.

REFERENCES

1 Health Education Authority (1995) *Healthlines*, Issue 27, November, 7.
2 Chandra, R.K. (1993) Nutrition and immunity: lessons from the past and new insights into the future. *American Journal of Clinical Nutrition* 53, 1087–101.
3 British Dietetic Association (1995) *Nutrition Intervention in Human Immunodeficiency Virus Infection*. Position Paper. BDA, Birmingham.
4 Macallan, D.C. *et al.* (1995) The energetic basis of weight loss in HIV infection. *New England Journal of Medicine* 333, 83–8.
5 Kotler, D.P. *et al.* (1989) Magnitude of body cell mass depletion and the timing of death from wasting in AIDS. *American Journal of Clinical Nutrition* 50, 444–7.

FURTHER READING

Health Visitors Association (1995) *Positive Practice: an HVA guide to caring for families and children affected by HIV/AIDS*. Details available from HVA publications, 50 Southwark Street, London SE1 1UN.

USEFUL ADDRESSES

The HIV Research and Information Exchange, Chelsea and Westminster Hospital, 369 Fulham Road, London SW10 9TR. Tel: 0181 746 5929/ Fax: 0181 746 5595. A charity funded centre providing access to worldwide data on HIV and AIDS research, treatment and care.

Appendices

Appendix 1

Sources of Further Information

GENERAL TEXTBOOKS ON NUTRITION AND DIETETICS

Garrow, J.S. & James, W.P.T. (eds) (1993) *Human Nutrition and Dietetics*, 4th edn. Churchill Livingstone, Edinburgh.

Shaw, V. & Lawson, M. (eds) (1994) *Clinical Paediatric Dietetics*. Blackwell Science, Oxford.

Thomas, B. (ed.) (1994) *Manual of Dietetic Practice*, 2nd edn. Blackwell Science, Oxford.

OTHER PUBLICATIONS

Foodsense Publications

These are a series of booklets on nutrition related topics produced for the general public by the MAFF Food Safety Directorate. They are available free of charge from: Foodsense, London SE99 7TT. Telephone orders: 0645 556000.

Current titles include:
Food Sense (PB0549)
Food Safety (PB0551)
About Food Additives (PB0552)
Understanding Food Labels (PB0553)
Food Protection (PB0554)
Healthy Eating (PB0550)
The New Microwave Labels (PB0779)
Food and Pesticides (PB0868)
Monitoring our Food and Nutrition (PB0896)
Understanding Radioactivity in Food (PB1212)
Natural Toxicants in our Food (PB1265)
Food Emergencies (PB1568)
Keeping Food Cool and Safe (PB1649)
Chemicals in Food – Managing the Risks (PB1695)
Food Allergy and other Unpleasant Reactions to Food (PB1696)
Microbiological Safety of Smoked Fish (PB0708)
Healthy Eating for Older People (PB1526)

The Food Safety Directorate also produces free Fact Sheets covering these and other subjects in more depth. Details of these can be obtained by telephoning the Consumer Helpline on 0345 573012 or by writing to MAFF Food Safety Directorate, Room 303a, Ergon House, c/o Nobel House, 17 Smith Square, London SW1P 3JR. Fax: 0171 238 6330.

HMSO Publications

Telephone orders: 0171 873 9090. General enquiries: HMSO Publications Centre, PO Box 276,

London SW8 5DT. Tel: 0171 873 0011.
Free catalogues of publications may be obtained from: HMSO Books, Publicity Dept B, St Crispins, Duke Street, Norwich NR3 1PD. Tel: 01603 695907.

Health Education Authority Publications

Details of Health Education Authority Briefing papers and other material are available from: Health Education Authority Customer Services Department, Marston Book Services Ltd, PO Box 87, Osney Mead Industrial Estate, Oxford OX2 0DT. Tel: 01865 204745.

British Nutrition Foundation Publications

Details of British Nutrition Foundation Briefing Papers and other material may be obtained from: The British Nutrition Foundation, High Holborn House, 52–54 High Holborn, London WC1V 6RQ. Tel: 0171 404 6504.

National Dairy Council Publications

The National Dairy Council produces a range of educational material for health professionals and the general public. Much of it is free of charge. Details can be obtained from: National Dairy Council, 5–7 John Princes Street, London W1M 0AP. Tel: 0171 499 7822.

Prescribing Publications

British National Formulary is produced jointly by the British Medical Association and The Pharmaceutical Society of Great Britain. A twice-yearly publication concerned with the prescribing, dispensing and administration of medicines.

MIMS – Monthly Index of Medical Specialities. A reference and prescribing guide for doctors in general practice.

USEFUL CONTACTS

British Dietetic Association, 7th floor Elizabeth House, 22 Suffolk Street Queensway, Birmingham B1 1LS. Tel: 0121 643 5483.

Health Education Authority, Hamilton House, Mabledon Place, London WC1H 9TX. Tel: 0171 383 3833.

Health Education Board for Scotland, Woodburn House, Canaan Lane, Edinburgh EH10 4SG. Tel: 0131 447 8044.

Health Promotion Wales, Ffynnon-las, Ty Glas Avenue, Llanishen, Cardiff CF4 5DZ. Tel: 01222 752222.

Health Promotion Agency for Northern Ireland, 18 Ormeau Avenue, Belfast BT2 8HS. Tel: 01232 311611.

Ministry of Agriculture, Fisheries and Food (MAFF), Ergon House, c/o Nobel House, 17 Smith Square, London SW1P 3JR. MAFF Helpline: 0645 335577.

MAFF Food Safety Directorate, Consumer helpline 0345 573012.

Appendix 2

Conversion Factors

IMPERIAL/METRIC CONVERSIONS

1 oz = 28.4 g (for convenience this is usually rounded to 1 oz = 30 g)
1 lb = 454 g (or 0.45 kg)
1 kg = 2.2 lb
1 stone = 14 lb or 6.36 kg
1 pint = 568 ml
1 litre = 1.76 pints ($1\frac{3}{4}$ pints)
1 inch = 2.4 cm
1 metre = 39.37 inches

DIETARY CONVERSION FACTORS

1 kcal = 4.18 kJ
1000 kcal = 4.18 MJ
1 MJ = 1000 kJ or 239 kcal

1 gram of protein provides   4 kcal (17 kJ)
1 gram of carbohydrate provides   4 kcal (17 kJ)
1 gram of alcohol provides   7 kcal (29 kJ)
1 gram of fat provides   9 kcal (37 kJ)

Minerals and trace elements are sometimes expressed in millimoles (mmol). This is equivalent to their atomic or molecular weight. Thus 1 mmol of sodium is equivalent to 23 mg sodium (its atomic weight).

To convert mmol to mg
Sodium	multiply by 23
Potassium	multiply by 39
Calcium	multiply by 40
Magnesium	multiply by 24
Phosphorus	multiply by 31

To convert mg to mmol, divide by the above factors.

Appendix 3

Abbreviations

ABV — Alcohol by volume, the alcoholic strength of a drink (sometimes written as % vol)

ACBS — Advisory Committee on Borderline Substances. ACBS approval means that a non-drug item can be prescribed by GPs

AIDS — Acquired immunodeficiency syndrome

BDA — British Dietetic Association or British Diabetic Association

BHA — Butylated hydroxyanisole, an antioxidant food additive

BHT — Butylated hydroxytoluene, an antioxidant food additive

BMI — Body Mass Index, a measure of obesity. BMI = Weight in kg/Height in metres^2

BMR — Basal Metabolic Rate, energy expenditure from metabolic and physiological processes (i.e. not including energy expenditure from physical activity)

BNF — British Nutrition Foundation

CHD — Coronary Heart Disease

COMA — Committee on Medical Aspects of Food Policy (a Department of Health expert committee)

DEXA — Dual X-ray Absorptiometry

DNA — Deoxyribonucleic acid

DRV — Dietary Reference Values, the set of standards showing nutrient needs of various sectors of the population

DHA — Docosahexaenoic acid, a long-chain n-3 polyunsaturated fatty acid important in retinal and central nervous system development

EAR — Estimated Average Requirement, the average need of a nutrient by a population

EPA — Eicosapentaenoic acid, a long-chain n-3 polyunsaturated fatty acid found mainly in fish oils which has antithrombotic effects

EPIC — European Prospective Investigation into Cancer

GLA — Gamma-linolenic acid, a long-chain n-6 fatty acid derived from linoleic acid with some anti-inflammatory properties. Evening primrose oil is a rich source of GLA

GP — General Practitioner

HBV — High Biological Value

HDL — High density lipoprotein, the type which transports cholesterol away from the tissues for excretion

HEA — Health Education Authority

HIV — Human immunodeficiency virus

HRT — Hormone replacement therapy

IBS — Irritable bowel syndrome

kcal — Kilocalorie, a unit of dietary energy. Popularly known as 'calorie'

kJ — Kilojoule, a unit of dietary energy

LCT — Long-chain triglycerides, most dietary fat is usually in this form

LDL — Low density lipoprotein, the type which transports cholesterol around the body and to the tissues

LRNI — Lower Reference Nutrient Intake, the

	amount of a nutrient which is sufficient for only 3% of a population
MAFF	Ministry of Agriculture, Fisheries and Food
MAO	Monoamine oxidase
MCT	Medium-chain triglycerides, a more easily absorbed form of fat
MIMS	Monthly Index of Medical Specialities. A reference and prescribing guide for UK doctors in general practice
MJ	Megajoule, equivalent to 1000 kilojoules (kJ)
MS	Multiple sclerosis
MSG	Monosodium glutamate
n-3 polyunsaturated fatty acid	A small proportion of dietary polyunsaturates derived from alpha-linolenic acid. Also called omega-3 polyunsaturated fatty acids
n-6 polyunsaturated fatty acids	Most dietary polyunsaturates (e.g. from oils and polyunsaturated spreads) are in this form. They are derived from linoleic acid. Also called omega-6 polyunsaturated fatty acids
NFS	National Food Survey
NHS	National Health Service
NMES	Non-milk extrinsic sugars, dietary sugars which are not an integral part of a food's cellular structure (excluding the free sugars naturally present in milk)
NSAIDS	Non-steroidal anti-inflammatory drugs
NSP	Non-starch polysaccharides, the scientifically correct term for dietary fibre
NTD	Neural tube defects, fetal malformations such as spina bidida
OA	Osteoarthritis
omega-3	polyunsaturated fatty acids usually abbreviated to n-3, see above
omega-6	polyunsaturated fatty acids usually abbreviated to n-6, see above
OPCS	Office of Population Censuses and Surveys
PAL	Physical Activity Level, a factor used to determine energy requirements
PEG	Percutaneous Endoscopic Gastrostomy
RA	Rheumatoid arthritis
RDA	Recommended Daily Amount or Allowance, the amount of a nutrient which covers the needs of 97% of the population. In the UK this is equivalent to the newer term RNI
RNI	Reference Nutrient Intake, the amount of a nutrient which is thought to be sufficient for the needs of 97% of the population
TVP	Texturised vegetable protein
VLCD	Very Low Calorie Diet
WHR	Waist-Hip Ratio

Appendix 4

Height, Weight and BMI Chart

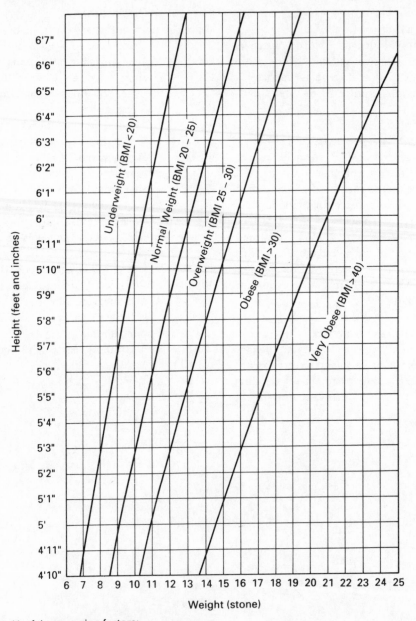

Useful conversion factors:

1 foot = 0.305 metres	1 stone = 6.356 kilograms
5' 0" = 1.52 m	10 stone = 63.56 kg
5' 6" = 1.68 m	15 stone = 95.3 kg
6' 0" = 1.83 m	20 stone = 127.1 kg

Index

LIVERPOOL
JOHN MOORES UNIVERSITY
AVRIL ROBARTS LRC
TEL. 0151 231 4022